To Kelli McCormack Brown,

classy and [illegible] colleague,

with a [illegible] and

all best wishes,

James Allegrante
2004

Kelli - Let this book & this thinking influence your practice & professional research. We're so pleased you value this historical document!

David Sleet
11/04

Derryberry's
Educating for Health

John P. Allegrante
David A. Sleet

Editors

Foreword by J. Michael McGinnis

Derryberry's Educating for Health

A Foundation for Contemporary Health Education Practice

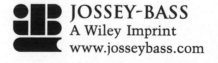

JOSSEY-BASS
A Wiley Imprint
www.josseybass.com

Published by Jossey-Bass
A Wiley Imprint
989 Market Street, San Francisco, CA 94103-1741   www.josseybass.com

Any views expressed in this publication do not necessarily represent the views of the
United States Government, and are not meant to serve as an official endorsement of any
statement to the extent that such statements may conflict with any official position of the
United States Government.

Copyright information continued on pp. 479–481.

Jossey-Bass books and products are available through most bookstores. To contact
Jossey-Bass directly call our Customer Care Department within the U.S. at
800-956-7739, outside the U.S. at 317-572-3986 or fax 317-572-4002.

Library of Congress Cataloging-in-Publication Data

Derryberry, Mayhew.
[Educating for health]
   Derryberry's educating for health : a foundation for contemporary health
education practice / [edited by] John P. Allegrante, David A. Sleet ; foreword by
J. Michael McGinnis.— 1st ed.
      p. ; cm.
   Originally published: Educating for health. New York, N.Y. : NCHE Press, 1987.
With new introd.
   Includes bibliographical references and index.
   ISBN 0-7879-7244-4 (alk. paper)
   1. Health education. 2. Public health.
   [DNLM: 1. Health Education—Collected Works. 2. Public Health—
Collected Works. 3. Research—methods—Collected Works. WA 7 D438d 2004]
   I. Title: Educating for health. II. Allegrante, John P. (John Philip), 1952- III. Sleet,
David A. IV. Title.
RA440.D47 2004
613'.07'1—dc22   2004004612

Printed in the United States of America
FIRST EDITION
PB Printing   10 9 8 7 6 5 4 3 2 1

Contents

DERRYBERRY'S EDUCATING FOR HEALTH

Part III: Establishing the Parameters of Health Education   215

Part IV: Community Health Education   261

To Charles N. Poskanzer and Ralph M. Grawunder

Foreword

Derryberry's Educating for Health: A Foundation for Contemporary Health Education Practice offers both a welcome celebration of the accomplishments in health education and an important toolkit for advances yet to come. Each of us benefits in our work from the priv-ilege of building upon foundations laid down by our predecessors. The beauty of this collection is the testimony it provides of the strength of those foundations.

For those of us who have spent time in federal service, reading through this anthology of Mayhew Derryberry's papers is a reminder of the extent to which federal initiatives in prevention policy are rooted in the pioneering work of Dr. Derryberry and the protégés and colleagues he recruited and taught. When Mayhew Derryberry moved, in 1937, from the health department in New York City to the federal Public Health Service, he was seemingly moving from the hurly-burly of the nation's most dynamic front line to an arena a step removed from the action. A federal disease prevention agenda was only beginning to emerge, and much of the nation's attention during this time was naturally focused on the problems of infectious diseases, particularly during childhood, which dominated the leading causes of morbidity and mortality until the middle of the twentieth century. In the preantibiotic era, sanitation—and its educational correlates—offered the only interventions, and the primary respon-sibility was at the local level.

At the time the U.S. Public Health Service was originally established, in 1798 when Congress created the Marine Hospital Service, its focus was largely on quarantine measures and the operation of a system of port-oriented hospitals for the commercial lifeblood of the country, the Merchant Marine Service. Derryberry's move to the federal level came as interest was growing in stronger federal leadership in disease control. The stage had been set by the 1909 recommendations of the Rockefeller Sanitary Commission and by early-twentieth-century initiatives targeting safer food and drugs and better maternal and child health.

With progress in reducing the disease burden and death rates due to infectious disease, with expanding sanitation efforts, with the introduction of vaccines and antibiotics, and with the increases in chronic diseases such as heart disease, cancer, and stroke, public and political demand for stronger efforts grew. The fledgling National Institute of Health (later National Institutes of Health) took on new importance as a source of insights for understanding newly recognized health threats and therapeutic potentials. The 1937 establishment of the National Cancer Institute was followed a decade later, in 1948, by the founding of the National Heart Institute (now the National Heart, Lung, and Blood Institute). The Communicable Disease Center (later the Centers for Disease Control and Prevention) was also established in 1948, building on the existing public health capacity and activities focused on malaria control. With the establishment of these federal health organizations, the role of the federal government as an agent of change in health was established, and the stage was set for broad-scale work on both the treatment and the prevention of disease and injury. With this role came the potential for leadership in elucidating the role of personal behavior in the causation of disease and injury, in deepening our understanding of the part played by health education in improving the public's health and safety, and in increasing our ability to provide such education.

Fortunately, Mayhew Derryberry was strategically positioned for this task. In 1941, Derryberry became chief of the newly formed

Division of Health Education in the Public Health Service and began assembling a team to engage the myriad issues intersecting at the nexus of behavior, social factors, and disease and injury. Many hold that it was at this time that Derryberry and his associates in the Division of Health Education laid the foundation for our modern efforts in health education policy, practice, and research. Much of the current work of health educators and other public health disciplines can be traced back to the earliest work and studies carried out by Derryberry and those who collaborated with him. Most notably, two social psychologists in the division, Godfrey Hochbaum and Irwin Rosenstock, conducted what is now the seminal study of the role of health beliefs in explaining utilization of public health screening services. This effort spawned development of the Health Belief Model and enhanced our understanding of health behavior for a generation to come.

With the enhanced understanding of the preventable nature of many health problems and the critical role of behavior that emerged from studies generated by the National Institute of Health during the 1950s and 1960s came new interest in health education during the 1970s. In 1973, President Nixon formed the President's Committee on Health Education to study the role of education in advancing the nation's health. Among other initiatives, the committee recommended that two parallel health education organizations be established, one internal to government and one external, to promote the involvement of the private sector in sponsoring the use of health education for better health. The Bureau of Health Education at the Centers for Disease Control served that role within government, and the National Center for Health Education (which assembled these and the original set of Derryberry papers) was formed to mobilize the private sector response.

Building on and drawing from the momentum of the president's committee, a number of related assessments were initiated to review the possibilities for stronger work in prevention, including stronger federal leadership. The most sustained of these assessments is perhaps the work launched in 1977 by then Health Education and Welfare (HEW) (now Health and Human Services) secretary Joseph Califano and his surgeon general, Julius Richmond, with the formation of the federal Task Force on Disease Prevention and Health Promotion, which I was privileged to chair in my capacity as HEW deputy assistant secretary at the time. That task force was charged with reviewing the possibilities for prevention, along with the activities of the relevant federal agencies, and recommending a series of program and budgetary enhancements to strengthen the work.

The 1978 report of that internal task force was entitled *Healthy People*, a name that was carried over to the following year with our 1979 release of *Healthy People: The Surgeon General's Report on Health Promotion and Disease Prevention*. It was our hope that this surgeon general's report would help draw the nation's attention to several important facts: (1) that the health of the American people had improved substantially, (2) that the gains were largely attributable to prevention, (3) that behavioral factors were perhaps the leading issues in the dominant health challenges of the day, (4) that health promotion and health education were therefore key to further progress, and (5) that the potential for further progress was so considerable that it might even be quantified. In respect to that final point, quantified targets were established in *Healthy People* for reducing, by 1990, the death rates for Americans at each major life stage: infancy, childhood, adolescence, and adulthood. In the following year, 1980, the report *Promoting Health/Preventing Disease: Objectives for the Nation* set out some 226 measurable targets for the year 1990 in health promotion, health protection, and clinical preventive services—targets in areas deemed important to achieving the overall reductions in deaths expressed in the *Healthy People* goals. Thus began the first iteration of the *Healthy People* process, a process now in its third decade with the publication of *Healthy People 2010*, many of the health education elements of which are traceable to the initiatives and legacy of Mayhew Derryberry.

The scope of progress spanning the nearly seventy years since Derryberry first started on the public scene is striking. We now know, through large-scale epidemiologic studies, that smoking tobacco is the leading cause of most lung cancers. We now know that elevated serum cholesterol, smoking, high blood pressure, obesity, and diabetes are key risk factors for developing cardiovascular disease. We now know that alcohol-impaired driving, failing to use safety belts, and speeding are the major contributors to motor vehicle injuries. And we now know the critical role that behavioral and social factors play as nonmedical determinants of disease. Most important, we are making significant progress against those factors.

We also know that in the relatively short span of our country's history, we have been fortunate to have had prominent leaders like Derryberry, who should be recognized for his leadership in catalyzing this nation's earliest efforts in heath promotion and disease prevention. Though the work is far from done—mention need only be made of the current burden of obesity trends, HIV infection, injuries, and addiction to recognize that fact—our progress has been great and our tools are more powerful because Mayhew Derryberry and the contemporaries he mentored had the foresight, the commitment, and the tenacity to change the landscape of federal policy. This volume will do much more than merely orient a new generation of public health education specialists to the work that provides the basis for much of contemporary health education practice. It will prompt a vital understanding of how people of unflagging courage, vision, and leadership can make a difference.

February 2004   J. MICHAEL MCGINNIS
                                    The Robert Wood Johnson Foundation
                                    Princeton, N.J.

Preface to the Original Edition

In the history of every profession one encounters individuals who have a dynamic impact on its character and direction. Sometimes they achieved such prominence by introducing new ideas or by the persistence with which they fought for their ideals in the face of rejection by peers. Others served as catalysts for ideas emerging from other disciplines. No matter how such individuals achieved their own success, they brought new insights to shape the profession's future irreversibly and forever.

Mayhew Derryberry, Ph.D., was this kind of leader. Anyone who educates for improved health practices can learn from Dr. Derryberry. The magnitude and timely relevance of his impact on health education and public health can best be appreciated by traveling back in time to see what health education was like when the theories, concepts, strategies, and methods that are taken for granted today were still unknown. Students in health education today learn about community organization, needs assessment, pretesting and evaluation of educational materials, program evaluation, group processes, behavioral science theories and models. All beginning students also focus on the role of attitudes and motivation. Their studies include the premise that people's behavior in the face of health hazards is determined by their personal, social, and cultural beliefs more than by medical history.

We accept without question that the scientific underpinning of health education is in the field of education and the social and behavioral sciences rather than in the health sciences. These concepts have their genesis in the careers of persons such as Mayhew Derryberry.

Dr. Derryberry's vision, firm convictions, persuasive leadership, and wide sweep of scientific and professional skills gave him a decisive role in broadening and enhancing the field of health education. A national and international trailblazer in health education, Dr. Derryberry directed the central health education unit of the U.S. Public Health Service during a very productive 27-year career. During this period, Dr. Derryberry, either individually or in collaboration with other eminent public health professionals, presented a number of papers on various subjects, including educational aspects of health services, involving the public in health decision making, influencing adult health behavior, and involvement of physicians and nurses in the communication process.

Several of us associated with Dr. Derryberry have worked to bring together a collection of his more significant papers. They not only serve as a tribute to his vitality, resourcefulness, and thinking but also provide a foundation for understanding the evolution and acceptance of concepts widely practiced today. This historical perspective of Dr. Derryberry's contribution to the profession has significance for the future growth and development of the next generation of health educators.

Dr. Derryberry was a leader in the period of intellectual ferment that began to take shape in the 1930s. A number of highly gifted and dedicated individuals contributed profoundly to the revolutionary changes that were taking place. Names like Nyswander, Morgan, Connolly, Rugen, Hiscock, and others are inseparably interwoven with significant developments in the health education field. Before them, the research and leadership of professionals such as Sedgwick, Winslow, and Turner helped to establish lasting legacies for those in or about to enter the public health education field. These people were illustrative of that creative period of time.

As a key participant, Dr. Derryberry encouraged and gave a sense of direction for demonstrating and testing revolutionary concepts in health education practices. Unafraid to take professional risks, Dr. Derryberry established demonstration projects and pilot studies, expanded research-potential through integration with other disciplines, and presented findings to various professional communities. Because of such efforts, Dr. Derryberry established a profound and lasting reputation in the public health field.

All this did not come easily. It was a long and sometimes difficult battle. There were many victories and some defeats. In the end Dr. Derryberry could look back and see a profession that had grown intellectually, methodologically, and ideologically. He saw a profession that was on the threshold of being recognized by other health and medical professionals as legitimate and significant.

These papers exist because of Dr. Derryberry's everlasting commitment to what has become the modern-day principle of feedback. He believed that it was necessary to put his ideas on paper so that the largest group possible could consider, discuss, and evaluate them. The technique of feedback requires an open mind, receptiveness to new ideas, and courage to take risks—attributes that Dr. Derryberry exhibited throughout his career as a public health researcher, leader, and teacher.

It is exciting to see how an idea is originally presented and how it can change over time. These papers show the evolution and development of community participation, communication strategies, evaluation, and a host of other components now taken for granted in health program development. Since the training of health educators was always near and dear to him, we hope that the next generation of health educators will draw inspiration and gain strength from Dr. Derryberry's papers.

We gratefully acknowledge permission given by various publishers to reprint the papers included in this book. As you read them, thinking about the ideas and judging their merits, remember that Dr. Derryberry would have been the first to ask: "What do you think of this? Will it work? What's a better way?" In order to better appreciate and respond to Dr. Derryberry's intellectual challenges, the papers have been arranged to reflect relevant issues. The short introductions to each chapter are designed to put the particular topic in proper perspective for present and future use.

Preface to This Edition

I was privileged to know Mayhew and Helen Derryberry, "Uncle Derry" and "Aunt Helen" to me, as a member of their extensive network of relatives. My brother and sisters and I, together with a whole host of second- and third-generation nephews, nieces, and cousins, were the beneficiaries of quality time spent with Helen and Derry at family gatherings, including graduations, weddings, and christenings, exotic Indian dinners prepared by Chef Helen (I still can recall the rebuke at my inappropriate review of her famous eggplant casserole), Cal football games, spontaneous bridge and other card games, and picnics (Helen and Derry loved picnics).

Through these events, we learned of and had an opportunity to meet many of Derry's professional colleagues from throughout the United States and beyond. We especially enjoyed meeting Derry's graduate students at Berkeley. We saw first-hand the magnitude of Derry's reputation and stature within the public health community as he mentored the next generation of practitioners.

Even though I always had an appreciation for Derry's work and accomplishments in the field, I did not comprehend the timeliness, sophistication, and depth of his research until I was asked by Helen to work with Clarence E. Pearson and the National Center for Health Education (NCHE). After Derry's untimely death, Helen devoted her time and resources to the project of publishing Derry's more significant papers, not only as a remembrance of his remarkable career but also to ensure that his research would not be lost to future generations of public health professionals. Helen's venture afforded me a unique opportunity to interface not only with Clarence and NCHE but also with those colleagues of Derry's and friends of Helen's—Cecilia Conrath Doak, Godfrey Hochbaum, and Jeannette Simmons—who likewise wanted to preserve Derry's valuable and relevant heritage and scholarship.

Through our collaborative efforts, the initial editorial committee, with Helen's constant oversight (she never forgot her days at *Harper's*), produced and published the original memorial to Derry. Helen was very proud of what we had accomplished. I know that she would be profoundly moved by the efforts of John Allegrante and David Sleet, as well as, again, NCHE, to revisit her dream of creating *Derryberry's Educating for Health*. John and David have validated our original efforts, for which we are eternally grateful.

On behalf of the family, and in loving memory of Helen and Derry, I want to express our heartfelt thanks to John, David, and NCHE for continuing the work launched by Helen as a testament to a person who touched so many lives, whether first-hand or as a result of his pioneering work in public health.

February 2004   WILLIAM D. TAYLOR, ESQUIRE
                                                   Sacramento, California

Acknowledgments to the Original Edition

So many professional colleagues, associates, and friends are responsible for this publication that I cannot begin to thank each and every one by name. Without your expertise, enlightened judgment, and perseverance this book would not have been published.

You have all contributed, each in your own way, toward fostering the philosophy and nurturing the spirit of health education represented in these papers. May the combined strength of our efforts renew our convictions and commitment to a better life for future generations.

Thank you, one and all.

1987   MRS. MAYHEW (HELEN) DERRYBERRY

Acknowledgments to This Edition

Although preparing an edited volume is not without its tribulations, this was a labor of love. But we know that it would not have been possible to undertake such a project without the efforts of many who gave generously of their time and thinking. Thus we owe a debt of gratitude to a number of individuals who have worked with us to make this book a reality.

We are especially grateful to J. Michael McGinnis, of the Robert Wood Johnson Foundation, who has followed in the footsteps of Mayhew Derryberry, serving through four successive presidential administrations (1977 to 1995) as assistant surgeon general, deputy assistant secretary for health, and director of the U.S. Office of Disease Prevention and Health Promotion, for contributing his elegant foreword to this book. A special note of thanks also goes to William D. Taylor, an attorney with Hanson Bridgett, Sacramento, California, Mayhew and Helen Derryberry's great-nephew, who was kind enough to contribute the new preface for this edition. It was Mr. Taylor, together with a writing team of Dr. Derryberry's closest colleagues and staff of the National Center for Health Education, including Helen Derryberry, who organized the original 1987 anthology, *Educating for Health: The Selected Papers of Mayhew Derryberry*.

Our thanks go to M. Elaine Auld, executive director of the Society for Public Health Education (SOPHE), and Rose Marie Matulionis, executive director of the Directors of Health Promotion and

Education (DHPE), formerly the Association of State and Territorial Directors of Health Promotion and Public Health Education (ASTDHPPHE), whose commentaries on Derryberry's contributions to the early organizational development of both SOPHE and ASTDHPPHE give testament to the vision and enduring legacy of leadership that he has left to these two important national professional associations and the profession as a whole. Similarly, we thank Linda E. Forys and Terri Lee Stratton, cochairs of the American Public Health Association Public Health Education and Health Promotion (PHEHP) Section Awards Committee, which bestows the Derryberry Award.

The field of health education is fortunate to have outstanding scientists and practitioners, many of whom have stood on the shoulders of giants like Mayhew Derryberry. Fortunately, a number of them graciously agreed to contribute to this book. We thank the living recipients of the Mayhew Derryberry Award—including Noreen M. Clark, Eugenia Eng, Martin Fishbein, Nicholas Freudenberg, Karen Glanz, Kate Lorig, Barbara K. Rimer, and David A. Sleet—as well as our colleagues James R. Sorenson and Lawrence W. Green—who joined Nicholas Freudenberg in writing on behalf of the deceased Godfrey Hochbaum, Marshall Becker, and Irwin Rosenstock. They all kindly contributed reflective commentaries that contain insightful tales and entertaining anecdotes about the life and legend of Mayhew Derryberry and his key contemporaries. Each of the commentaries provides fitting tribute to the man, his principles, and his profession, and serves to further contextualize his enduring legacy for the next generation of health educators.

In addition, we gratefully acknowledge Richard K. Means, professor emeritus at Auburn University, author of a brief biographical essay about Derryberry that appeared in "Key Leaders in Health Education: A Century of Commitment," a volume in *The Eta Sigma Gamma Monograph Series*. We have drawn extensively on this essay, which provided an invaluable point of departure in recounting Derryberry's career. We also thank Ann Nolte, professor emeritus and historian of health education at Illinois State University, who helped us to track down one of the few remaining photographs of Derryberry, which Becky Smith, executive director of the American Association for Health Education, then rescued for us from the association's archives.

Others helped us organize ideas for this book. We extend a very special thanks to Ray Marks, a 2000 SOPHE/CDC Fellow in Unintentional Injury Prevention and our research associate at Teachers College, Columbia University, for contributing the discussion questions that appear at the end of each chapter and for her tireless efforts in assisting us with every aspect of this project. Her commitment, careful and erudite attention to editorial detail, and management of the innumerable logistics associated with manuscript development and production were crucial in facilitating our work, and without this assistance, we think it is safe to say, this book would not have been completed.

We are fortunate to have worked with an outstanding editor at Jossey-Bass, Andrew Pasternack, whose appreciation for the history of health education and confidence in us were invaluable to moving this book project forward. He played an especially critical role during the early phases of the project in helping us to conceptualize the idea and then coaching us on how to most effectively organize the manuscript. In addition, Jossey-Bass production editor Gigi Mark, editorial assistant Seth Schwartz, and assistant manager of marketing Jessica Egbert were also exceptionally supportive; they too have our deepest appreciation. And we thank our anonymous reviewers, whose comments early in the process of developing the manuscript influenced our thinking about how best to organize and integrate new material.

We acknowledge and thank Elizabeth Fee, chief of the History of Medicine Division at the National Library of Medicine, who provided valuable advice on the issue of language and historicity; Stephen J. Greenberg, coordinator of public services at the History of Medicine Division, who was kind enough to research the archives

at the National Library of Medicine for additional papers by Derryberry; Constance B. Oberle, Cadwalader, Wickersham & Taft, who
provided legal counsel on copyright and other issues on behalf of
the National Center for Health Education; and Robert "Rocky"
Schwarz, manager of the Word Processing Center at Teachers College, Columbia University, and his team, including Gina Lee and
Frances Hill, who scanned and digitized text from the original book
manuscript; Constance Tsai and I-Shien Lei, who worked to secure
the necessary copyright permissions; and Betty Engel, who reproduced the figures and tables from the original manuscripts.

We thank the National Center for Health Education, who, with
generous support from the Metropolitan Life Insurance Company,
published the first anthology. We are especially grateful to
Clarence E. Pearson, former staff member of the President's Committee on Health Education and former president of the National
Center for Health Education, who procured for us one of the few
remaining copies of the 1987 edition. We also owe a special debt of
gratitude to Teachers College, Columbia University, and the U.S.
Centers for Disease Control and Prevention, without whose support this new volume would not have been possible.

Finally, we would be remiss if we did not thank our respective
wives, Andrea Allegrante and Louise Gobron, as well as Jason Allegrante, who have encouraged and supported us in working on
this project when we might otherwise have been working on a family project.

February 2004

JOHN P. ALLEGRANTE
New York, New York
DAVID A. SLEET
Atlanta, Georgia

The Editors

JOHN P. ALLEGRANTE is senior professor of health education at Teachers College, Columbia University, and president and CEO of the National Center for Health Education. He holds appointments as adjunct professor of sociomedical sciences at the Mailman School of Public Health of Columbia University and adjunct professor of behavioral science in medicine at the Weill Medical College of Cornell University. His current research interests include developing and testing novel behavioral and educational strategies that can improve health behavior and health outcomes in people with chronic disease. Allegrante is a contributing author to *Critical Issues in Global Health* and is the author of numerous other book chapters and many journal articles in health education and health promotion. A past president and Distinguished Fellow of the Society for Public Health Education, he is currently associate editor of *Health Education Research*. He received the Distinguished Career Award from the American Public Health Association (APHA) Public Health Education and Health Promotion Section in 2003.

DAVID A. SLEET is associate director for science in the Division of Unintentional Injury Prevention at the U.S. Centers for Disease Control and Prevention (CDC). He also holds adjunct appointments at the Rollins School of Public Health of Emory University and at the University of New Mexico, University of Tennessee, and

Curtin University in Perth, Australia. Before joining CDC, Sleet was a research psychologist at the U.S. National Highway Traffic Safety Administration in Washington, D.C., and for twenty-six years was a professor of public health and health science at San Diego State University. He has published more than 150 articles related to injury prevention, health promotion, disease prevention, and community health. A Fellow of the American Academy of Health Behavior, Sleet received the APHA Mayhew Derryberry Award in 1999 and the Association of State and Territorial Directors of Health Promotion and Public Health Education Award for Health Promotion and Health Education Advocacy in 2001. He and his team at CDC won the 2001 Health and Human Services Secretary's Award and the 2003 National Highway Traffic Safety Administration Administrator's Award for Distinguished Service for Research.

The Contributors

JOHN P. ALLEGRANTE is professor of health education at Teachers College, Columbia University, and president and CEO of the National Center for Health Education.

M. ELAINE AULD is executive director of the Society for Public Health Education.

NOREEN M. CLARK is Marshall H. Becker Professor and dean of the University of Michigan School of Public Health.

EUGENIA ENG is professor of health behavior and health education at the University of North Carolina School of Public Health at Chapel Hill.

MARTIN FISHBEIN is Harry C. Coles, Jr. Distinguished Professor of communication at the Annenberg Public Policy Center, the Annenberg School for Communication at the University of Pennsylvania.

LINDA E. FORYS is director of health education for Harris County Public Health and Environmental Services, Houston, Texas.

NICHOLAS FREUDENBERG is Distinguished Professor and director of the Program in Urban Public Health at Hunter College of the City University of New York.

KAREN GLANZ is professor of behavioral sciences and health education and a Georgia Cancer Coalition Distinguished Scholar at the Rollins School of Public Health at Emory University.

LAWRENCE W. GREEN is a Distinguished Fellow at the Centers for Disease Control and Prevention in Atlanta and visiting professor of behavioral sciences and health education at the Rollins School of Public Health of Emory University.

KATE LORIG is research professor of medicine at the Stanford University School of Medicine.

ROSE MARIE MATULIONIS is executive director of the Directors of Health Promotion and Education.

BARBARA K. RIMER is Alumni Distinguished Professor of health behavior and health education at the University of North Carolina School of Public Health at Chapel Hill.

DAVID A. SLEET is associate director for science in the Division of Unintentional Injury Prevention at the National Center for Injury Prevention at the Centers for Disease Control and Prevention in Atlanta.

JAMES R. SORENSON is professor of health behavior and health education at the University of North Carolina School of Public Health at Chapel Hill.

TERRI LEE STRATTON is a senior health education specialist with the California Department of Health Services.

Derryberry's
Educating for Health

INTRODUCTION

Introduction and Overview

John P. Allegrante and David A. Sleet

This book updates *Educating for Health: Selected Papers of Mayhew Derryberry*, an anthology originally published in 1987 by the National Center for Health Education in New York. It occurred to us in planning this book that more than a few people would ask, Why reissue a book that was originally published almost two decades ago when so much in the world has changed? Part of the reason is the same reason why undergraduate students at some of America's colleges and universities still read the "Great Books," because some insights and ideas transcend change and the passage of time. It is precisely because so much has changed in the world in the last twenty-five years that writings like these, which have enduring value, should be preserved and revisited by subsequent generations.

There are also several more immediately practical reasons why we believe this new volume, *Derryberry's Educating for Health: A Foundation for Contemporary Health Education Practice*, not only will be of historical interest to the current generation of scientists and practitioners in the field of health education but will also extend the legacy of Mayhew Derryberry's work to the next generation of behavioral scientists and health educators.

To begin with, Derryberry was the first director of health education in the U.S. Public Health Service and an extraordinary figure in the annals of the field of health education. From that position he made significant contributions and developed and described a unique perspective on the potential value and role of health education that no other individual had developed or had written about before with such authority and clarity. Second, historical perspective informs contemporary research and practice. The principles Derryberry pioneered in establishing for the field of health education—today a science-based profession more than merely craft—have stood the test of time. The work with which he occupied his time provides the foundation on which our generation has built its efforts to advance the health of the public through education. Finally, because an entire generation of Derryberry's contemporaries are, sadly, now beginning to depart, we felt it important, indeed urgent, to reestablish his legacy for a new generation of students and practicing professionals.

The Man, His Life, His Times

In the pantheon of health education, Mayhew Derryberry stands out as a leader of uncommon vision and uncommon action. He was born December 25, 1902, in Columbia, Tennessee, where he spent most of his youth. He was educated at the University of Tennessee and earned a bachelor of arts degree with majors in chemistry and mathematics in 1925. In 1927, he earned a master of arts degree in education and psychology at Teachers College, Columbia University, where he is likely to have been influenced by the philosopher and renowned founder of progressive education John Dewey, the educational psychologist Edward L. Thorndike, and both Thomas Denison Wood, the "father of health education," and Jesse Feiring Williams, a prominent professor of physical education. Derryberry received his Ph.D. degree in health and physical education from New York University in 1933, studying at that institution with a number of the early leaders in the field.

Derryberry's formal higher education thus took place toward the middle of the Great Depression and before World War II. Moreover, his professional preparation took place well before the creation of the many federal health-related institutions of the postwar era in which he would later work and play key leadership roles. But he was fortunate to have studied with some of the giants of the field, apparently leaving his years of professional education with a cosmopolitanism, which, together with important understandings and skills, would serve him and the profession well into the future.

In 1926, while he was a research assistant at New York University, he began his career with the American Child Health Association, where he was associate director of the ten-year School Health Study, one of the first large-scale studies to examine the health status of the nation's schoolchildren and evaluate school health programs. His early writings suggest that it was through this work that he became aware of the impact of childhood diseases on subsequent human development and learning and of the evident, but largely undocumented, disparities in health status this created, particularly for African Americans. He remained with the American Child Health Association until 1933 and rose to the position of associate director of research before leaving for the New York City Health Department, where he held the position of secretary to the sanitary superintendent until 1937. During those years he became an advocate for school health programs and wrote a series of distinct but related papers on child health that were published in the *Child Health Bulletin* and in several other prominent journals.

In 1937, Dr. Derryberry moved to the nation's fledgling National Institute of Health and U.S. Public Health Service in Washington, D.C., where he served as a senior public health analyst and chief of the Health Education Studies Section in the Division of Public Health Methods. It was at the Public Health Service, on the stage of national government service, that he began to play out what was perhaps the most extraordinary phase of his long and productive career. In 1941, Derryberry was named chief of the newly formed Division of Health Education of the Public Health Service and held that position until his retirement in 1963. During this period he catalyzed some of the earliest studies of human health behavior, with Godfrey Hochbaum, Andie Knutson, Howard Leventhal, and Irwin Rosenstock. All of these men were social psychologists and all had been influenced by the early work of the famous social psychologist Kurt Lewin. Together they pioneered in developing an applied theory of what motivated human health behavior, the Health Belief Model. And because their initial thinking about the Health Belief Model was grounded in observations they made about the public's use and acceptance of community screening programs, they recognized early on that questions generated from reflective practice needed to drive research and that research needed to inform both public health practice and policy.

During his years with the Public Health Service, Derryberry was also active in several professional associations, holding key leadership roles with the American Public Health Association (APHA), the Society for Public Health Education (SOPHE), and the Association of State and Territorial Directors of Health Promotion and Public Health Education (ASTDHPPHE), now the Directors of Health Promotion and Education (DHPE). He served as chairman of the APHA Committee on Planning Health Education and later as chairman of the APHA Public Health Education Section (now the Public Health Education and Health Promotion Section). He was also a founding member of SOPHE in 1950 and served as the new organization's second president in 1951–1952. In addition, he helped to organize and launch ASTDHPPHE and was involved in the International Union for Health Education (now the International Union for Health Promotion and Education). He was subsequently honored for his many contributions to these organizations when SOPHE gave him the Distinguished Fellow Award in 1970 and when the APHA Public Health Education and Health Promotion Section acknowledged him posthumously by establishing the Mayhew Derryberry Award in 1981. (The first recipient was one of Derryberry's first protégés, Godfrey Hochbaum.)

Dr. Derryberry held academic appointments on the faculties of the University of California at Berkeley and the University of Minnesota, where, as the reader will learn, he taught and mentored numerous students who themselves went on to key leadership roles in health education research and practice. During his long career he also proved to be a gifted speaker and prolific writer. His first publication, in 1931, was a monograph he coauthored with George Palmer and Philip Van Ingen, titled *Health Protection for the Preschool Child*. He went on to write approximately eighty journal and newsletter articles, the last of which was published in 1977. In between he wrote another sixty-four unpublished papers and addresses that identified methods, discussed the qualifications of the public health workforce, and dispensed advice and wisdom on an astonishingly wide range of topics: for example, immunizations, the nutritional status of children, measurement and statistical methods, the relationship between social factors and health, and program evaluation. Because his writing was both trenchant and prescient, many of his papers have left an indelible mark on the profession and are still considered classics. (See Appendix A for a listing of both his published and unpublished papers.)

Derryberry ended his twenty-six-year career in federal government service in 1963, when he departed for an assignment as a U.S. Agency for International Development (USAID) family-planning adviser to India, just as President Johnson's Great Society programs— civil rights, Medicare, and the War on Poverty—were being proposed by Congress, programs that would help spawn health education's modern emphasis on the role of the community. An important legacy of his work was that it engaged behavioral and social scientists in the problems of public health and elucidated the valuable role that health education can play to improve human health. Writing in *The Eta Sigma Gamma Monograph Series* issue "Key Leaders in Health Education: A Century of Commitment," Richard Means, professor emeritus at Auburn University and a historian of the field of health education, has said: "Many remember 'Derry' as a modest and quiet person, yet one not reluctant to speak out on important issues and firm in his beliefs. Over the years, he exerted strong leadership in numerous capacities which extended to the international level. His influence was tremendous during what might be called the formative years of modern health education in schools and at the public health level" (Means, 1990, p. 19).

Derryberry died at the Public Health Service Hospital in San Francisco on December 24, 1979, at the age of seventy-seven. He was survived by his lifetime partner and wife, Helen F. Derryberry, who died in 1988. Writing in the *American Journal of Public Health*, where Derryberry's obituary appeared in the association news in April 1980, William Griffiths, Malcolm Merrill, and Dorothy Nyswander—all contemporaries and longtime colleagues of Derryberry—wrote that "'Derry,' as Dr. Mayhew Derryberry was known to thousands of his public health colleagues, probably did more to develop and enhance the profession of public heath education than any other single individual" (Griffiths, Merrill, & Nyswander, 1980, p. 445).[1]

Organization of This Book

We have organized this book into two major sections. The first section, which immediately follows this introduction, contains reflective essays on the life, times, and contributions of Derryberry, written by almost all of the living recipients of the APHA Public Health Education and Health Promotion Section's Mayhew Derryberry Award. These individuals have made outstanding contributions to the profession of health education, and many have engaged in a lifetime of work that has resulted in the construction of necessary bridges between social science and its application to applied research and practice in health education. Several recipients of the award—Godfrey Hochbaum, Marshall Becker, and Irwin Rosenstock—are now deceased. We invited James Sorenson, Lawrence Green, and Nicholas Freudenberg (an award recipient himself) to speculate on how these deceased recipients' work had been influenced by Derryberry. Many of our invited contributors spoke admiringly of Derryberry and told us how much they had learned from reading his original papers during the formative stages of their own career development. The result, we hope you will agree, is a set of remarkable essays that convey not only a sense of the man and the intellectual challenges of the times in which he lived and worked but also the ways in which his pioneering contributions constitute an important historical thread that continues to connect the work of health educators and behavioral health scientists from one generation to another.

Because Derryberry's leadership and vision contributed to the founding and early organizational development of ASTDHPPHE (now DHPE)and SOPHE, we also invited commentaries from the current executive directors of both organizations. These essays reveal Derryberry's contributions to the early development of both professional organizations, and therefore we hope the book will be used by DHPE and SOPHE, as well as by academic professional preparation programs, to orient students and new professionals to the profession and its history. In addition, a brief history of the Derryberry Award, contributed by the current cochairs of the awards committee of the APHA Pubic Health Education and Health Promotion Section, provides a backdrop to the contributions by the Derryberry Award winners.

The second section, *Derryberry's Educating for Health*, contains the original text of the 1987 six-part volume, *Educating for Health: Selected Papers of Mayhew Derryberry*. Part One is titled "Linking Statistical Methods to Health Education"; Part Two, "Education: A Challenge to All Health Professions"; Part Three, "Establishing the Parameters of Health Education"; Part Four, "Community Health Education"; Part Five, "Influencing the International Health Field"; and Part Six, "Research in Public Health Issues." Each part contains between three and seven of Derryberry's most significant papers—each treated as a chapter—several of which were coauthored with prominent collaborators. Although Derryberry's writing was shaped by the often turbulent context of the middle decades of the twentieth century, the principles he elucidated endure to this day. Thus what is so remarkable in reading these chapters is just how well the concepts proposed stand the test of time. We believe that this is because Derryberry, early on, conceptualized the field so well and understood—perhaps better than any of his contemporaries—what the enduring principles of health education practice would and should be well into the future.

Finally, a note about the original text and its historicity. Derryberry wrote many of his most important papers during the 1950s, 1960s, and 1970s, a period of rapid and remarkable social and scientific ferment in the United States. He and the editors of the journals in which he published adhered to conventions in the use of language that were acceptable during their time but would not be so today. Although we have decided to retain most of the original text of Derryberry's papers to preserve its historical authenticity for posterity, we have taken the liberty to selectively edit some of his writing for this collection. Thus we have corrected words that had been misspelled in the original anthology and have updated the spelling of certain words, punctuation, grammar, and other conventions of usage to make these items consistent with modern standards.

We hope that as a result of reading and discussing this book both the current and next generation of health education specialists will better appreciate the roots of the science and professional practice that characterize health education today, for the principles that Derryberry first elucidated are still relevant to the contemporary issues and challenges that face the field of health education.

Audience and How to Use This Book

Derryberry's Educating for Health: A Foundation for Contemporary Health Education Practice is primarily intended for both undergraduate and graduate students who are undertaking professional preparation in health education for practice in school or community settings. We envision this book being especially useful as a supplemental text in foundational or introductory courses. In addition, the book should be valuable as an essential primary text for courses and seminars that deal directly with the history and development of public health and particularly the field of health education and health promotion. Thus we hope that current practitioners, faculty and students in professional preparation programs, and historians of public health will think of this book as a key reference in the historical development of the field of health education—especially in relation to the evolution of theory-based practice and the relevance of the behavioral and social sciences to public health.

We believe that an effective way to use this book is to read Derryberry's original chapters and then reflect about the relevance to contemporary health education practice of the issues and challenges he addressed. Because the field has changed so dramatically in the years since the publication of his original papers and even since the publication of the first anthology, students and professionals should be encouraged to connect Derryberry's work to that of present-day practice. Here are some general questions that might prompt that connection:

- What were the social conditions of the time that influenced Derryberry's thinking on how to improve health status, and how are they similar or different from conditions today?

- What were the leading causes of morbidity and mortality during the 1950s, and how have these indicators of health status changed in the last fifty years?

- What were the challenges Derryberry faced in his work, and how do his writings suggest he dealt with them?

- How has the role of the behavioral and social sciences in health education changed since Derryberry's time?

- What lessons can be learned from Derryberry's early contributions that apply to contemporary health education practice?

- What federal initiatives in health education are needed now to continue the progress we have made in public health since Derryberry's leadership of the Public Health Service?

In addition to these broad questions, we have supplied a series of specific discussion questions at the end of each chapter. These questions are designed to facilitate dialogue about connections between then and now and about the nexus between theory and practice.

Note

1. We have drawn extensively on the two previously published biographical essays discussed here and listed in the References. Please see these essays for further details about Derryberry's life and career. Although the essential facts are consistent across these two essays, the *American Journal of Public Health* essay gives Derryberry's year of birth incorrectly as 1901. The correct year is 1902. In addition, we have written a substantially abbreviated version of Derryberry's biography, which, along with excerpts from one of his papers that was originally published in *Public Health Reports* ("Today's Health Problems and Health Education," which appears as Chapter Eleven in this book), appeared in the Voices from the Past department of the March 2004 issue of the *American Journal of Public Health*, which is also listed in the references below.

References

Allegrante, J. P., Sleet, D. A., & McGinnis, J. M. (2004). Mayhew Derryberry: Pioneer of health education. *American Journal of Public Health*, 94, 370–371.

Griffiths, W., Merrill, M. H., & Nyswander, D. B. (1980). Association News. Mayhew Derryberry, Ph.D., 1901–1979. *American Journal of Public Health*, 70, 445–446.

Means, R. K. (1990). Mayhew Derryberry. In A. Nolte & M. K. Beyrer (Eds.), Key leaders in health education: A century of commitment. *The Eta Sigma Gamma Monograph Series*, 8, 18–19.

Commentaries from the Profession

The Public Health Education and Health Promotion (PHEHP) Section of the American Public Health Association (APHA) and the Mayhew Derryberry Award

Linda E. Forys and Terri Lee Stratton

The Public Health Education and Health Promotion (PHEHP) Section of the American Public Health Association (APHA) is delighted with the publication of *Derryberry's Educating for Health: A Foundation for Contemporary Health Education Practice*. It represents "getting back to basics" for all in the field of health education and health promotion.

In order to honor and remember the work of Dr. Derryberry, who had also served as chair of the APHA Public Health Education Section, the PHEHP Section established the Mayhew Derryberry Award in 1981 to recognize the contributions of outstanding behavioral scientists to the field of health education (see Appendix B). This award has so far recognized thirteen exceptional individuals: Godfrey Hochbaum (1981); Marshall H. Becker (1982); Noreen M. Clark (1985); Jeanette Simmons (1991), Karen Glanz,

Frances M. Lewis, and Barbara K. Rimer (1992); Kate Lorig (1993); Irwin M. Rosenstock and Nicholas Freudenberg (1994); Eugenia Eng (1998); David A. Sleet (1999); and Martin Fishbein (2003).

Each of these award recipients (with the exception of Jeanette Simmons and Fran Lewis) or his or her surrogate has graciously contributed reflections on Derryberry's life and his influence on the field. Whether you know about or never knew about Derryberry, you will take pleasure in reading what the award recipients have to say about him. Like many of you, some of these recipients had never before read some of the writings printed in this book. Hence the APHA PHEHP Section applauded the idea that this book be made available for all to read.

The chapters in this book offer important documentation that health education did not grow up in a vacuum. Its concepts and practices have always involved a contemporary response to the constantly evolving challenges in public health. We can see in Derryberry's work how theory emerged as an important underpinning for public health education and how theory interacting with practice produces better results. This book reminds us that even old ideas were once new, and some ideas are timeless. Mayhew Derryberry's work has stood the test of time.

APHA's Public Health Education and Health Promotion Section expects to continue giving the Mayhew Derryberry Award as a tribute to the man and his extraordinary influence on the field. The award also stands as a reminder that we value, as Derryberry did before us, the application of behavioral and social science theory in public health education. The PHEHP Section invites nominations and applications each year (usually to be submitted by April 30) and makes the award at the end of the year, in November, during a special PHEHP awards luncheon at the APHA annual meeting. To learn more about the Derryberry Award, go to www.jhsph.edu/hao/phehp/.

The Association of State and Territorial Directors of Health Promotion and Public Health Education (ASTDHPPHE) and the Enduring Legacy of Mayhew Derryberry

Rose Marie Matulionis

The Association of State and Territorial Directors of Health Promotion and Public Health Education (ASTDHPPHE) was founded in 1946 as the Conference of State Directors of Public Health Education, a joint effort between directors of health education in state health departments and deans of health education in schools of public health. The formation of the conference was supported by Mayhew Derryberry, then chief of health education with the Public Health Service (PHS). It was Dr. Derryberry's vision that the creation of this organization would strengthen state public health education program goals and objectives and develop a network for the sharing of program efforts, ideas, and materials. In addition, Derryberry was interested in strengthening the practice of public health education through regional PHS offices.

Today ASTDHPPHE, which was recently renamed and now called the Directors of Health Promotion and Education (DHPE), represents fifty-five directors of health education and health promotion units of state health departments and the health departments of the District of Columbia, Puerto Rico, the Virgin Islands, Guam, and American Samoa, as well as several directors of the health education units of Indian Health Service area offices. DHPE also has approximately 140 associate members and members emeritus.

We have Dr. Derryberry to thank for the enduring influence that DHPE members have had on public health, for without him, ASTDHPPHE might not have been formed and certainly would not have matured into what is today DHPE. We held our twenty-first annual conference in 2003, attracting upward of 500 professional health educators, health promotion professionals, and other public health professionals. Today, the Centers for Disease Control and Prevention (CDC) and DHPE cosponsor the National Conference on Health Education and Health Promotion. Our association is 225 members strong and enjoys wide and continuing support from many of the various divisions, centers, and institutes at the CDC, as well as from the National Institutes of Health and numerous private companies and foundations. Although our individual commitment to educating for health has certainly grown, our collective commitment has really blossomed.

Dr. Derryberry's important writings, reflected in this volume, remind us of the roots of health education and health promotion. Revisiting his thinking about prevention also reminds us of the importance of our work and the value of public health education. What was important then is still important now—only we have better tools and tactics to succeed.

The Society for Public Health Education (SOPHE) and the Enduring Legacy of Mayhew Derryberry

M. Elaine Auld

The Society for Public Health Education (SOPHE) is an independent, international professional association comprising a diverse membership of health education professionals and students. SOPHE promotes healthy behaviors, healthy communities, and healthy environments through its membership, its network of local chapters, and its numerous partnerships with other organizations. With its primary focus on public health education, and through its network of twenty-three chapters across thirty-two states, western Canada, and northern Mexico, SOPHE provides leadership through standards for professional preparation, research, and practice; opportunities for professional development; endorsement of a profession-wide code of ethics; and advocacy for policy and legislation affecting health education and health promotion. The mission of SOPHE is to provide leadership to the profession of health education and health promotion, to contribute to the health of all people through advances in health education theory and research, to foster excellence in health education practice, and to encourage public policies conducive to health. Founded in 1950, SOPHE is a 501(c)(3) professional organization and is the only professional organization devoted exclusively to public health education and health promotion.

From its inception, SOPHE has been fortunate to have had outstanding leaders from every corner of the field of health education. Mayhew Derryberry was among the visionary founding members of SOPHE. At the society's first meeting, in St. Louis in 1950, he served as president-elect on the first executive committee, along with Clair E. Turner, SOPHE's first president; Levitte B. Mendel, vice president; J. Louis Neff, secretary; and Ruth E. Grout, treasurer. (Membership dues were only $5!)

Derryberry became SOPHE's second president, taking office in 1951, and was instrumental in growing the organization's fledgling membership. At the third annual meeting, in 1952, Derryberry used his presidential address to warn the SOPHE membership of what he saw as five potential pitfalls: systematized and packaged thinking, undue administrative structure, use of esoteric language, habituated behavior, and emphasis on research at the expense of good practice. His presidency and subsequent leadership roles in SOPHE spanned over two decades, earning him profession-wide accolades and respect across public health disciplines. He was awarded the Distinguished Fellow Award—SOPHE's highest honor—in 1970, joining a pantheon of SOPHE leaders who have shaped the field in the service of the public's health for over half a century. He continued to lead and inspire the profession by serving on the editorial board of SOPHE's first journal, *Health Education Monographs*, from 1976 until 1978.

Without the dedication, commitment, and vision of Mayhew Derryberry, SOPHE might not be the force in public heath education that it is today. This volume is a tribute to the enduring legacy of Derryberry's principles of health education, which can be found to this day in the scientific sessions and continuing education programs of SOPHE's annual and midyear meetings; in its premier journals, *Health Education & Behavior* and *Health Promotion Practice*; in its high standards and efforts to catalyze the exchange between research and practice; and in its leadership in advocacy for a healthier world.

Commentaries by
Derryberry Award Winners

The Influence of Mayhew Derryberry on Godfrey Hochbaum

James R. Sorenson

I had the good fortune of entering our profession when the works of Mayhew Derryberry and of Godfrey Hochbaum had begun to have impact on the field of health education. These works provided guidance for those of us committed not just to understanding, in a theoretical sense, the health of the public, but also to improving it, in a practical sense. And it was in pointing out the necessary marriage between theory and practice that both Derryberry and Hochbaum strengthened the field of health education. Additionally, these scholars, among others, brought to our field the recognition that the behavioral sciences could provide a rich context, in terms of theories, methods, and perspectives, for improving the health of the public. The evaluation of health promotion programs and the development of theory-informed programs are both essential to a more scientific and effective health education effort. Finally,

Godfrey Hochbaum was at the time of his death professor emeritus of health behavior and health education at the University of North Carolina School of Public Health at Chapel Hill.

while acknowledging the role of social and environmental factors in health promotion, they focused largely on the individual and particularly on the role of human motivation and beliefs in health behavior. Their legacy resides in literally hundreds of studies and interventions that give us insight into these factors in health and provide us with more effective health education approaches.

What an exciting time it must have been at the Public Health Service (PHS) when Derryberry, Hochbaum, and Irwin Rosenstock were there together. It is not surprising that something as seminal as the Health Belief Model saw its origins in such a context. There can be little doubt that these pioneers brought the behavioral sciences into public health and influenced not only one another's work but the future of health education. In the acknowledgments to his seminal report *Public Participation in Medical Screening Programs: A Sociopsychological Study*, Hochbaum (1958) notes the contributions to this work of both Derryberry, who was then chief of the PHS Division of Health Education, and Rosenstock, who was then chief of the Behavioral Studies Section in Derryberry's division. Reading this now famous PHS publication one is struck by how contemporary the thinking is. This may simply be a reflection of how embedded the constructs and assumptions of the Health Belief Model have become in our profession's mind-set and how robust they have proven to be over the years. It is clear in this report that Hochbaum and others recognized that the findings could provide insight not only into why people did or did not participate in tuberculosis screening but also into similar behavior for a spectrum of other screening programs.

I had the good fortune of being able to incorporate into my professional work the contributions of both Mayhew Derryberry and Godfrey Hochbaum, and I had in addition the distinct pleasure of both meeting and working with Godfrey. It is a cliché to speak of a person as a legend in his own time, but in Godfrey's case the description was true. I first met him when I was being interviewed for chair of the Department of Health Behavior and Health Education at the University of North Carolina at Chapel Hill. Before meeting Godfrey I had thought there was something awkward, if not backward, about my being interviewed by him to be his chair. As he did with everyone, he immediately put me at ease with his charming demeanor and accent along with his intense personal interest in my work and the department. A couple of years later I had the combined pleasure and frustration of coauthoring a paper with Godfrey. Kate Lorig was also an author. Godfrey, the first author, and I began by meeting for breakfast to discuss ideas and develop a manuscript outline. At our second meeting Godfrey arrived with three or four typed pages, single-spaced, of one idea after another for the manuscript. He did this for all our subsequent meetings, even when we, or at least I, thought we had narrowed the focus of the paper. The pleasure was in working with someone so committed to health education and so full of ideas. The frustration was that I simply had difficulty keeping up with his flow of ideas. This paper (Hochbaum, Sorenson, & Lorig, 1992), which is among Godfrey's last publications, reflected his commitment to using theory to inform and improve health education programs. It also revealed Godfrey to be a professional open to all ideas, not committed solely to the Health Belief Model. These were traits he shared with Derryberry. Hochbaum was adamant that theory is only a tool and that if the field is to move forward we need to look as much to our practice colleagues and their approaches as to the academics and their often more formal theories. In either case, both Derryberry and Hochbaum believed that we must use theory to guide our efforts.

At the remembrance service for Godfrey and his wife, Lori, on September 22, 2000, I was struck by a set of common themes as I read the many written comments about this complete professional from former colleagues and students. There was no question among these writers about his contributions to our field, not just as one of the originators of the Health Belief Model but also as one who had a broad impact on the philosophy and even the ethics of the field. Most noted that Godfrey enjoyed, even in retirement, a good debate over the proper focus, purpose, and approach of health education, a passion he shared with Derryberry as well. His willingness to debate was not the result of a combative nature. Rather it was grounded in strong beliefs about our profession and its ultimate importance. Moreover, as with Derryberry, on a personal level, the themes of a kind, enthusiastic, and generous man emerged many times over. These attributes, combined with his professional contributions, resulted in a professional career of great importance, not only historically but for its influence on the future as well. Derryberry would have been proud.

References

Hochbaum, G. M., Sorenson, J. R., & Lorig, K. (1992). Theory in health education practice. *Health Education Quarterly, 19*, 295–313.

Hochbaum, G. M. (1958). *Public participation in medical screening programs: A sociopsychological study*. PHS publication no. 572. Washington, DC: U.S. Government Printing Office.

The Mayhew Derryberry Legacy and Marshall Becker

Lawrence W. Green

The late Professor Marshall H. Becker received the Mayhew Derryberry Award after following, almost unconsciously, in "Derry"'s footprints for many of his professionally formative years. Marshall would have heard of Derryberry from Irwin M. "Rusty" Rosenstock, Marshall's Ph.D. program mentor, during their years together at the University of Michigan School of Public Health. Rusty was a wonderful

---

Marshall H. Becker was at the time of his death professor of health behavior and health education at the University of Michigan School of Public Health.

storyteller, Marshall an avid student of personalities in the field, and Derry a larger-than-life object of stories to be told. Rusty surely regaled Marshall with research and theory stories from the Derryberry-Hochbaum-Rosenstock collaborations on why people seek preventive services. Rusty and Godfrey Hochbaum were members of Derry's research staff in the Division of Health Education of the U.S. Public Health Service. Among these stories were also surely ones about the origins, development, and evolution of the Health Belief Model, incubated during the late 1950s as Derry's staff, first Hochbaum, then Rosenstock and others, took the emerging conceptual model from one health problem to another, adapting it until it seemed to take on a relatively stable and generalizable form, with its essential features of beliefs in susceptibility, severity, and benefits of action, that every student and practitioner of health education since has learned and probably memorized.

But Marshall was not one to be satisfied with essential features, as readers will know from his subsequent, enormous stamp on the Health Belief Model. He left Rusty's tutelage at the University of Michigan in 1969 for an assistant professorship in the Department of Behavioral Sciences at the Johns Hopkins University School of Hygiene and Public Health (now the Johns Hopkins Bloomberg School of Public Health). Here his genealogy gets entangled with mine. I had completed my MPH and DrPH degrees in health education at the University of California at Berkeley in the late 1960s, when Derryberry was in his post–Public Health Service retirement years and serving as a full-time lecturer there. Even then, he was always available as an adviser and sage. I joined him on the Berkeley faculty for two years after completing my doctorate and then went on to Johns Hopkins in 1970. At Hopkins, I was a year behind Marshall, and in a different department, housed a few floors below him, in the School of Hygiene and Public Health. If Marshall had hoped to escape Derryberry stories, he was trapped. It was apparently his fate.

In the decade of the 1970s, Hopkins enabled Marshall to conduct extensive and definitive validation studies of the Health Belief

Model, studies that Derryberry actively supported. Marshall extended the model in ways that strengthened its theoretical grounding and its fit with socially relevant conditions surrounding health decisions and behavior. Together with Lois Maiman he developed instruments to provide standardized measures of the Health Belief Model, and tested their psychometric properties on adults, children, and the parents of children. We collaborated on one paper, presented at the American Association for the Advancement of Science and published in the *International Journal of Health Education*. In 1974, as editor of *Health Education Monographs*, I persuaded Marshall to be the guest editor for an issue devoted to the theoretical grounding of and cumulative research on the Health Belief Model. This was such an enormously popular issue that the publishers put it out subsequently as a separate book for wider classroom consumption. Marshall subsequently took the reins for editing what became the *Health Education Quarterly*, now *Health Education and Behavior*, a journal of the Society for Public Health Education (SOPHE).

We had these limited collaborations, linking health education and behavioral science, but mostly we swapped stories about our understandings—mine from Derry and his from Rusty—about the early development and evolution of the Health Belief Model and about Derryberry's famous Division of Health Education in the Public Health Service, with its legendary research unit filled with behavioral scientists. I had one more connection to Derryberry that added to the lore. I had been in the first health education Commissioned Officer Student Extern Program (COSTEP) of the U.S. Public Health Service Corps in 1962, not long after the early studies with the Health Belief Model had been published. My assignment was in the San Francisco regional office, but I had my first-ever trip east of the Mississippi River when the COSTEP participants were brought together in Washington, D.C. Here we met the federal health educators, whose names were often mentioned in our graduate courses, including their boss, the larger-than-life Mayhew Derryberry. We met some of the behavioral scientists, although not the mythical Hochbaum and Rosenstock. Marshall filled in the behavioral scientists' picture for me, as I often filled in the Derryberry and health education pictures for him.

Marshall's acceptance of the Mayhew Derryberry Award from the Public Health Education and Health Promotion Section of APHA, together with his gigantic contributions to the stewardship of the SOPHE journal, made him a virtual health educator. Derryberry had been chair of the Public Health Education Section of APHA and a founding member and second president of SOPHE (1951–1952). His vision in building the research team that produced the original Health Belief Model and his contributions to this research and earlier research enterprises would qualify him equally as a virtual behavioral scientist. The intertwining of the careers and contributions of these two giants in the health education literature with the small glimpses I had of these connections in my interloper role gives me a sense of participation in a significant period of scientific and theoretical grounding of health education practice.

Mayhew Derryberry Whispering in My Ear

Noreen M. Clark

Great public health leaders shape not only their own time; their legacy continues to shape times to come. True leaders fight conventionally accepted but ineffective practice. As a result a visionary leader is almost by definition a bit out of step with his or her contemporaries. The trick is to be in close enough formation with others to have one's ideas accepted and sufficiently out in front to see the direction to take. The best leaders think deeply about an issue. They go beyond the apparent answer that although relatively easy to apply won't go to the heart of the problem. Thinking deeply, being slightly out of step, and harnessing the energy for change is the powerful legacy that describes Mayhew Derryberry.

Mayhew Derryberry was more than smart; he was thoughtful and fearless in delving to root causes. Even a quick review of this volume's chapters confirms this observation. He was one of a small group of people working at the time who saw that the social and behavioral sciences constitute the theoretical foundation for health education practice. We take this notion for granted nowadays. However, when Derryberry was doing his work, these two arenas of public health were isolated from each other, both in academic institutions and in the field of practice. Just look at his writings on social and behavioral factors in health, and you'll see how he laid out the road map for creating more effective interventions.

He was also one of the first to articulate the potential impact of health education. He saw that enriching practice with theory and conducting evaluative research that would separate effective from ineffective approaches would enable health education to assume a powerful place in public health and health care delivery.

He provided compelling examples to show that the real health educators and managers of health are families. He made the case that therefore a primary function of health educators and other health professionals is to position and enable individuals to control their own circumstances. Our job is to help families and communities find effective solutions to their health problems. This behavioral approach was not a popular idea in an era when the professional educative role stopped at providing information and facts. Further, to suggest that health professionals other than health educators had an educative role was a brave proposition in his time. Even now it is hard for some to accept his notion that a central obligation of the health educator is to help other professionals be optimal educators.

He articulated in compelling ways the need for health care providers to communicate sensitively and effectively with patients—seeing communication between the two as fundamental to maintaining or acquiring good health. If you need an example of the subtlety of his observations, see his telling description of the way in which referring a child for routine medical testing can lead his parent to believe the child has a serious health problem, disrupting both family life and good clinical practice (see Chapter Five in this volume).

Dr. Derryberry's legacy has had a profound impact on my own work. My focus on self-regulation as the driving factor in learning to solve a health problem was shaped by his emphasis on behavior (both individual and social) as the crucial center of change. His emphasis on patient-centered communication and effective interaction between clinician and patient is fully consistent with my view of how people are empowered to manage their chronic illnesses. His focus on evaluation research as the key to better practice has guided my interest in assessing interventions. I like to think that the programs developed by my research group—for example, the Open Airways Program for children with asthma, the "Take PRIDE" Program for older adults with heart disease, the Physicians Asthma Care and Education Program (PACE) for pediatricians— are embodiments of Derryberry's teachings.

Frequently, I remind myself how important it is to think deeply about the public health problems we are facing. From time to time I consciously reflect on how my work might affect those who will follow after me, and increasingly I'm not worried when I'm a bit out of step with my colleagues on important issues. At such times I believe that Mayhew Derryberry is whispering in my ear.

Research and Practice: The Inspiration, Vision, and Leadership of Mayhew Derryberry

Karen Glanz

Consider this profile of a leader in public health and health education: someone whose dissertation research reported on a study of more than 95,000 families in over a hundred cities; someone with a solid command of statistics, social psychology, sociology, anthropology, and health services and the ability to integrate them seamlessly; and someone with skills as an articulate speaker and teacher, who traveled in the United States and internationally to advocate for delivery of community-responsive and needs-based public health programs to improve the quality and quantity of healthy life.

Such a leader has forged important trails in health education, but he is not a Renaissance man of the twenty-first century. All these talents and accomplishments describe Mayhew Derryberry. The majority of his written works were completed in the decades from the 1930s to the 1960s, without the modern tools of statistical software packages, desktop PCs, mobile phones, the Internet, voice mail, or even a fax machine. The temporal context makes his contributions and his vision all the more remarkable.

I did not know and never personally met or saw Mayhew Derryberry, but he influenced my approach through his writings and through his impact on his junior colleagues in the Public Health Service and during his career as a university professor. I consider myself a third-generation beneficiary of "Derry"'s leadership in health education. My mentors and their colleagues—Irwin "Rusty" Rosenstock, Jack Kirscht, Marshall Becker, and Godfrey Hochbaum—passed on to me their enthusiasm for applying behavioral sciences research to public health problems. Like Derryberry, they recognized the importance and challenge of studying and using knowledge from disciplines that are not obviously central to health and medicine. In the late 1970s, I did my graduate studies at the University of Michigan in one of the first programs to deliberately train behavioral scientists for careers in public health education. My commitment to a career that would blend theory, research, and practice found a home in public health that never quite fit into the "pure" biomedical sciences or behavioral sciences.

As a pioneer in the field of health education, Derryberry set the stage for embracing a broad emphasis on social determinants. Over the past forty years, outstanding leaders in health education have repeatedly stressed the importance of political, economic, and social factors as determinants of health. This view was sometimes lost in the emphasis on information dissemination that too often came to be thought of as "health education." What seemed like the new idea of taking a social perspective in lieu of an individual behavioral emphasis (that is, blaming the victim) is not new at all but periodically needs to be revived. In 1960, Derryberry noted that "health education . . . requires careful and thorough consideration of the present knowledge, attitudes, goals, perceptions, social status, power structure, cultural traditions, and other aspects of whatever public is to be reached" (see Chapter Sixteen).

In reading this collection, I am struck by the emphasis on developing a conceptual approach to understanding health behavior and formulating consumer and professional education. This has always been an important challenge and one that persists—not to find any one formula, recipe, or even model to understand behavior but to continually examine and reexamine what motivates the health-related actions of individuals and families. The idea that health is an instrumental value—a means to an end, and not an end in itself—for most people directs us to study people's values and attitudes. The systems approach articulated by Derryberry set the stage for today's emphasis on the common reliance on settings, such as schools and workplaces, for delivering health education.

An emphasis on the continuous cycle of problem diagnosis, program design, and evaluation runs through Derryberry's writings. Likewise, he depicted the big picture of health improvement and disease reduction as a cycle of interacting types of endeavors, including fundamental research, intervention research, and application and program delivery. These ideas are the basis for major health promotion and disparity-reducing initiatives today.

Importantly, Derryberry reminded us not to mistake effort for accomplishment. I learned this distinction unequivocally as a student of Rusty Rosenstock, who likened a public health program to a bird. He admonished that we spent too much time counting "wing-flaps" and not enough time examining whether the bird had reached its destination. He assured me that if my objectives were to gain experience, I could not help but meet them, but that all the effort would not be worthwhile if I didn't also get better at doing something of value!

Thus, as this collection points out, evaluation is central to the endeavors we persist at but so is creativity. Derryberry wrote of evaluating health education exhibits shown at the New York World's Fair in the 1960s. When my parents took me to that amazing window on the world of the then present and future, little did I know that I was brushing shoulders with the work that would later guide my own path, and that of my students and colleagues, for decades to come.

Derryberry and the Roots of Modern Health Behavior Theory

Barbara K. Rimer

This wonderful collection of writings from Mayhew Derryberry has the effect of taking us back in time—to a very different time and place and yet one that also is very familiar. Several of the chapters were written right around the time I was born—over fifty years ago. It was a time in the United States in which the communicable diseases were only just becoming less of a threat while the chronic diseases were becoming more of a threat. It was a time when even public health officials did not universally accept the relationship between smoking and lung cancer, a time in which the Pap test was just becoming widely available for the early detection of cervical cancer and mammography was not a household word. It was before the civil rights movement and the women's movement had become major forces for change in America. And the Internet was a distant galaxy. It is another universe and yet one very reminiscent of our world today.

What is striking and almost disconcerting is how much Derryberry's words foreshadow today's themes in health behavior and health education. This collection reminds us with these words just how important it is to understand our history. I want to focus briefly on a few of the important themes that Derryberry developed or about which he wrote. Most of them are familiar to today's health education professionals and students, but I suspect their historical evolution is not so widely appreciated. They include understanding teachable moments; educational diagnosis; the roots of the social ecological model; the need to select educational methods based on the needs of populations; the importance of communication and of conducting research on messages, senders, receivers, and relevant communication characteristics; and the importance of the groups to which one belongs as a source of one's health-related beliefs and behaviors. Derryberry wrote about basic behavioral research as akin to basic research in the other sciences. He also wrote persuasively about the need for good evaluation and not allowing data collection to become an end in itself. He wrote about evidence, and he wrote about the importance of building a compelling research base in health education. Moreover, he is one of the first people of whom I am aware to have written about informed decision making, going beyond mere informed consent. His writing was clear, succinct, and well organized, allowing the reader to grasp the main points without having to labor over the text. One cannot read his words without being awed by the breadth of his knowledge and interests and his vision. I never met Mayhew Derryberry, but I sure wish I had.

Derryberry wrote about the interrelatedness of cultural, economic, psychological, racial, social, and psychological factors. He said, for example, "Agencies engaged in promoting the welfare of society can accomplish their objectives most efficiently when they adjust their programs to meet the needs of the cultural, social, and economic status of the particular group with which they work" (see Chapter One). He identified the major elements of what we refer to today as the social ecological model.

He recognized that although sick people are often highly motivated to follow medical advice, people who are well may be far less ready to change their behaviors, especially when those behaviors bring satisfaction today. Derryberry saw that although conquering the communicable diseases might require a single action on a person's part, chronic diseases and injuries required more complex and repeated actions, including the self-initiated actions of the people involved.

Understanding the central position of the learner is as important today as it was in 1939 when Derryberry wrote "How to Influence Health Behavior of Adults" (see Chapter Nine). In this same work, he wrote about fear appeals and suggested that fear appeals that merely raise anxiety have no place in the strategy mix of health educators. But he said that it is acceptable to use fear appeals when there is a specific behavior that can obviate the fear, for example, obtaining a smallpox vaccination to reduce the likelihood of developing the disease. The recognition that there are circumstances under which it is acceptable to induce fear may be seen as presaging the important work led by Levanthal, Hochbaum, Rosenstock, and others to encourage people to get X-rays to screen for tuberculosis and to seek tetanus boosters. Despite Derryberry's sage advice about fear appeals more than sixty years ago, we still battle against the improper use of fear in public health campaigns today.

I was especially awed by Derryberry's way of characterizing health education as "applying [a] basic body of knowledge about the ways in which people acquire information, develop attitudes, and change their behavior about health," which he compared to the process of applying the body of knowledge from the biological sciences in medical diagnosis (see Chapter Ten). He went on to discuss the importance of diagnosing health education situations and selecting interventions based on the particular situation, and criticized those who choose all-purpose methods without understanding the specifics. He wrote that "[a]ll too many people regard health education as a pharmacy of methods and materials when actually it is the compounding of these ingredients—the analytical process— that is most important" (see Chapter Thirteen). In this way, he fore-shadowed Green and Kreuter's important work in formulating and formalizing the process of educational diagnosis, as part of the PRECEDE Model.

Dr. Derryberry wrote a lot about communication, and clearly, he was influenced by the scholarship of the day in this area. He fol-lowed research in a number of communication-related areas and applied the findings to health education. He wrote that

> Success in handling new public health demands of the second half of this century requires that we become much more precise and adept in an old technique— communications. We must improve communication from scientist to scientist, from scientist to practitioner, among practitioners who are working together, and from practitioners to those who benefit from our services.
>
> We can begin by learning and putting into practice the existing research on the communication process [see Chapter Seventeen].

It may be surprising to learn that Derryberry wrote these words in 1938! He speaks to us today, and we should heed his words, includ-ing his message to focus not only on methods but on the intended receivers.

To say that Derryberry foreshadowed much of modern health behavior is to take nothing away from those who followed. Rather it is to draw attention not only to our shared historical roots but also to a man who clearly was both of his time and ahead of ours. The readers of this important volume will appreciate Mayhew Derryberry as a man of his time and beyond his time. I, for one, am grateful for his contributions and feel that I have been given an incredible gift by this packaging of his work.

Nurse Lorig and Dr. Derryberry

Kate Lorig

In the mid-1960s I was a Peace Corps nurse organizing public health programs in southern Chile, and I had written to the University of California at Berkeley inquiring about the MPH program in health education. In due time a letter arrived signed by Mayhew Derryberry. He advised me that since I was a nurse I would be better off applying for the MS program at the University of California at San Francisco School of Nursing. Little did I know this was to be the theme of our fifteen-year relationship. Being compliant, I did as suggested and pursued a degree in nursing. But I did meet "Derry," as I took all my electives in health education at Berkeley.

My early memories are of him teaching common sense. The theory stuff I just did not understand. It was thirteen years later that I again tried for a degree in health education. By this time Derry had retired but faithfully came to our Friday doctoral seminars. At first he was a bit standoffish: after all I was still a nurse, and as I learned, Derry did not much like nurses. In seminars his emphasis was always on the use of theory. We did extensive readings in the early social psychologists. Talcott Parsons was one of his special favorites. The more I came to know Derry, the more I learned of his special wisdom that came from long practice and experience. I also began to know the man. He told the story of the evening he was to meet a friend and fellow academic at a well-known restaurant. The maître d' thought it was some type of a joke when Dr. Derryberry asked if Dr. Radelfinger had yet arrived.

It was also during this time that Derry started his own unique exercise program. Being impressed by some of the early data on goal setting, he decided to walk every street in San Francisco. Every day or two he would set out for a new adventure, after which he would mark another few blocks off his map. We often talked of what he found, interesting people, fruit stands, or restaurants. Even in his last years Derry was interested in everything and everybody around him.

What I remember most, and also what marks one of the most important days in my life, came just a few months before his death. He was in his usual place at our doctoral seminar. I had just presented some thoughts about my dissertation. After the seminar he said, "You know, you're all right for a nurse." This was high praise indeed from one of our founding fathers.

Derryberry: A Twentieth-Century Man for All Seasons

Nicholas Freudenberg

This compilation of published and unpublished work of Mayhew Derryberry provides a compelling portrait of health education theory and practice in the United States in the middle two quarters of the twentieth century. I want to highlight some of the beliefs and values that informed Derryberry's work and then explore their relevance for health educators in the first part of the twenty-first century. At the same time, I want to acknowledge the contributions to health education of Irwin M. "Rusty" Rosenstock, for many years a colleague of Derryberry at the U.S. Public Health Service. Rosenstock, who died in 2001, was a developer of the Health Belief Model and the cowinner of the 1994 Derryberry Award. (Irwin M. Rosenstock was at the time of his death professor emeritus of health behavior and health education at the University of Michigan School of Public Health.)

The last century may be remembered as the century of science. Not only were scientific principles and methods applied to all sectors of human activity—from sexual behavior to industrial production— science was also used to understand all dimensions of our planet, outer space, and the composition of life itself. Derryberry—and

Rosenstock—shared this abiding interest, applying new scientific knowledge to health education and human behavior. Derryberry's essays demonstrate his wide knowledge in medicine, epidemiology, psychology, sociology, and anthropology, to name a few, and his passion for using new findings to inform public health practice. Rosenstock and his colleagues developed the Health Belief Model in the 1950s in part to explain the failure of many people to participate in screening and prevention programs. Like Derryberry, Rosenstock was especially interested in studying what motivated people to take action on health, in order to develop more successful health campaigns.

Like many other twentieth-century American social scientists, Derryberry and Rosenstock were primarily interested in the individual within society. Both acknowledged the important role of social factors and the influence of the health care system, but the main goal of much of their work was to understand how to help individuals take action to improve their own health. This focus distinguishes Derryberry's and Rosenstock's work from the efforts of sociologists of the previous century and from more recent research that emphasizes the structural determinants of population health.

Another characteristic of Derryberry's approach to public health is pragmatism. Although he was certainly familiar with current theory in social psychology, sociology, and anthropology, his essays demonstrate a refreshing ability to roll up his sleeves to tackle the daily problems that confront public health practitioners. Unfettered by the academic ideologies that came to characterize some of late-twentieth-century social science, Derryberry was able to bring a fresh mind to each problem, to listen carefully to the various stakeholders, and to let evidence guide practice.

Finally, Derryberry and Rosenstock exhibited quiet optimism, a belief that government could and should identify and solve health and social problems. Their work in the Public Health Service helped to build a solid foundation for federal involvement in public health. Derryberry's commitment to patient, community, and provider education showed a faith in democracy, a belief that informed citizens could make good decisions for themselves and their communities.

In some ways Derryberry lived in a simpler, less morally perilous time. He wrote before Watergate, before tobacco company executives admitted they knew of but had lied about tobacco's lethal properties, before the September 11, 2001, attack on the World Trade Center and the Pentagon, before some politicians shut down the federal government in order to achieve their political goals, before the United States withdrew from many international treaties. The cynicism and fear that permeate political discourse in the United States today would no doubt have displeased Derryberry. Perhaps his pragmatism and decency would have helped us to find ways out of these present-day horrors and to uncover new paths to better health.

Today, in the early twenty-first century, faith in science seems more problematic, more fragile than it once was. True, discoveries in genetics, new antiretrovirals, and new information technology promise future improvements in health. But it can also be argued that science has also produced weaponized anthrax, smart bombs, and the thousands of petrochemical products that threaten our lives and our environment. Science is no longer viewed as the inevitable partner of public health. Rather it can be a force for good or evil, and learning to distinguish between the two adds one more task to the public health professional's function.

Another change in our view of public health is the growing importance of policy as a determinant of health. Derryberry was of course aware of this influence and carefully studied how institutional policies facilitated or hindered individual action for health. But in the last few decades, public health researchers have again called attention to the profound impact of health care, environmental, corporate, and tax policies on the health of the public. While working on Capitol Hill, testifying in court, or demonstrating in the streets may have been unfamiliar to Derryberry, one senses he would have celebrated these additional tools that health educators can bring to their task of health promotion.

Reading the essays of Mayhew Derryberry and Rusty Rosenstock should remind us health educators of two basic but contradictory truths. On the one hand our work is always grounded in a specific time and place. These two individuals studied the health behavior of Americans in the middle of the twentieth century, and their work is inextricably bound to the then-prevailing beliefs, ideologies, and perceptions. On the other hand public health and health education are motivated by certain enduring values. The chapters in this volume illustrate Derryberry's commitment to using evidence to guide practice, engaging a range of participants in the planning and implementation process, working across disciplines and sectors, and defining our roles in relationship to emerging needs. By reminding us of the roots of our profession, Derryberry helps us reaffirm these basic values.

Footprints on the Path to Social and Behavioral Change

Eugenia Eng

The footprints left by Mayhew Derryberry on the field of health education are indelible. The path he forged for health education to merge with the behavioral sciences is now paved and well marked by the agencies, scientific journals and anthologies, awards, and professional organizations that his work has inspired. His groundbreaking work with the Public Health Service moved the field of health education away from an intimate kinship with the field of education's cognitive learning theories and principles of teaching. Instead, Derryberry's vision and leadership moved health education toward becoming an instrument of social and behavioral change, concerned with enabling individuals, their families and communities, and the institutions serving them to ensure the conditions necessary for people to be in good health. The Society for Public

Health Education's mission was shaped by Derryberry's commitment to contribute to the health of all people through advances in health education theory and research, excellence in health education practice, and the promotion of public policies conducive to health.

Of special significance is the impact of individuals he mentored, such as Godfrey Hochbaum and Irwin Rosenstock, on generations of faculty and students at schools of public health. In 1971, Hochbaum was among the first faculty recruited by Guy Steuart when Steuart assumed the position of chair of the Department of Health Education at the School of Public Health of the University of North Carolina, where I teach. Hochbaum was trained in psychology and was among the first hired by Derryberry to join the Public Health Service's Division of Health Education. Hochbaum's study of tuberculosis-screening behavior took the innovative approach of focusing on people who sought, rather than turned away from, X-ray services (Hochbaum, 1958). The Health Belief Model, which emerged from his findings, serves as a touchstone for the field of health education on how and why a psychosocial model of health actions should be examined for its contributions to our understanding of preventive and sick role behaviors (Janz & Becker, 1984).

Like Hochbaum, Steuart's training was also in psychology. In South Africa, Steuart joined a team of physicians, led by Sidney Kark, to develop a model of comprehensive health care that would attend to improving the social, economic, and political conditions necessary for people to be in good health. Steuart's findings on the structure and function of kinship and friendship groups in a Zulu community's natural helping system led the team to begin examining associations between social relationships and health (Steuart & Kark, 1962/1993). The team's work in linking medical science to the social and behavioral sciences is recognized as the genesis for social epidemiology (Trostle, 1986), community-oriented primary care (Connor & Mullan, 1982), and the lay health advisor intervention strategy (Eng & Parker, 2002).

After joining the University of North Carolina, Steuart and Hochbaum began examining factors that hinder or facilitate behavioral change, which are not only beyond the health educator's control but may also be beyond the control of the individual. Their intellectual debates, in the form of memos circulated among faculty and students, were aimed at stimulating a climate for engaging in critical thinking, asking important questions, and generating new ideas about ensuring the conditions for people to be in good health. For example, their debate on the concept of informed choice asked whether it is wisdom or folly for the field of health education to claim responsibility for behavioral outcomes: "Whether the goals are in terms of behavior, cognition or affect, . . . [behavioral] change or maintenance, the influence that health educators might bring to bear must surely be tied to scientific knowledge . . . [which] will lie in medicine, epidemiology, clinical psychology, psychiatry, [and] environmental science, . . . not to mention, the perceptions of the people themselves of what they need and want" (Steuart, 1981, p. 3).

Steuart and Hochbaum's debates, however, did not arise out of concern for the viability of their profession. Rather, like Derryberry (1952), they were fully aware of the potential dangers to be found in research and practice based on packaged thinking. Moreover, Hochbaum (1981) believed that "[a]ny profession ceases to be viable when its basic tenets turn from hypotheses to dogma" (p. 32). They were concerned with any hint of retreating from the rapidly expanding complexities and uncertainties of health as a social concern. Building on Derryberry's thinking, Hochbaum's and Steuart's combined lifetime contributions to the field have moved its research agenda, programs of professional action, and teaching to

Recognize that an individual's cognition, affect, and behavior are not contained in a sealed-tight bubble

Work with units of practice, well beyond the individual, to effect behavioral change, by engaging directly with families, social networks, communities, and organizations to effect social change

View the forces of culture, economics, and political power as critically germane to the promotion of health for all people

Offer opportunities for agencies, communities, and investigators to take a partnership approach to research in which all partners contribute their expertise and share responsibility and ownership to enhance understanding of health disparities, and apply this knowledge to interventions to improve the health and well-being of communities

As we enter this new millennium it is not surprising to find that competence in understanding the behavioral and social factors of health is a core requirement for schools of public health and professional preparation programs in community health education seeking to be accredited by the Council on Education for Public Health. This recognition and requirement for behavioral science training in public health is in part a reflection of Derryberry's influence, his own research and writings, and those of his colleagues and the students and researchers he trained and mentored so well.

These recognitions are befitting for our field and profession. Derryberry redirected the path of public health action squarely toward behavioral change. Of equal significance is that this path was built on our foundations in community organizing and social justice (Derryberry, 1960; Nyswander, 1966). Hence it is not surprising that national and international attention to eliminating health disparities is being informed by our wide-angle lens on research and practice, which engages vulnerable communities in partnerships with agencies and universities to investigate and address social determinants of health in order to achieve social change (Steuart, 1985; Eng & Parker, 1994; Israel, Shultz, Parker, & Becker, 1998).

References

Connor, E., & Mullan, F. (1982). *Community oriented primary care*. Washington, DC: National Academy Press.

Derryberry, M. (1952). *Presidential address to the Society of Public Health Educators.* Washington, DC: Archives of the Society for Public Health Education.

Derryberry, M. (1960). Health education: Its objectives and methods. *Health Education Monographs, 8,* 5–11.

Eng, E., & Parker, E. A. (1994). Measuring community competence in the Mississippi Delta: The interface between program evaluation and empowerment. *Health Education Quarterly, 21,* 199–220.

Eng, E., & Parker, E. A. (2002). Natural helper models. In R. DiClemente, R. Crosby, & M. Kegler (Eds.), *Emerging theories and models in health promotion research & practice* (pp. 126–156). San Francisco: Jossey-Bass.

Hochbaum, G. M. (1958). *Public participation in medical screening programs: A sociopsychological study.* PHS publication no. 572. Washington, DC: U.S. Government Printing Office.

Hochbaum, G. M. (1981). *Behavioral change as the goal of health education.* Unpublished manuscript, University of North Carolina, School of Public Health, Department of Health Education.

Israel, B. A., Shultz, A. J., Parker, E. A., & Becker, A. B. (1998). Review of community-based research: Assessing partnership approaches to improve public health. *Annual Review of Public Health, 19,* 173–202.

Janz, N. K., & Becker, M. H. (1984). The Health Belief Model: A decade later. *Health Education Quarterly, 11,* 1–47.

Nyswander, D. (1966). The open society: Its implications for health education. *Health Education Monographs, 1,* 3–13.

Steuart, G. W. (1981). *To Be or Not to Be: That Is Not the Question.* Unpublished manuscript, University of North Carolina, School of Public Health, Department of Health Education.

Steuart, G. W. (1985). Social and behavioral change strategies. In H. T. Phillips & S. A. Gaylord (Eds.), *Aging and public health.* New York: Springer.

Steuart, G. W., & Kark, S. (1993). Community health education. *Health Education Quarterly Supplement 1,* S29–S47. (Originally published in S. L. Kark & G. W. Steuart [Eds.], [1962], *A practice of social medicine: A South African team's experiences in different African communities* [pp. 65–90], Edinburgh and London: E & S Livingstone).

Trostle, J. (1986). Anthropology and epidemiology in the twentieth century: A selective history of collaborative projects and theoretical affinities, 1920 to 1970. In C. R. Janes, R. Stall, & S. M. Gifford (Eds.), *Anthropology and epidemiology.* Boston: Reidel.

Mayhew Derryberry: A Career in Changing Health Behavior

David A. Sleet

Between the covers of this volume, the reader will find material on health education and behavioral science written by a giant in the field. The chapters in this book present a unique account of the early modern history of our thinking about health behavior and public health, personal observations from experimental settings and the field, comments from the lecture hall at society meetings and practitioner gatherings, and reflections on health education practice and the personal experiences of Mayhew Derryberry during his thirty-six years of service to the profession of health education.

William Foege, director of the Centers for Disease Control and Prevention from 1977 to 1983, said in his commencement address to the graduates of the Rollins School of Public Health at Emory University: "You've been warmed by fires you did not build; drank from wells you did not dig. Now you must feel the need to build new fires, and construct new wells." Mayhew Derryberry was like that. He built many fires and dug many wells for health education and inspired others to do the same.

In preparing this commentary I asked several colleagues who knew or worked with Derryberry to reflect on their memories of him. David Sencer, director of the CDC from 1965 to 1977, recalled that

> [Derryberry's] brother was a malariologist for TVA [Tennessee Valley Authority]. TVA had a large medical and entomology department that pioneered in environmental control of mosquito populations. One of the early things that Derry did that I remember was to surreptitiously record medical residents instructing diabetic patients on diets, insulin and general care. It was a

nightmare! After he retired from Public Health Service he was a USAID advisor to the Government of India for family planning. While in India, Derry refused to live in State Department furnished housing and lived in a Moslem section of the City, where he made many friends and learned about the local community. When the weather got too hot, he and his wife would sleep on the roof, like everyone else in the community.

Another long-time associate of Derryberry was William Carlyon, director of health education at the American Medical Association from 1972 to 1987. He remembered Derryberry's influence on the study of health behavior:

Dr. Derryberry dedicated his career to influencing health behavior. From 1933 to 1977, he helped the profession answer the question 'What educational methods work, with what kinds of people, to produce what kinds of actions?' He fully realized before any of the rest of us, that these are dynamic interrelationships, which must be the subject of more careful research and evaluation. Practitioners must use the fruits of this research to improve health education and public health practice.

Finally, Lawrence W. Green, a distinguished fellow at CDC and former director of the CDC Office on Smoking and Health, recalled:

[Derryberry] was bald as an eagle and imposing in his stature, energy and authority. He addressed us informally and gave us a history of the PHS and the health education presence in the PHS. He inspired in me a sense of national possibilities for health education if our generation could put it on a more solid scientific footing and at the same time keep the faith in our principles, some of which would not lend themselves easily to scientific measurement and evaluation. He and his wife Helen also hosted us occasionally at their Berkeley apartment and made us feel very much a part of their extended health education family.

In each of these accounts, one sees Derryberry as a man with a strong purpose and professional commitment but also as a person who was profoundly humane, likeable, and committed to the greater good of the community.

Derryberry always stressed that health education must avoid simplistic approaches to changing the complex behavioral, social, environmental, and cultural forces influencing health decisions. Health education, which once consisted mainly of inspirational messages on leaflets and posters, became increasingly sophisticated under Derryberry's leadership as he began to apply theoretical constructs from the behavioral sciences.

His writings on the difficulty of individual and community change resonate to today's public health challenges. He had no ready solutions back then, nor do we today. But by illuminating the complexity of the behavior-change process, he raised not only the vision of what is possible but also the specter of how difficult it would be to achieve. In all of this he was telling us to pay attention to theory and to what the study of human behavior in other fields had to teach us.

Mayhew Derryberry and those who followed him in federal service left their fingerprints on the Public Health Service—the fingerprints of behavioral science. CDC, for example, today supports several hundred research studies on behavioral science and public health and actively supports the Behavioral Science Working Group, which includes representatives from nearly every part of CDC.

The fields of behavioral medicine, health psychology, and behavioral safety are three of the outgrowths of Derryberry's efforts to legitimize behavioral approaches to public health. There are also strong remnants of his early influence in many of today's professional organizations such as the Society for Prevention Research, the Society of Behavioral Medicine, and the American Psychological Association's Division 38–Health Psychology. The NIH Office of Behavioral and Social Science Research and the recent Institute of Medicine reports *Promoting Health: Intervention Strategies from Social and Behavioral Research* (2000) and *Health and Behavior: The Interplay of Biological, Behavioral, and Societal Influences* (2001) attest to the scientific value of behavioral and social sciences in public health—something Derryberry labored hard to establish. It may have taken a long time for public health to incorporate Derryberry's concepts and practical knowledge, but its having done so has resulted in enormous advances in public health research and practice.

The chapters in this book illustrate Derryberry's command of health education. Back then he could not have imagined how health education would be transformed by the Internet, telematics, and medical informatics. These new strategies for knowledge management and communication offer empowerment through knowledge, a concept in which Derryberry strongly believed. This transformation has brought opportunities to health education of which he could have only dreamt.

He also could not have imagined the public health problems we face today, such as bioterrorism, emerging infections, and the critical role of health communications in dealing with public health emergencies. But it is clear today, as it was to Dr. Derryberry fifty years ago, that there is no magic bullet for achieving public health— that public health is a marathon, not a sprint. Derryberry walked slowly but persistently toward the goal of changing health behavior and establishing health education as a valuable and respected discipline. He provided an important scientific basis for our work today and, more clearly than anyone else, gave meaning to Lewin's phrase, "there is nothing more practical than a good theory."

References

Institute of Medicine. (2000). *Promoting health: Intervention strategies from social and behavioral research*. Washington, DC: National Academy of Sciences.

Institute of Medicine. (2001). *Health and behavior: The interplay of biological, behavioral, and societal influences*. Washington, DC: National Academy of Sciences.

Mayhew Derryberry: A Man I Would Have Liked to Have Known

Martin Fishbein

Although I did not know Mayhew Derryberry personally, this remarkable volume of his collected works makes it clear that I, like all other behavioral and social scientists interested in the public's health, owe him a huge debt of gratitude. Not only was Dr. Derryberry instrumental in getting the federal government to pay attention to the behavioral and social sciences but throughout his career he championed health education and emphasized the importance of prevention. Perhaps most important, he recognized the role of behavior and behavioral change as critical determinants of many of our most pressing health problems. For example, as early as 1947 he pointed out: "There are two important phases of the health education program. There is the initial task of securing public support for the concept that protection and improvement of the health of the people is a social responsibility. . . . The second, larger and more difficult task is to accomplish the changes in individual behavior that will result in improvement of personal and family health" (Derryberry, 1947, p. 1629; see also Chapter Twenty-Three).

Derryberry was convinced that education and communication could influence behavior, but he was also aware that bringing about such change would be a difficult and challenging task. "Health education is concerned with effecting improved health attitudes and behavior in the general public. Accomplishment of this goal requires careful and thorough consideration of the present knowledge, attitudes, goals, perceptions, social status, power structure, cultural traditions, and other aspects of whatever public is to be reached. Only in terms of these elements can a successful program be built" (Derryberry, 1960a, p. 9; see also Chapter Sixteen).

Although I have always been interested in the relations between attitudes and behavior and although some of my early work included attempts to predict and understand some health-related behaviors (for example, engaging in premarital sex, the use of contraceptives, and the use of seatbelts), it was not until the AIDS epidemic that I truly became involved in health promotion and disease prevention. Once it was determined that AIDS (or more correctly HIV) was transmitted through sexual and drug use behaviors, it was clear to me that those of us involved in studying behavior and behavioral change had a real obligation to try to prevent the spread of this deadly disease. Although I did not know it at the time, I was about to accept Derryberry's challenge to "research workers in human behavior to test out some of their theories in the area of health behavior" (Derryberry, 1960b, p. 169; see also Chapter Twenty-Nine).

But even more important than simply testing the applicability of theory for predicting and understanding health-related behaviors, the real challenge was to demonstrate the usefulness of theory in designing and developing effective health behavior change interventions. As Derryberry (1960b) put it, health education must also be "interested in research on the effectiveness of efforts to bring about change" (p. 164).

Because many others have already documented Dr. Derryberry's many accomplishments, I will not try to repeat them here. Instead, I would like to take this opportunity to reinforce Derryberry's position that the work of behavioral and social scientists is critical to advancing the nation's health. As Derryberry often argued, behavior is the key to health. For example, in the area of HIV prevention, it is not who one is but what one does that determines whether one will or will not be exposed to, or transmit, HIV, the virus that causes AIDS. Clearly, if we could convince everyone not to engage in unprotected sex with others who are HIV positive or whose HIV status is unknown and if we could convince all injecting drug users not to share injection paraphernalia and to always use a new or sterile needle, the AIDS epidemic would soon be behind us. Similarly, if we could convince everyone to exercise regularly and to eat a healthy diet (and make it possible for them to do so), the incidence and prevalence of many chronic diseases would be greatly reduced. In addition, if we could convince women over forty to have regular mammograms and men over fifty to have a colonoscopy every five years, many breast, colon, and prostate cancers would be detected early (or, at least in the case of colon cancer, prevented), and with early diagnosis and treatment, disease mortality would be greatly reduced.

But how do we develop communications or other types of interventions to increase the likelihood that people will engage in these health-related behaviors? Clearly, the more we know about the determinants of any given behavior, the more likely we are to be able to provide information or develop other types of interventions to effectively influence that behavior. Fortunately, the social and behavioral sciences have come a very long way in identifying the determinants of any given behavior. Indeed, there are now a number of empirically supported theories of behavior and behavioral change (for example, the Health Belief Model; social cognitive theory; the theory of reasoned action; the information, motivation, and behavior model; protection motivation theory; and the theory of planned behavior). To a certain extent, by identifying a critical set of variables that are assumed to underlie intentions and behavior, each theory provides some diagnostic tools necessary for behavioral understanding. As Derryberry so eloquently pointed out: "Health education requires diagnosis of the particular situation before methods are chosen" (Skinner & Derryberry, 1954, p. 1107; see also

Chapter Ten). "Just as physicians are expected to perform diagnostic tests before treating a disease and epidemiologists to spend the necessary time in diagnosing the problem of an epidemic before instituting community treatment, so the public health field has a right to expect from the health educator a diagnostic approach to the field of human behavior" (McKeever & Derryberry, 1956, p. 57; see also Chapter Twenty-One).

Common to all of the theories described here is the notion that an individual's behavior ultimately rests upon an underlying set of cognitions or beliefs. By properly applying theory as a diagnostic tool, one can identify a small set of beliefs that discriminate between those who are and are not performing a given behavior. And it is these beliefs that need to be addressed if one wishes to reinforce or change a person's intentions to perform the behavior in question. But Derryberry also pointed out that one person's (or population's) reasons for performing (or not performing) a given behavior may be very different from another person's (or population's) reasons. That is, he clearly understood that these underlying beliefs (and in particular the beliefs that discriminate between those who do and those who do not perform the behavior) are likely to vary, not only from behavior to behavior but also from population to population. Fortunately, when properly applied, almost all behavioral theories are both behavior and population specific. However, to properly apply these theories, one must understand them, know how to operationalize them, and know how to implement them. And these competencies are most likely to be held by people trained in the behavioral and social sciences.

It is important to recognize, however, that although we have come a long way in learning how to identify the critical beliefs underlying any given (health-related) behavior, the real challenge for health education, and for behavioral and social scientists, is figuring out how to provide people with the necessary information to change or reinforce these beliefs, thus allowing them ultimately to arrive at a decision to engage in healthy behaviors or to avoid engaging in behaviors that are likely to place them at a health risk. Although our theories of behavioral prediction are quite well established and empirically supported, our theories of communication and message (or intervention) design are still rather primitive. Indeed, I think it's safe to say that we know very little about why a given individual will or will not accept a given piece of information. I have long felt that one of our most pressing problems is to develop theories to help us understand the factors that influence message acceptance (or rejection).

Note, however, that communications and most other types of informational interventions do not directly change behavior; instead, their immediate impact is on beliefs. Changes in beliefs may lead to changes in many other variables, such as attitudes, perceived norms, and self-efficacy, and changes in these variables may ultimately lead to changes in intentions and behavior. Although our theories of behavioral prediction have given us quite a good understanding of the relations among beliefs, attitudes, norms, self-efficacy, and intentions, we have just begun to develop theories linking intentions to behavior. Why is it that although most people act in accordance with their intentions, there is almost always a substantial minority of people who are either unable or unwilling to do so? How can we increase the likelihood that people who have formed health-protective intentions will in fact act upon them? Another challenge for behavioral and social scientists is to better understand the intention-behavior relationship.

It is worth noting that these challenges are not really new. Throughout his career, Dr. Derryberry recognized and wrote about most of the issues that continue to confront health education. Although public health education has come a long way in the past twenty years, many of Derryberry's challenges to behavioral and social scientists have yet to be met, and they remain pressing issues in the battle to improve the public's health. After reading this volume, I can only say that I would like to have known Mayhew Derryberry.

References

Derryberry, M. (1947). The role of health education in a public health program. *Public Health Reports, 62,* 1629–1641.

Derryberry, M. (1960a). Health education—Its objectives and methods. *Health Education Monographs, 8,* 3–9.

Derryberry, M. (1960b). Research: Retrospective and prospective. *International Journal of Health Education, 3,* 164–169.

McKeever, N., & Derryberry, M. (1956). What does the changing picture in public health mean to health education in programs and practices? *American Journal of Public Health, 46,* 54–60.

Skinner, M. L., & Derryberry, M. (1954). Health education for outpatients. *Public Health Reports, 69,* 1107–1114.

DERRYBERRY'S
EDUCATING FOR HEALTH

Part I

Linking Statistical Methods
to Health Education Practice

Overview

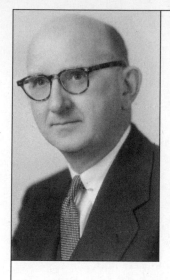

During Mayhew Derryberry's first years at the Public Health Service he worked as a statistician, dealing with various issues including infant mortality rates, medical judgments about malnutrition, school health services, qualifications of various health personnel, measurement of midwives' knowledge and practices, and health education. The chapters in Part One demonstrate one of Dr. Derryberry's primary contributions to health education practice—showing the importance of, and developing methods for, employing a statistical basis for determining physical, psychological, sociological, and educational needs. They also tie together these different types of needs to illustrate that no one set or type of data is itself sufficient to address health problems in each area. Rather, various types of data must be interrelated in health education practice. Today practitioners accept without question this foundation for program planning. However, fifty years ago the linkage of demographic data to health education program planning was nonexistent.

The six chapters constituting Part One have two dominant themes: first, the use of statistical methods to obtain the educational data necessary to improve health services and, second, the strong influence of attitudes and beliefs in shaping human behavior.

Chapters One and Two are among the earliest studies to document how psychological and sociological influences affect human behavior in preventive health programs. In the second chapter not only the clients are studied but also the providers of service. Derryberry emphasizes that learning and subsequent behavior are affected by negative or positive attitudes held by both providers of service and the public. For example, Derryberry suggests that the success of a child immunization program depended on how the *parents* perceived the subject. In addition to describing the nature of a particular health problem, he recommends what needs to be done to address the particular condition.

The contents of the third chapter, focused on the knowledge and practices of midwives, had a bearing on most of the subsequent training programs for midwives. Published in 1936, this work predates the quality-control thinking of the 1970s. It reveals how strongly Derryberry felt about tying knowledge and performance together—a belief he practiced throughout his career.

Dr. Derryberry's early work on weight and skeletal build of children revised the criteria for measurement of school-aged children and revolutionized some School Health Service programs. Chapters Four and Five amplify his commitment to what we today would call a "systems approach to education." He stresses that the interrelated contributions of parents, teachers, and administrators are essential if children are to be effectively educated about health. He shows that attitudes and behavior are influenced by the way messages are delivered and the way people perceive and receive them. Thus, rather than relying solely on "instruction" time to achieve our purpose, we must view the services, policies, and procedures in the school environment as influencing learning together.

The last chapter in Part One addresses the importance of education in well-baby clinics. In the 1930s, there was a strong effort to provide preventive health services separately, apart from therapeutic clinics. Derryberry's analysis of the clinic visit points to the role of education in prevention and shows how to make such a visit a significant learning experience.

These early writings show the entrance of Dr. Derryberry into the public health field, his interest in and commitment to service, and his deep conviction that providers of service must become sensitive to the multiple needs of clients.

1

Social and Economic Factors Associated with Health Protection for the Preschool Child

Agencies engaged in promoting the welfare of society can accomplish their objective most efficiently when they adjust their programs to meet the needs of the cultural, social, and economic status of the particular group with which they work. Both the educational and service angles of welfare programs should be planned to overcome the handicaps of prejudice, ignorance, and poverty.

Purpose of the Investigation

The present study was focused on the influences of some of the social forces on the amount of preventive medical service preschool children receive. Four preventive health measures were investigated: health examinations, dental health examinations, vaccination against smallpox, and immunization against diphtheria. The sociological factors included economic status, cultural level, race, and such social and cultural factors as are represented in the birthplace of the parents. The problem, then, was the determination of the relationship of the above sociological forces to each of the four health measures.

Originally published as the abstract of Mayhew Derryberry's thesis submitted in partial fulfillment of the requirements for the degree of doctor of philosophy in the School of Education of New York University, 1933.

Collection of Data

The data were obtained in 156 cities with a population over 20,000
and include 95,032 families representing 145,720 children under
six years of age.[1] Each family was interviewed by a local representative according to a prescribed technique. Evidence on the nativity and race of the parents was obtained in addition to information
concerning the utilization of preventive health service. Other social
and cultural factors included illiteracy, number of preschool children in the family, per capita effective income, economic status as
rated by superintendents of schools, proportion of married women
gainfully employed, and population of the city.

Analysis of Data

Four types of sociological influence were considered: (1) the influence of the family—its cultural, religious, economic, and traditional
background; (2) the influence of race; (3) the influence of the medical and public health attitude; and (4) the influence of the sociological distinctions between cities. The study of the first three factors
was based on the comparison of relevant percentages. The fourth
influence was analyzed by the method of multiple correlation.

The conclusions on the influence of the family are based on the
following types of evidence: (1) the proportion of preschool children who have had each health measure by nativity stock; (2) the
proportion of children of mixed nativities who have had each
health measure; (3) the distribution of health measures by nativity
groups; (4) the proportion of children in each of five economic
groups who have had each health measure by nativity groups;
(5) the proportion of children of each age who have had each service by nativity groups; and (6) the proportion of children in families of one, two, and three children who have had each measure.

The medical and public health attitude is shown by: (1) the
probabilities of vaccination if a child is immunized and vice versa,

(2) the probabilities of immunity measures for one child when the sibling has had the services, and (3) intercorrelation of the standing of cities in each measure. The influence of race is shown by a comparison of the percentage of white and African American children who have had each health service in the different sections of the country and in given economic status groupings.

Multiple correlations of the nativity composition, percent African American population of the city, per capita effective income, percent illiterate, and proportion of married women gainfully employed on each health service furnish the basis of the conclusion on the effect of the sociological distinctions between cities.

Conclusions

1. Differences in the culture, traditions, and customs of immigrants from various countries are largely responsible for varying amounts of preventive service for the preschool child.

2. Children of native-born and northern European parents receive more health supervision but less protection from smallpox and diphtheria than do the children of southern European parents.

3. Among the several nativities studied, there are three types of customs toward the age at which immunity against smallpox and diphtheria is given. The Russian, Polish, Austrian, Hungarian, and German parents immunize the very young children. The native-borns and Canadians wait until preparation for school stimulates the practice. The Italians and Irish do not choose a specific age as the time for immunizing and vaccinating their children.

4. Individuals who are sufficiently liberal-minded to choose a mate from a nativity different from their own are likely to favor preventive medical service for their children even though their own nativity group is prejudiced. This

is especially true of families where both parents are from different foreign countries. They give more service to their children than any other group.

5. The economic status of the family conditions the amount of preventive medical service children receive. However, the influence is much more potent among some nativities than others.

6. The coincidental occurrence of smallpox vaccination and diphtheria immunization in the same children is very low. Suggested causes for this condition are: (a) agencies engaged in prophylaxis are not stressing vaccinations for the younger children, and (b) no efficient educational program on the value of immunization and vaccination accompanies the prophylactic procedure.

7. There is very little agreement among health agencies concerning the relative emphasis that should be given to the four preventive health measures.

8. In general African American preschool children receive less service than white children. However, for some measures and for some sections of the country, the African American receives more service than the white.

9. Among children of the same economic level, the differences in service between white and African American children are much less marked.

10. The nativity composition of a city is an important factor in determining the amount of preventive health service preschool children of that city receive.

11. Cities having large groups of their population with low intelligence and cultural levels tend to have more vaccinations and immunizations. Fewer of their children benefit from the examination measures.

Recommendations

1. Programs for promoting health protection for the preschool child should be formulated to meet the needs of the social groups they intend to serve. For example, the Russians, because of their traditions and culture, are favorable to preventive health service, and, therefore, not nearly so much energy is needed to promote this service among them as is needed among the Polish and Canadian groups. Among the native group, activity should be increased to overcome the prejudices toward early immunity from communicable diseases. Among the Italian and Polish groups, the value of securing medical and dental advice before trouble arises should be urged.

2. Any evaluation of the efforts of a city in its public health work to increase the amount of preventive service for preschool children should take into account the prejudices and attitudes of the social groups on which the effort has been expended. For example, there is a vast difference between the amount of work involved in the attainment of a given amount of service among a Russian group and that involved in reaching the same goal among a Polish group. A mere gross evaluation, therefore, would not give due credit for this wide difference in effort and would not constitute a correct evaluation.

3. The economic distinctions shown in terms of the economic rating and the number of preschool children in the family challenge public health to remove the inequalities of service in the different groups. This should be accomplished both by the education of the parents in the value of the services and by an increase in facilities so that service is provided for those who desire it but are handicapped by their economic limitations.

4. Agencies responsible for administering measures for the prevention of contagion should insist that a smallpox vaccination

be given in conjunction with immunization against diphtheria and vice versa.

5. There is no better time to impress a parent with the value of a practice than at the time the service is being given to one of the children. It is therefore recommended that more time and attention be given to the education of the parent at the time a preventive service is rendered. If the education is effective, the cost of other forms of propaganda and education will be reduced.

6. Race should not limit the protection that is given to children. More adequate preventive service should be extended the African American child, especially in the South.

Discussion Questions

1. According to Derryberry, how can agencies engaged in promoting the welfare of society accomplish their objectives most efficiently?

2. Why do you think there was so little agreement among health agencies concerning the relative emphasis that should be given to preventive measures, for example, immunizations, during Derryberry's era?

3. What were some of the recommendations made by Derryberry that might still be useful today in delivering preventive services such as vaccinations?

Note

1. The data were gathered by the Committee on Medical Care for Children of the White House Conference on Child Health and Protection. The gross amount of preventive service given in the various cities of the country and in the country as a whole was reported by George T. Palmer, Mayhew Derryberry, and Philip Van Ingen in *Health Protection for the Preschool Child* (New York: D. Appleton-Century Company, 1931).

2

Medical and Public Health Attitude Toward Smallpox Vaccination and Diphtheria Immunization

O ne of the objectives of public health work is the control of communicable diseases. Two of these diseases, smallpox and diphtheria, have their greatest mortality among preschool children. For each an effective preventive is known. Yet the White House Conference Survey[1] showed that among the preschool children of 156 cities, only 21 percent had been vaccinated against smallpox and an equal percentage had been immunized against diphtheria. Such low percentages prompted an investigation of the attitudes of the immunizing agencies toward these two measures. No attempt is made here to determine the attitude of the private practitioner as opposed to the public health agencies. Rather, it is the purpose of this paper to examine indirectly the manner in which the immunizing agencies are functioning and to indicate from the results obtained some of the possible weaknesses of the present procedures.

Attitude Toward Early Vaccination and Immunization

Although 21 percent of all the preschool children have been immunized against diphtheria and the same percentage have

Coauthored by George T. Palmer and Mayhew Derryberry. Originally published in the *New England Journal of Medicine*, August 30, 1934, *211*(9), 413–415. Reprinted with permission.

been vaccinated against smallpox, only 11 percent of the group have received both of these protective services. Even among children ready for school entrance (the five-year-olds), the proportion protected against both diseases is only 22 percent of those who have had vaccination and 32 percent of those who have had immunization. Such a comparison reveals that 50 percent (22 out of 44) of the five-year-old vaccinated children have been immunized, and 66 percent (22 out of 32) of the immunized five-year-old children have been vaccinated. In other words, the probability of a five-year-old child being vaccinated, if he has been immunized, is about one and one-third times as great as his chances of being immunized if he has been vaccinated.

But these probabilities are not the same for the lower age groups. In fact the situation is quite the reverse. Among the younger children, the probabilities of immunization among vaccinated children are much greater than the probabilities of vaccination if a child has been immunized. This difference is at a maximum at one year of age (see Figure 2.1).

These facts reveal very clearly an attitude of the agencies administering the immunity measures. They are more interested in protecting the young child from diphtheria than they are in vaccinating him against smallpox.

When a young child comes in for vaccination, his chances for both vaccination and immunization are considerably greater than when he comes in for immunization. In other words, the prophylactic agencies, whether they be private or public, are not pushing vaccination and immunization to the same degree. If it is true that smallpox vaccination is being taken too much for granted, then here is reflected an attitude among the public health agencies that needs to be corrected.

This discrepancy between the interest in vaccination and immunization is further confirmed when we consider the relative amount of protection of each type that different children in the same families have received. Of 5,591[2] families in which there are two chil-

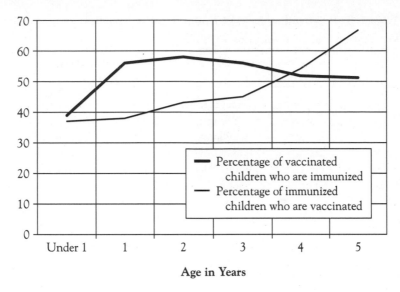

Figure 2.1. Relative Public Health Emphasis on the Immunity Measures at Each Age.

dren of different ages under six, there are 333 in which the younger child has been vaccinated when the older sibling has been immunized and 449 in which the younger child has been immunized when the older child has been vaccinated. Among 3,086 families with three children of different ages, the corresponding figures are 292 and 398, respectively. When these comparisons are made by specific ages (using the age of the younger child for purposes of classification), the same conclusions hold (see Table 2.1).

It is evident from these data that the attitude of the agencies responsible for administering immunity measures is less favorable toward vaccination of the young child than toward immunization.[3] Naturally we should expect public health agencies to promote the newer measures of immunization against diphtheria, but it hardly seems efficient to concentrate on the prevention of diphtheria and tend to neglect the prevention of smallpox. Even though the incidence of smallpox has been reduced to a very low point, is it likely

Table 2.1. Relative Emphasis of Public Health Agencies on Vaccination and Immunization of Siblings.

	Families with Two Children		Families with More Than Two Children	
Age of Younger Child	Percentage of Younger Children Vaccinated When Older Sibling Is Immunized	Percentage of Younger Children Immunized When Older Sibling Is Vaccinated	Percentage of Younger Children Vaccinated When Older Sibling Is Immunized	Percentage of Younger Children Immunized When Older Sibling Is Vaccinated
Under 1	3	7	3	5
1	18	26	12	23
2	26	41	24	32
3	39	39	32	36
4	45	42	38	46

that this low level can be maintained if widespread vaccination among young children is not continued?

Health Education Coincident with Vaccination and Immunization

Vaccination against smallpox and immunization against diphtheria need not be merely services rendered to the family by a health agency. They may be, and should be, educational experiences for the parent in the value of such services. This occasion of contact with the family would seem to offer an opportunity of emphasizing more effectively the meaning of a health protection practice than would general publicity at other times.

To what extent, then, are our health agencies engaged in such a program of effective education? We may obtain some index of the degree to which such a program is functioning by the extent to which families with more than one child protect all their children when one child has been protected. If efficient education accompanies immunization, then the protection for the older child would be associated with protection for the younger child and vice versa. Once convinced of the value of the service, the parent would insist on the service for all children without further social urging. On the other hand, if the immunization process is merely a health service to the family with no parental education associated with it, then the younger child would not always be protected when the older sibling had had the service, for the protection might have been given the older child before the younger child was born.

With these considerations in mind, we selected from the families with two children all those in which the older child had been protected from diphtheria. We then determined the proportion of these families in which the younger child had been immunized against diphtheria. We next selected from the families with two children all those in which the younger child had been immunized and determined the proportion of these in which the older sibling had been immunized.

Among the 1,711 families in which the older child had been immunized, only 771 or 45 percent of the younger children were so protected. On the other hand, among the 793 families in which the younger child had been immunized, 771 or 97 percent of the older children had been protected. The corresponding percentages for vaccination against smallpox were 31 and 96, respectively.

Such wide discrepancies as these would not occur if the agency responsible for administering the immunity measures were efficiently educating parents to understand the advantages of early protection against these two communicable diseases. If the procedure of efficient education were followed, then families in which an older child was protected would also have the younger child protected. But these discrepancies occur in every age combination for both vaccination against smallpox and immunization against diphtheria. Not only do the discrepancies occur in every age group, but they increase as the differences in age between the children become greater (see Table 2.2).

Table 2.2. Protection for Both Children in the Family When One Child Has Been Protected.

| | Families with Two Children in the Family Percentage of Children Protected | | | |
| | Older, When Younger Is Protected Against: | | Younger, When Older Is Protected Against: | |
Difference in Age	Diphtheria	Smallpox	Diphtheria	Smallpox
1 Year	98	94	71	56
2 Years	98	98	58	40
3 Years	96	94	37	23
4 Years	92	95	20	15
5 Years	100	60	7	2

| | Families with Three Children in the Family Percentage of Children Protected | | | |
| | Older, When Younger Is Protected Against: | | Younger, When Older Is Protected Against: | |
Difference in Age	Diphtheria	Smallpox	Diphtheria	Smallpox
1 Year	98	96	61	50
2 Years	98	97	50	34
3 Years	99	98	19	13
4 Years	100	100	4	1
5 Years	*	*	0	0

* In none of the families having a five-year-old and a child under one were any of the latter immunized or vaccinated. Therefore, these proportions were indeterminate.

These figures indicate clearly that immunization against diphtheria and vaccination against smallpox are services rendered to the family without the accompaniment of effective education in the importance and value of such procedures. In other words, the immunizing agency tends to protect all the children that are in the family at the time one is protected, but does not instill into the parent a conviction of the value of the service so that immunization and vaccination will be demanded by the parent for the next children born into the family.

Summary

1. The coincidental occurrence of smallpox vaccination and diphtheria immunization in the same children is very low. About one out of ten of our preschool children are protected from both diphtheria and smallpox.

2. Two causes suggested for the low amount of complete protection are the following:

    a. Agencies engaged in administering the immunity measures are not stressing vaccination for the younger children.

    b. No efficient educational program on the value of immunization and vaccination accompanies the immunizing procedure. It is more in the nature of a health service rendered to the family.

Discussion Questions

1. What does Derryberry suggest is an often overlooked yet potentially valuable educational opportunity for the parent in vaccination and immunization services?

2. What were some of the documented reasons why the coincidental occurrence of vaccination and immunization were so low in Derryberry's experience?

3. How do you think this situation has changed today?

Notes

1. The study is based on the data collected during the White House Conference and reported in G. T. Palmer, M. Derryberry, & P. Van Ingen in *Health Protection for the Preschool Child* (New York: D. Appleton-Century Company, 1931). The study was financed by the Follow-Up Committee of the White House Conference.

2. These represent only native-born families in two extreme economic status groups. The extra burden of the work involved prevented a more inclusive amount of data. The conclusions are substantiated in each economic status and in each size of family.

3. The replies of 2,374 medical men to a questionnaire sent out by the White House Conference Committee on Medical Care for Children confirm this conclusion. The men to whom the questionnaire was sent were either practicing pediatrics or especially interested in pediatrics. Ninety-one percent of them state that they "specially urge" immunization against diphtheria and 7 percent state that they "do not suggest vaccination unless parents ask for it." Yet 82 percent of the doctors report that "nearly all" the parents are favorable toward vaccination, and only 52 percent of the doctors report "nearly all" parents are favorable toward immunization.

3

The Development of a Technique for Measuring the Knowledge and Practice of Midwives

Improvement in the care given women during the maternity cycle is, and has been for the past decade, an important objective of public health service.[1] The procedures followed to obtain this objective have varied in the several sections of the country because of the differing conditions prevailing in the various localities. In the rural sections of the southern states, one of the elements to which consideration must be given in effecting any progress in improving maternity and infant hygiene is the education and supervision of the African American midwife, who at the time of delivery is frequently the sole attendant of a maternity case.

In many of the southern states, public health authorities have realized the need for improving the midwifery service and have instituted programs with that objective in view, but the procedures incorporated in these programs are extremely varied in the several states as well as for the different counties within a given state. In some states the permits are granted to midwives solely on the basis of a local doctor's recommendation; in other states intensive group instruction is given at midwife classes before the midwives are given their permits, and then later nursing visits are made for supervisory purposes; in other states permits are granted without any previous

Coauthored by Mayhew Derryberry and Josephine Daniel. Originally published in *Public Health Reports*, June 12, 1936, *51*(24), 757–771. Reprinted with permission.

instruction, and the only education and control of the midwife consists of frequent visits by the nurse, coupled with supervisory
antepartum and postpartum visits with the midwife to her patients.

Certainly some of the many procedures now being practiced
must be more effective than others. If it were known which ones
yield the best results, then definite progress could be made toward
improving all programs for control of the midwife. The question
then is: Which of the present existing procedures secure the best
midwifery service with the minimum of public expenditure? The
Office of Studies of Public Health Methods of the United States
Public Health Service, long interested in evaluation studies of public health procedures, recently began a study of the problem for this
very purpose of determining which procedures have been most
effective in producing competent midwife service. Such an evaluation, when completed, may well be considered a sound basis for the
construction of efficient programs for controlling midwives in
the rural sections of the South.

Method of Evaluation

It is axiomatic that any procedure is effective to the extent that it
produces results. For this evaluation of programs of midwifery supervision and control, it is assumed that communities in which midwives are practicing the procedures outlined in the manuals of
midwifery practice issued by the respective state health departments
have been more in control over midwives than communities in
which the midwives are not following accepted obstetrical practice.
The aim will be to discover the methods of selection, instruction,
supervision, and control of the midwives used in those counties that
have capable midwives as opposed to the methods employed in
those counties where the quality of the midwife practice leaves
much to be desired.

The evaluation, then, may be conceived in terms of four distinct
steps of procedure:

1. Construction and preliminary trial of a test for the measurement of a midwife's knowledge and practice.

2. Development of a means of discovering and recording all those administrative procedures of a health department concerned with the control and supervision of midwives.

3. With the techniques developed in steps 1 and 2, the measurement of a sampling of midwives in each of a number of communities and the recording of the health departments' activities for those communities.

4. Relating the quality of service rendered by the midwives in each community to the type of midwife control used in that community, thus precipitating the methods of control that have been effective in producing a high quality of midwife service.

These steps are somewhat discrete procedures and must be taken consecutively in the order named. What follows herein is a report of the experimentation that was conducted in completing the first step of the project. It describes in detail the experimental derivation of a technique for measuring midwife information and practice.

Records of the actual procedures followed by a midwife in her antepartum, delivery, and postpartum care of a number of maternity cases would constitute an ideal measure of the quality of maternal service given by that particular midwife. From such records one could ascertain the extent to which the midwife was following the techniques prescribed in the midwifery manual.

To obtain unbiased observational records of midwives in their routine activities, however, is almost impossible. If midwives know that they are being observed, they are likely to omit certain things that they would otherwise do and follow more closely the prescribed procedures. Furthermore, the observation of each of a number of midwives for several maternity cases necessitates an unreasonable amount of time and expense. It is essential, therefore, to develop some other method that will give an index of the quality of care given by a midwife—in other words, some measure that will distinguish midwives who practice good techniques from those who follow poor and even bad practices. This index should reflect distinctions in the quality of service rendered by different midwives rather than attempt to measure directly the ability of each midwife to meet emergencies, or their understanding of the maternity cycle.

Any index that is devised must be objective; that is, the index must be of such a nature that the results obtained are not dependent upon the individual who uses the index. Midwives who register as superior midwives when this index is applied by one examiner should also register as superior if measured by some other examiner.

The index must also be representative of the actual information and conduct of the midwife. It must be shown to be indicative of the variations in the quality of service that the various individual midwives give. Those midwives who pay no attention to accepted methods of cleanliness and prescribe for their patients all sorts of home remedies, many of them based on superstitions, must register low on the index as compared with those midwives whose routine procedures conform to the pattern set forth in the midwife manual.

After careful consideration had been given to a number of possible methods of developing an index with these characteristics, the personal interview was selected as the method most likely to yield the desired results in the practical situation. Accordingly, an extensive form, containing some 66 objective standardized groups of questions on midwifery information and practice was constructed. These questions were focused on the general subjects of equipment, prenatal care, complications of pregnancy, delivery care, complications of delivery, and postpartum care of both the mother and the baby. Information was sought on both good and bad practices under each of these general headings.

The questions were framed in a variety of ways in the attempt to elicit the truth. The fact that a midwife may know the correct procedure is no assurance that she follows that procedure. Insofar as possible, the questions were asked in terms of behavior rather than information. Often questions on the same practices were asked in more than one connection in the hope of arriving more nearly at the actual practice. For example, each of the following questions was asked in an attempt to identify those midwives who practice vaginal examinations:

- Have any of your cases insisted that you make a vaginal examination? (If yes) What did you do? (If no) What would you do?

- What can you find out from an internal examination?

- Does it help you to make an internal examination?

Since the African American midwife is very susceptible to suggestion, many of the questions were stated negatively, thus causing her to defend the proper procedure. For example, note the following sample questions:

- Do you remind the expectant mothers that they should eat enough for two people?

- When you get water from a good deep well, do you bother to boil it? (If yes) Why?

The first drafted interview was subjected to a preliminary trial, and after a few slight revisions, no further changes were made before the preliminary data were gathered.

Evidence for the Interview Form

In the beginning of the study, advantage was taken of the fact that the Office of Child Hygiene Investigations had been conducting an intensive study of the midwives in a county in Virginia. The nurse who had been conducting that study was engaged to initiate and carry on the field work in connection with the development of the index. Midwives were interviewed by the nurse, using the objective inter-view form, in the county in which she had been working, as well as in two adjoining counties, one of which was in North Carolina.

The geography and population of the three counties are markedly similar. All three of the counties are strictly rural in that their largest town has a population of around 2,000. The African American population slightly outnumbers the white, and midwives deliver approximately 60 percent of the total births in two of the counties and 25 percent in the other county. Most of the midwives are African American, past middle age, unable to read or write, and live on small farms more or less isolated from one another. Since transportation is difficult, they seldom visit outside their immedi-ate neighborhood.

Concerning the supervision that has been given the midwives, there are wide differences among the counties. In county A, there had been no county health unit prior to January 1, 1935, and con-sequently the only supervision and education given had come from a nurse in the state health department. She made an annual super-visory visit to the county but, because of her extensive territory, could not give intensive supervision (such as home visits and demonstration antepartum and postpartum home calls) to the mid-wives of any one of the several counties under her jurisdiction. In county B, supervision of midwives was begun in 1922 by the state health department. In 1924, when a full-time county nurse was employed, she assumed this responsibility. The program has been interrupted for short periods several times, but the supervision of the midwives of this county has been much more intensive than in county A. In county C, the midwives were under continuous inten-sive supervision from 1923 to 1932 by a nurse employed as the county public health nurse. She visited the midwives in their homes frequently, inspecting their equipment, accompanied them on calls to their patients, and demonstrated the prescribed techniques of antepartum and postpartum care. Since 1932 the supervision has been under the state department of health. A state nurse holds annual classes, performs bag inspection, and issues the annual licenses.

In counties A and B the midwives are given a permanent license, but in county C only an annual license is issued. This latter procedure allows for more effective control, since the weeding out of the worst midwives from the group occurs annually.

To obtain data on the adequacy of the interview form, 20 midwives were interviewed in county A, 34 in county B, and 26 in county C, making a total of 80 midwives interviewed.

Scoring the Interview Forms

When the interviews had been completed, the responses to each question were given a numerical value, and the sum of these values for each midwife represented her score. The correct response to each question, with one or two exceptions, was given a score of 1. For example, if the answer to the question "What food other than breast milk do you give the baby?" was "Boiled water," the question was given a score of 1. Such responses as "sugar bubby" and "water with a pinch of soda and sugar" were scored 0. A minus score of 2 was given if the midwife believed in such superstitions as "burnt feather under the nose," "snuff in the face," or "eating raw red onion" as methods of hurrying up the birth of the baby.

Objectivity and Reliability of the Interview Form

It was impractical to determine, empirically, the objectivity of the interview form by having two interviewers question the same group of midwives and then compute the degree of agreement between the results obtained. But the very nature of the questions, which were always asked in the same way, and the fact that the interviewer always recorded the total response given argue the objectivity of the method.

A large number of questions were included to ensure some representation of each of the many phases of midwife practice and knowledge. Of course, all possible questions were not asked, nor would it have been possible to ask questions about every phase of midwifery care. But proof that the questions included are representative of the quality of information and behavior peculiar to each midwife is furnished from an internal analysis of the data. By randomly dividing the entire battery of questions into two groupings and then scoring the two separate sets of questions, two scores were obtained for each midwife—one on each half of the material. A comparison of the relative standing of each midwife on one set of questions with her relative standing on the other set of questions indicates the accuracy of the distinctions made by the interview form. If the midwives who make relatively high scores on one-half of the questions also make relatively high scores on the other half, and if those who score low on one set also score low on the other set, then it can be assumed that the interview form contains an adequate number of questions, for the same distinctions are made between the midwives irrespective of which set of questions is used. Also it may be safely inferred from such analysis that the addition to the interview form of other questions of similar nature would not materially affect the distinctions between the midwives shown by the entire set of questions used. An index of the degree to which the same distinctions are made using the two halves of the material is afforded by the correlation between the two sets of scores (Table 3.1).[2] The extent to which the total material makes reliable distinctions between the midwives is shown in the last column of Table 3.1.

The correlation of .95, representing the reliability of the entire battery of questions, indicates clearly that the interview form as constructed makes reliable distinctions between the midwives and that the questions are representative of some common factor. Since all the questions are based on midwifery information and practice, it may be assumed that the common factor is quality of midwife service.

Table 3.1. Reliability of the Midwife Interview Form (correlations between scores on one-half of the interview form with scores on the other half of the interview form).

Source of Data	Number of Cases	Correlations One-half with one-half	Reliability of total material*
County A	20	.90	.95
County B	34	.90	.95
County C	26	.84	.95
Total	80	.90	.95

* Figures in this column represent the correlation that would be expected between the entire set of questions and another set of questions of equal number and reliability. They are obtained using Spearman's formula

$$r_x = 2r_h \div 1 + r_h$$

where r_x is the reliability of the total test and r_h is the correlation between the scores on two halves of the test. From Henry E. Garett, *Statistics in Psychology and Education* (New York: Longmans, Green Co., 1926), p. 271.

Validity of the Method

Is the assumption that this index is a measure of the quality of midwife service and of the knowledge that midwives have valid? Several types of data were used to prove the validity of the index. The first was a comparison of the midwives from the three counties. Since, by definition, the midwives in county A had considerably less supervision than the midwives in county B, and those in county B had somewhat less intensive supervision than those in county C, we would expect the midwives in county A to be inferior to the two other groups and the midwives in county C to be slightly better than those in either group A or B. If the technique actually reveals differences in midwives that are produced by supervision, then the scores of the midwives in county A should be lower than the scores of the midwives of the other two counties.

It is evident from the distributions of the scores of the midwives in the three counties (Table 3.2) that the scores in county A are not as high as the scores in the other two counties and that the scores in county B tend to be lower than those in county C. In terms of average scores, there are about 22 points of difference between group A and group B and the same number of differences between group B and group C. In terms of median scores, the difference is even greater.[3] The distinctions between groups of midwives made by the interview form corresponded with the differences that are known to exist. As a measure to distinguish extreme groups, the interview form is therefore valid.

Ratings of the ability of the midwives in county B, made by the nurse who had had intimate contact with these midwives for a

Table 3.2. Distribution of Scores on the Midwife Interview Form for the Three Counties Included in the Study.

Midwife Interview Score	Frequency of Occurrence of Each Score in:		
	County A	County B	County C
150–159	0	2	2
140–149	1	2	8
130–139	1	3	5
120–129	1	5	3
110–119	1	3	3
100–109	1	5	1
90–99	1	5	2
80–89	2	4	2
70–79	3	4	0
60–69	6	0	0
50–59	3	1	0
Total	20	34	26
Mean Score*	84.2	106.4	128.0
Median	74	101	137

* These means were computed from the raw ungrouped data.

period of 7 months, served as the second criterion for the establishment of the validity of the interview form. The nurse who made the ratings had just completed an intensive study of these midwives, during which time she had talked with them in their homes, had watched the majority of them at both antepartum and postpartum visits, and in three instances had observed the midwives during deliveries. The 34 midwives were independently rated on a scale of from 1 to 10 on 2 separate occasions. The correlation between the two sets of ratings is .94.[4] The correlations between each of the two ratings and the scores on the interview form are .84 and .86. Considering the unreliability of subjective ratings, these correlations indicate a fairly high degree of validity for the discriminations made by the interview form.

As previously suggested, the ideal criterion would be complete actual records of the kind of prenatal, delivery, and postnatal care that each midwife habitually gives. Observations of the midwives, however, would not reveal this, for if the midwife knew the proper procedure, she would very likely follow it in the presence of the nurse, although she might behave in an entirely different manner were the nurse not present. Then, too, to obtain such observations is practically impossible in a rural community where distances are great and where facilities for communication are limited.

An attempt was made, therefore, to discover further the kind of care the individual midwives give by questioning the mother concerning the prenatal care and by questioning the attendant at the birth, other than the midwife, in regard to the delivery and postpartum care.

It was soon discovered that little or no prenatal advice was being given. Many of the cases did not engage the midwife in advance; and even when they did, the midwife seldom visited an expectant mother. Consequently, questions about what advice had been given by the midwife were often embarrassing to the mother. In view of this difficulty and the fact that none of the midwives in county B, where it was possible to do this intensive investigation, gave anything like adequate prenatal service to their patients, the questions on antepartum care were discontinued.

However, during the limited time of the preliminary experiment, information on delivery and postpartum care was obtained on a total of 56 mothers whose homes were visited by the field worker after the babies had been delivered by midwives from county B. Both the other attendant at the birth and the mother herself were questioned concerning the way in which the midwife prepared for and conducted the delivery, how she cared for the baby, and what intrapartum and postpartum care she gave the mother. It is, of course, difficult to judge the quality of a midwife on the reports of her activity as given by the patient and the attendant. In 17 of the 56 cases the midwives arrived after the baby had been born. For such cases, questions on preparation and delivery did not apply. In 6 cases the doctor was called in by either the midwife or the family, and in these cases the delivery care and postpartum advice were given by the physician.

In many instances the mothers did not know whether the midwife had carefully washed her hands before delivering the baby, whether "drops" had been put in the baby's eyes, or whether many other of the accepted techniques had been followed. The difficulties in this type of material make direct evaluation impracticable unless a large number of postpartum reports can be obtained for each midwife. In the period covered by this study, it was impossible to secure more than 3 cases for any one midwife, and this number was possible for only 11 midwives. Two cases were obtained for each of 9 midwives, and there was only one case for each of 5 others. The remaining midwives in the group studied did not attend a birth during the study period.

Although the delivery and postnatal data are not sufficiently complete to serve as a criterion for a direct validation of the midwife interview form, there are a few distinct differences in score on the midwife interview that are associated with specific practices revealed by the postpartum interview. For example, midwives who had scores of 130 or above (the average score for the 25 midwives for which postpartum interviews were obtained was 112) made an average of 4.3 return postpartum visits, whereas those who made scores of 100 or below made only 1.9 postpartum visits. Midwives who make high scores on the midwife interview tend to give more continued postpartum care than midwives who make low scores. A number of other comparisons, given below, indicate that the midwives who are reported as following accepted techniques make slightly higher scores than those who did not follow prescribed practices.

The average score for the 15 midwives who did nothing to speed up the birth of the baby was 116; for the 6 who gave quinine, camphor in hot water, parched eggshell tea, or greased "privates" (the perineum), the average score was 103.

The mothers interviewed were sure that 9 of the midwives used either a sterile cloth or a special dressing on the cord. The average score for these 9 was 119. The average for the 15 who used cotton, a scorched rag, or a clean rag was 108.

The evidence was fairly conclusive that 3 of the midwives did not wash their hands more than once during the delivery. Their average score was 94, as opposed to an average of 117 for the 19 who were reported to have washed their hands a number of times.

The mothers attended by 7 of the midwives reported that they were advised to bathe their breasts and nipples in boric water to prevent soreness. The average score for these 7 midwives was 129, while for the 14 who either gave no advice at all or advised greasing with lard, camphorated oil, or mutton suet and sage, the average score was 105.

Vaginal examinations were performed by 9 of the midwives according to the statements of the patients they attended. The average score for these 9 was 110, as compared with 114 for the 13 midwives who were reported as not performing vaginal examinations.

Fifteen midwives made sure that the mother was bathed before the baby was born. Their average score was 119. This is considerably higher than the average score of 103 for the 7 who did not take this precaution.

The 18 midwives who advised their patients to bathe the field with Lysol water each time after the pads were changed had an average score of 118, whereas the 6 who did not advise this hygienic precaution score only 92.

The differences between the averages are slight and, because of the small number of midwives included in each sample, are not statistically significant. However, the fact that in every case the acceptable practice is associated with the higher score indicates that the interview technique does distinguish the more competent midwives from those who are ignorant, untrained, and followers of superstition.

Abbreviation of the Interview Form

As previously stated, the experimental interview form contained a large number of questions to ensure a wide representation of the elements of midwifery knowledge and practice. In the field the interviewer found it long and tedious to administer. Often the midwife became bored and restless, thereby increasing the difficulty of completing the interview.

If the form were to be practical for extensive use, the number of questions included needed to be reduced in order to eliminate the fatigue of both the interviewer and the person interviewed, and to increase the number of interviews that could be conducted during the day.

The primary basis for eliminating questions was the diagnostic significance of the separate questions. The diagnostic significance of an item depends upon two factors: (1) The frequency with which the question is answered correctly and (2) the degree to which the item distinguishes the good midwives from the incompetent. Certainly a question that 90 percent or more of the midwives answer correctly cannot be very valuable as an item that distinguishes good midwives, for the responses given by the good midwives do not differ from the responses given by those lacking ability. For instance; all but five of the midwives mentioned "slapping the back," "hot and cold water baths," or "artificial respiration" as methods for starting the baby to breathe. Since practically all the midwives, good and poor, knew at least one of these acceptable methods, this question was eliminated. Likewise, all questions that were answered incorrectly by over 90 percent of the midwives were excluded.[5] Of the 219 items originally included, 27 were excluded on this criterion.

Furthermore, to be truly discerning, an item must be answered correctly more frequently by the good midwives than by the poor ones. It has already been shown that those midwives who make high scores on the total interview form perform a better quality of service than those who make low scores; therefore, the value of any item may be judged by separating the midwives into two groups, according to the way in which they answer the item, and comparing the total scores (scores obtained on all the questions of those midwives who answer the particular item correctly with the total score of those who answer incorrectly). If a correct reply is more often associated with a high total score, and an incorrect reply more frequently accompanies a low total score, then that item or question may be considered of value, for it distinguishes good midwives from poor ones. Take the following question: "Do any of your cases ever engage you in advance? Does it make any difference whether they do or not? What?" In response to this question, 27 midwives stated that they urged their cases to engage them early in order that they might discover danger signs or the need for a doctor.

The average score for these 27 midwives was 135, whereas the 53 who did not mention this reason for early engagement averaged only 94. Moreover, very few of the midwives who answer the question incorrectly make higher scores than those who answer this question correctly, and vice versa, as may be seen in the first two histograms in Figure 3.1. This question is therefore highly diagnostic, for the midwives who answer it correctly make much higher scores than those who do not answer it correctly.

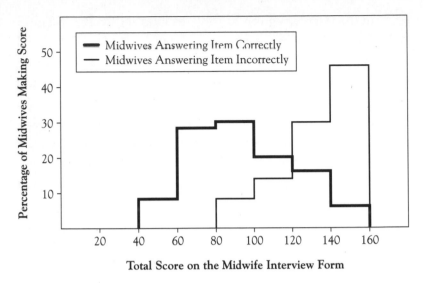

Figure 3.1. An Example of a Good Diagnostic Item.

Contrast with the above the results on the following question: "What kinds of food should an expecting[6] mother eat?" Cereal was mentioned by 29 midwives. Their average total score was 110. The average score of the 51 who failed to mention cereal as desirable food was 107. The difference is negligible. The histograms showing the distribution of scores for these two groups (as shown in Figure 3.2) are almost identical. The question is useless in distinguishing the good and poor midwives, and it was excluded from the final test.

Each of the remaining 192 items was subjected to this type of analysis. To take into account both the overlapping of scores and the difference between the mean scores of the midwives who answered an item correctly and those who answered it incorrectly, an index of the significance of each item was computed.[7] A distribution of these indices of significance is given in Table 3.3. In the final selection only the items with significance of 3.0 or more were retained.

In addition to the exclusion of items of low diagnostic significance, elimination was made of those questions that had proved dif-

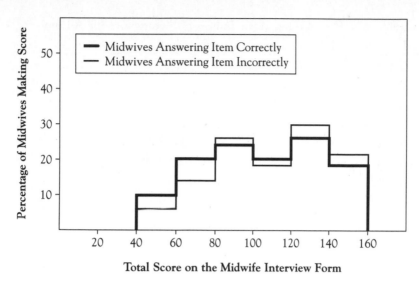

Figure 3.2. An Example of a Poor Diagnostic Item.

ficult to administer in the field, and also the items that had presented difficulty in the scoring.

There were only 14 items of real significance that had proved difficult to administer or score. The majority of the items with such difficulties had already been excluded by the previous analysis. The very fact that the midwives could not easily understand an item, or that the responses to an item were sometimes ambiguous, tended to lower its diagnostic value.

As result of the 3 types of exclusion just described, the original 219 items were reduced to 126, which can be grouped into 41 questions.

Evidence for the Abbreviated Interview Form

As assurance that the abbreviation of the interview form has not destroyed its value, both the reliability and the validity of the test were recomputed. When the scores for one-half of the questions are

Table 3.3. Distribution of the Indices of Significance for All the Items in the Midwife Interview Form.

Index of Significance	Frequency of Occurrence	Index of Significance	Frequency of Occurrence
0–0.9	17	6.0–6.9	26
1.0–1.9	17	7.0–7.9	7
2.0–2.9	18	8.0–8.9	9
3.0–3.9	29	9.0–9.9	3
4.0–4.9	39		
5.0–5.9	27	Total	192

correlated with the scores for the other half of the questions, the resulting correlations indicate that the test is still sufficiently extensive to be representative of the quality of midwife service. The same distinctions between the midwives are made irrespective of which group of the questions is used.

The average score on the abbreviated form for the midwives in county A was 50.4; in county B, 65; and in county C, 85. A comparison of the differences between these averages with those obtained using the original form shows that the same distinctions between the counties have been preserved in abbreviating the interview form.

The correlations of the two sets of ratings by the nurse with the scores on the abbreviated test in county B were .83 and .85. These correspond favorably with the previous correlations of .84 and .86. It is safe to say that abbreviating the test has not lessened its value as a measure of the quality of midwife service (see Table 3.4).

Summary

From a large battery of questions on midwifery practice and knowledge, an interview form has been constructed as an index of the quality of service a midwife renders when she attends a maternity case. The technique has been shown to be a reliable and valid mea-

Table 3.4. Reliability of the Abbreviated Midwife Interview Form.

Source of Data	Number of Cases	Correlations	
		One-half with one-half	Reliability of total material*
County A	20	.93	.96
County B	34	.88	.94
County C**	26	.77	.87
Total	80	.90	.95

* Obtained by using the Spearman correlation formula; see Table 3.1.

** The scores for the midwives in this county are much more homogeneous than the scores for the midwives in the other 2 counties. The reliability of the test is lowered by the low standard deviation. The standard deviation of the scores for counties A and B is 10 and for county C is 8.

sure of the service given by an individual midwife. Therefore, the degree of success or failure of any given program of midwifery control can be judged using this interview form.

In addition to its usefulness as a method of evaluating public health effort, the technique will serve to select the better midwives. Nurses in their supervisory programs can interview the midwives in their community and determine those who need the most supervision and teaching. Midwives who score extremely low can be eliminated by taking away their licenses. Those with high scores need not be checked so often. The supervisory time will thus be focused on those midwives needing the most help, who may reasonably be expected to profit therefrom.

The interview form was developed as a first step in the evaluation study of various public health procedures used in the control of the midwife in the southern states. Future studies contemplate completing the evaluation by carrying out the three remaining steps described in the beginning of this paper. A technique for registering the administrative procedures followed by health departments for the education, supervision, and control of midwives will be constructed. Utilizing this technique, the health department practices for a number of counties in which the modes of midwife control are different will be recorded, and a number of midwives in each of these counties will also be measured using the midwife interview form. From the relationships between these two sets of data, it will be possible to determine which procedures are effective in producing a high quality of midwife service. Programs of midwifery control can then be constructed to include procedures of tested effectiveness.

Discussion Questions

1. Why did Derryberry feel so strongly that midwifery practice and its evaluation was so important?

2. What strategies and consecutive steps did he suggest for evaluation processes in this realm?

3. What further methods did he recommend be taken before such an evaluation could proceed?

4. Discuss the relevance, in your view, of some of the recommendations he made for future evaluative studies in this sphere.

Notes

1. From the Office of Studies of Public Health Methods in cooperation with the Division of Domestic Quarantine and the Office of Child Health Association to the U.S. Public Health Service for the purpose of conducting this study. Grateful acknowledgment is made to the State Health Department of Virginia and to the State Board of Health of North Carolina for the privilege of working in the respective counties and for a list of the midwives and their addresses, thus facilitating the collection of data. In connection with this paper, the reader is referred to "The Rural Midwife: Her Social and Economic Background and Her Practices as Observed in Brunswick County, Va.," *Public Health Reports*, 50, 1807–1815 (December 27), 1935.

2. The correlation was computed using the Pearson product moment formula:

$$r_{zy} = \Sigma xy \div N\sigma x\sigma y$$

3. The difference between the means of group A and group B, and the difference between the means of group B and group C, are reliable differences. The standard deviation of the first difference is 7.6 and of the second difference is 5.9.

4. One would ordinarily expect a correlation of unity between the 2 sets of ratings by the same person. The fact that the correlation is not unity is partial explanation for the low correlations with the scores on the interview form.

5. This criterion for exclusion should not be taken to mean that the information or activity covered by a question that over 90 percent fail is unimportant, but rather that the question is not useful in making distinctions between the midwives.

6. The correct term here is "expectant," but the midwives use "expecting," and the questions are stated as nearly as possible in their "language." Many other expressions in the interview form were stated in terms used by the midwives without regard to their grammatical accuracy.

7. The significance of each item is the relation of the difference between the mean scores of the midwives in the two categories (those who answered the item correctly and those who failed the item) to the standard deviation of that difference. The formula is

$$\text{Index of Significance} = (M_1 - M_2) \div \sqrt{\sigma^2 m_1 + \sigma^2 m_2}$$

where M_1 is the average score of the midwives who responded to the item correctly, M_3 is the variability of M_1; M_2 and M_3 are similar constants for the distribution of scores for those midwives who answer the item incorrectly.

4

Appraising the Educational Content
of a Health Service Program

The White House Conference "Report on the School Health Program" enunciates a number of fundamental guiding policies. Many of these have had their influence on the school health programs of the country. The subject of this chapter is prompted by the acceptance of one of these principles, which is: "The health program of the schools should be definitely and fundamentally educational in nature and scope."

In using the term "health service program" we are including the following activities: (1) medical and dental examination programs with the subsequent follow-up of cases with physical defects; (2) those activities carried on for the purpose of preventing the spread of communicable diseases; (3) the first aid and emergency treatments; and (4) the special advisory functions of the doctor and nurse relative to adjustments in the school routine to benefit children with certain physical handicaps, such as cardiac disorders, and hearing and vision defects.

What are the educational values one might expect from a health service program? We must know these before proceeding to any

Coauthored by Mayhew Derryberry and George T. Palmer. Originally published in the *American Journal of Public Health*, May 1937, 27(5), 476–480. Reprinted with permission.

appraisal. Biologically defined, education is a change in the organism resulting from activity. From this standpoint, the health service program has an educational influence on all those who participate in it. There are changes not only in the child but in all others concerned— the parent, the teacher, the nurse, the principal, the physician, the dentist, and the dental hygienist. Changes that take place may be desirable or undesirable. Are any of our programs conducted in such a way that educational values, such as favorable attitudes and proper health habits, result? Or are we merely paying lip service to an ideal and possibly developing unfavorable attitudes toward medical service and advice? The answer to these questions rests on a critical evaluation of our procedures. The first essential in evaluating a program is to define its objectives specifically. Unless we know exactly what we are trying to achieve, measurement is impossible. Values must be measured in terms of the degree to which specific objectives are attained.

Some of the desired educational values for the *child* are:

1. A favorable attitude toward professional medical and dental care.

2. An appreciation of the value and importance of early medical advice and the dangers of self-medication and over-the-counter drugstore prescribing.

3. Information concerning the transmission of communicable diseases, methods of protection, and proper health behaviors relative to their control.

4. The development of good health habits. The advice received from professional personnel at the time of the examination should be a potent influence toward improving the health behaviors of the child.

5. A respect for the achievements of medical science and an appreciation of the work that is continually being attempted in connection with the control of disease.

Not only does the school health program have a responsibility to the child, but if it is to achieve one of its main functions, namely, the amelioration of handicaps among the children served, then it must educate the *parents* in a number of important ways. These are:

1. It should produce a better understanding of the child not only with respect to his physical needs but also to his mental and social needs. Either at the time of the examination or in the course of the follow-up, the specific needs of the child should be made clear to the parent.

2. It should inform parents concerning the medical facilities of the community and how they can best be used. It should also teach both parents and children how to appraise the various types of so-called medical facilities, or, in other words, how to separate the quacks from reputable and acceptable facilities. Too often, the program concentrates on the attainment of only one of the desirable results—the correction of a defect—and ignores the concomitant bad result that accrues from the way in which the attempt at correction is made. The purchase of glasses from the ten-cent store is sometimes considered a correction by the parent.

3. It should develop among parents a favorable attitude toward the school, so that they will think of it as a place where they can go for friendly advice concerning their child instead of waiting for the school to come to them.

4. From the program, parents should develop a favorable attitude toward all preventive measures, such as immunizations and vaccination, early care of colds, and so on. The emphasis upon perfect attendance has done much in a negative and undesirable health education way. There are times when children ought to be absent.

Since the *teacher* is a participant in the school health program, we may also expect her or him to reap certain educational values. These are:

1. A better understanding of the handicaps of children in general and of her children, in particular. If the teacher assumes certain responsibilities for screening out children who should be seen by physicians as early as possible and if she is present at the examination of those children, then she feels that she has a responsibility for the health of the children in her room. On the other hand, if the medical service is conducted without the teacher, she learns that someone else has the responsibility for the health of the children and that it is not her function.

2. An improved knowledge of the meaning of certain physical symptoms and behaviors that she may observe in her children.

3. A more thorough understanding of the home conditions of the children whose homes are visited by any of the school health personnel. How many school nurses report back to the teacher on the home environment of a child they have visited so that proper curriculum and other adjustments can be made?

4. A knowledge of how to utilize the services of the other members of the school health staff in understanding her own children. In a properly coordinated program the teacher should learn when to rely on her own judgment and when to call upon the physician or nurse and how to utilize their time to the best advantage.

During the *nurse's* participation in the program, certain educational values should also accrue to her. One of these should be an appreciation of the fact that children are more than objects with physical defects that must be corrected, and that her job is a teaching job with the parent more than a coercive job of getting children under medical care. To this end the nurse must learn the scholastic and social problems of the child as well as his physical condition. As a second educational value the nurse should learn that she is a part of the total situation and that the work that she does and the records that she keeps are merely a means to an end rather than an end in themselves.

In a properly functioning school health program, the *principal* also is a participant and as a result of his participation there are certain educational outcomes that should be expected. First of all, he should gain an appreciation of the need for administrative adjustment for children with specific handicaps. The principal should also learn the limitations of a school medical examination. It is impossible under the present organization of the school medical service to give periodic health examinations to all of the children. School medical examinations cannot be as accurate as we would hope because the previous history of the child is seldom available. Therefore, we cannot expect the physician to give the type of medical service that might be expected from a private physician with his own patients. These limitations should be recognized by the principals in order that demands will not be made upon school physicians to do the impossible.

These are some of the many educational outcomes that may be expected from a well-rounded program of school health service. How can we evaluate the extent to which these outcomes have been attained?

In the past, expert opinion has frequently been used in the evaluation of various public health programs. By this method an individual (or a group of individuals) studies the program, its objectives, the administrative organization, and the activities carried on. From this study the experts state in more or less qualitative terms their opinions concerning the effectiveness of the program in achieving its objectives. There are several dangers in this method of evaluation. First, the estimate of the success of the program depends upon the expert or experts who make the evaluation. If a physician evaluates the program, his judgments will be largely based upon the adequacy of the examination, the length of time that it takes to make it, and the relative number of children so examined. It is probable that he will give less attention to the follow-up and educational activities in the program. If, on the other hand, the evaluation is made by a health education expert, much more emphasis will be placed upon the educational content of the curriculum and the extent to which the examination is used as a teaching experience.

Realizing these dangers inherent in evaluation by expert opinion, those who critically study public health procedure have turned to appraisal forms and rating scales as methods of overcoming some of the bias likely to result from expert opinion. Such appraisal forms consist of a number of items that experts agree should be present in a good health program. Specific numerical values are granted for the presence of each of the items in the appraisal form, and the evaluation is made by summing up the scores for each of the items carried on in the program. This largely eliminates the failure to obtain a comprehensive picture of a school health program. It likewise eliminates the errors that arise because of the difference in emphasis that various experts attach to particular activities. It does not, however, remove the difference in standards in the observation. For example, items in an appraisal form such as "Provision for integration of health topics with other subjects of the curriculum" and "Satisfactory evidence of special adjustment of school regime to meet needs of children with heart defects" are specific items. But the decision as to whether the adjustment of the school regime is satisfactory or whether the integration of health topics into the curriculum is provided for will depend upon the standard used by the evaluator to judge satisfactoriness and integration. Furthermore, these appraisal forms place their emphasis upon administrative practices rather than upon results. A school that is following all the prescribed procedures would be evaluated as having a very acceptable program even though many of the objectives listed are not being obtained. Despite these limitations, appraisal forms have been very useful. They have called attention to many of the lacks in school programs, and this has frequently led to improvements.

An adequate evaluation depends on the measurement of the actual results obtained. Do children who have been under a given health service follow preventive measures? Do they realize the values of early medical advice and the dangers of self-medication? Do they go to a dentist regularly? Answers to such questions should be the essence of a proper evaluation.

However, it is not easy to obtain answers. To do so requires measurement of knowledge, attitudes, and behavior of children, of parents, of teachers, of nurses, of physicians, and of principals. Only a few of the measurements needed to provide answers to these questions have been devised. Their construction is a long, careful research problem in itself. Therefore, we cannot be expected to describe comprehensive measurements suitable for evaluating present health service programs. All we can now do is outline the criteria for such measurements.

First, the measurements must be objective. They must be so constituted that the results obtained by one evaluator will be the same as those obtained by any other evaluator in the same situation. If this condition is not met by the measurements, the results obtained are indicative of the person who made the evaluation, and not of the program. Evaluations based on individual subjective judgments are especially faulty when judged by this criterion.

Second, the test items must be indicative of the total objective rather than a measurement only of the particular items included. Suppose we were measuring the extent to which the program had produced in the children favorable attitudes toward health behaviors. It would, of course, be impossible to measure the children's attitudes toward every possible health behavior. Therefore, the materials chosen for measuring children's attitudes must be so selected that they represent more than just the particular items included. In other words, if another section of the materials were used, the same distinctions in the children's attitudes would be obtained. Those in the public health field have been too prone to place significance on the answers to individual questions. The psychologists ask a group of questions bearing on the point at issue and judge the mass effect of the replies. We must become accustomed to using questions and answers as indices and not for their individual significance. Answers vary too much with the way questions are asked. We must get at the truth by indirect rather than by direct approaches.

Third, the measurements used must be truly indicative of the degree to which the objectives have been achieved. Satisfying this criterion is particularly difficult because many of the most important educational values of the health service program do not exhibit themselves until later in life. For example, one of the most important outcomes should be an appreciation of medical supervision and a tendency to seek medical advice on health problems. Direct measurement of the attainment of that objective cannot be made until several years after the child has been exposed to the program. Therefore, any immediate evaluation of attainment must be by indirect measurement of a child's behavior under artificial situations; but this indirect measurement must first be shown to be indicative of the actual subsequent behavior of the child—otherwise the evaluation is not valid.

The health service program can be definitely and fundamentally educational. We may think that the direct, immediate, and only outcome of an examination is the correction of defects. Occasionally it may be, but in many instances the specific physical condition disclosed in an examination is relatively minor. It is merely a practical demonstration of a desirable procedure. The school medical service cannot be at a child's beck and call every minute. The service must teach something. If it does not teach something that the child can use later, it is merely palliative, and little progress is to be expected.

We are not getting all the educational value possible out of the health service program. We are too impatient; our objective is too limited; our eyes are too narrowly focused on the defect. We do not want to slow up the examination to talk to children or to parents. It cuts into our number of examinations. This is a mistake. We must raise our eyes to the longtime educational outcomes of the health service experience. The tooth that we repair today is just one little experience. The school cannot accept the responsibility for all future repair work. The aim should be to get the child and the family to accept the responsibility in the future for their own good and of their own volition.

Once the educational values are utilized in the school health program, then evaluation is worthwhile to guide procedures. Accurate appraisal is a slow, painful process, but it is worth the effort. We must seek the aid of experts in psychological measurement to do the pioneering research in the construction of measuring instruments. Practical evaluation procedures must await these preliminaries.

Discussion Questions

1. How did Mayhew Derryberry define education in the biological sense?

2. From this standpoint, how did he see the educational influence of a health service program?

3. What are some of the desired educational values he described for the child?

4. Do you agree or disagree with these viewpoints? Why? Why not?

5

The Physician's and the Nurse's Part in Health Education

Health education has been claimed to be one of the major functions of each professional group engaged in the school health program. The physicians contend that they should do health education because they know the subject matter; the teachers claim that health education is their function because they know the method; the nurses maintain that they are the logical ones to teach health because, in addition to knowing sufficient subject matter and to having acquired some technics of presentation, they know the families and are in intimate contact with them. Implied in all these contentions is the concept that health education is primarily a matter of instructing parents and children on health subjects. The idea seems to be that if the proper professional worker gives instruction to those needing it, desirable results are assured. But the bare statement of the spoken or written word is not the sole means of bringing about the changes in attitude and behavior that we are trying to effect through our health education. *How* a statement is spoken or written may have far more significance for the person addressed than actually what is said. Actions, too, often confound the words accompanying the action so that the individual may learn something

Coauthored by Mayhew Derryberry and Dorothy Nyswander. Originally published in the *American Journal of Public Health*, October 1939, *29*(10), 1109–1113. Reprinted with permission.

altogether different from what was intended. So instead of discussing the controversial question of whether health teaching should be done by the physician, by the nurse, or by the teacher, we have chosen to focus attention on the educational possibilities that are inherent in many of the administrative procedures and policies that are part and parcel of our school health programs.

As a background for this discussion, it might be well to recall some of the factors with which all of us are familiar that influence *what* and *how* people learn. First, one seldom learns just one thing from even a single experience. Ordinarily a number of things are learned from the same situation. A child not only learns that his skin infection is impetigo when the doctor or nurse examines it and gives him the information; but depending upon the way he is told and the circumstances under which he is told, he may learn that accidental infections occur that do not reflect upon his home life, that the doctor and nurse are his friends, that they will protect him from embarrassment in the presence of his friends and classmates, and that they will help him to get well. On the other hand, he may learn that the physician and nurse have no concern for his feelings, for they do not hesitate to tell him in the presence of other children that the infection is associated with dirt or that he is unfit to be with his friends; he may even get the implication from conversations that he overhears in the medical room between doctor, nurse, and teacher that his home is responsible for his condition. Thus, in the latter case, he learns to fear the medical room and to resent these people who attack his fortress of inner security—his home.

Children and adults, who after all follow very much the same principles in learning, undergo at least three definite forms of change in each learning situation: (1) they learn the words that were spoken; (2) they learn to react emotionally to the way the total situation was handled; and (3) they learn what action to take in the future to obtain any satisfactions that were present or what to do to avoid any unpleasantness that was inherent in the situation. Thus a wealth of attitudes, biases, hates, fears, and prejudices are developed in every individual, and these are often found to have their origin in situations where the obvious intention of the teaching was far different.

Corollary to this principle is the fact that it is not necessary that something be done to or for an individual in order that he may learn. He frequently learns when we as teachers think we have done nothing to or for him. This is particularly true with reference to the development of attitudes. Providing a comfortable, quiet place where a mother may sit to discuss the health problems of her child with the doctor, conserving the mother's time through carefully planned appointment systems, and so on, are examples of situations in which parents learn to appreciate the school health services, whereas failures to keep appointments with parents or children, advising them to go to clinics where the waiting list cannot possibly admit another person, and giving a medical examination without an explanation to the parent of what was or was not found are very likely to develop in the parents and children negative attitudes that often seem irrational to the staff.

In the light of the certainty with which learning other than that specifically intended takes place in various situations, let us examine some of the school health procedures to discover the possibilities for both positive and negative education that they present.

First of all, both the initial and every other contact of a parent or child with the physician and nurse are fraught with educational possibilities. Usually the first contact of the parent with a physician or nurse is a note either requesting the parent to take his child to a physician or an examination or inviting him to be present at the school examination of the child. Do physicians and nurses analyze such messages sent to the home to see that they accomplish the real objectives of the school health service? Is the manner in which the note is sent and the wording of it such that the parents are convinced that the request is made because the school has a vital interest in the child's health, or do the parents learn from the note that the school health service is merely carrying out a routine service without much thought as to the circumstances governing the lives of the family?

To make the point more concrete, consider the following extreme example, which is an actual case. "Come to school at 9 A.M. to see me," signed "School Nurse," was hurriedly written on a scrap of paper left undated, folded, and given to a boy with the command, "Take that home to Mother." If such a note survives the usual vicissitudes of messages given to little boys and reaches its destination, is it likely to start a chain of events in which the parent will understand that a specific problem is to be discussed with her; will she keep the appointment with the nurse and expect professional guidance that she may trust?

Consideration for the way in which notes are worded, who sends them home, and the method of sending them has been experimentally shown by the New York City study to influence the response obtained. One type of note resulted in a 30 percent response from the parents. A more carefully planned note caused 85 percent to respond to the message sent home.

The next most common experience of the parent and child with the school health service from which much positive or negative health takes place is the visit to the medical room to see the doctor or nurse. Even the room itself can affect the parents' and children's attitudes toward and conceptions of the school health service. If the medical quarters are clean, well lighted, and well ventilated; if they have adequate room for all those who are visiting at one time; and if there are sufficient chairs for those who must wait for short periods; other things being equal, favorable attitudes toward the health work of the school will be developed. But if, as so often happens, the physician and nurse must work in a niche in a corner or in an empty classroom vacated because of its lack of light, the unlikely stage set will not promote a confidence in medical service or build a respect for the confidential, trustworthy relationships between patient and physician that we claim we are trying to build up.

Although the physical layout of the medical quarters and the comforts or inconveniences that the child and parent experience while waiting in them have important influence on learning, the treatment accorded them by the doctor and nurse during the examination and accompanying interview is far more potent in determining what they learn. Are they greeted courteously? Are explanations made carefully if unexpected delays occur? Is the mother made to feel that her presence is not only welcome but important? These are the factors that build attitudes. This, of course, is no new thought, for all school health workers have stressed the possibilities for educating both parent and child at the time of the medical examination. But in our observations of some of the examinations in various school systems, we have been led to wonder if the possibilities for learning the wrong attitudes and the wrong health behaviors from our routine procedures have been fully recognized.

Do we always recognize that the things we do not tell the parent, but that are implied by our actions, lead him to form many erroneous convictions and may bring about negative attitudes toward the school health service? Perhaps an extreme situation will emphasize this point. Consider the mother who observes the examination with a stethoscope of the chest of her only child. The doctor listens, listens again, frowns, and listens again. He has the child lie down on a couch and listens several times, shakes his head, then listens a second time with the child standing. The mother, suspecting something, anxiously asks, "What is the matter, Doctor?" Not wishing, without a cardiograph and more adequate examination, to make a diagnosis of the heart murmur he has heard, the doctor answers, "The nurse will tell you what to do." The nurse, according to the prescribed policy, gives the mother a printed slip and says in a routine fashion, "Take this slip with you and take John to your private physician. Don't worry about it." The mother looks at the slip. On it is written "cardiac" with a question mark after it.

Now more concerned than ever, having no family physician and having received no instruction in the selection of one, the mother finds a doctor's sign on the way home and decides to take Johnny there that night. The doctor, after no more careful examination than was given at the school, tells her that Johnny has a little heart murmur but it amounts to nothing. He further tells her that the school should have told her that it was nothing at the time.

Now what did that mother learn? First of all, she learned that the school physician did not tell her all he knew. She also learned that the private physician had little respect for the school physician and the way he handled the situation. She learned to pay little attention to the advice and instruction from the school medical service. She may have learned that the school health service made her spend money for an examination that she would not have spent if she had not come in contact with it. Nor did she have the positive learning experience of finding out what a good cardiac examination is like. On the other hand, she went through an experience with considerable negative emotional content and will no doubt tell it over and over to other mothers who have children in school. Thus, she becomes a negative agent of health education, not because of instruction that was given to her but because the school doctor in examining her child followed prescribed medical technics but overlooked the effect of those technics on the personalities with which he was dealing.

In recounting this incident, we are aware of the pressure placed upon physicians and nurses to examine a large number of children within a very short time. We are also aware of the many restrictions that policies place upon them with reference to usurping the functions of the private physician. However, we have given the incident in the extreme to show how negative health education may result if proper consideration is not given to the attitudes and ideas that are outcomes of the procedures we use.

If the parent has not been present at the examination and some condition needing medical attention has been found, opportunities for negative or positive education occur in the follow-up procedures. The methods used may include a note to the parent, a home visit by the nurse, a consultation in school, or contacting the child in school. Whatever the procedure, the information given should be positive and backed by sufficient reason to convince the parent that medical care is needed. All of us are familiar with the situations frequently arising during the follow-up, when the private physician or clinic disagrees with the findings of the school physician. It is recognized that disagreements in diagnosis are sure to arise, but do we consider what such disagreements teach the families with which we are working? Too often we concern ourselves only with the administrative relationships that hamper our work and fail to recognize the effect of such situations on those who are the objects of our endeavor.

The description of these difficulties by no means suggests the solution. It does, however, point out the possibilities for negative education presented by the school health service, and what may be learned as a result of some of the administrative procedures and policies under which the school physician and nurse must work. Although we are not in a position to suggest the proper procedures, it is our conviction that administrative policies and procedures should be influenced far more by the ideas and attitudes they engender in the parents and children than by immediate administrative exigencies of the situation.

In summary, then, there are many situations in the school health program involving the physician and the nurse that abound with teaching possibilities. If in these situations the procedures followed by the physicians and nurses bring pleasant experiences to the parents and children and satisfy their wants and needs, much good health education will result; favorable attitudes toward proper attention for the immediate health problem as well as toward the future use of medical care will be built up. If, on the other hand, the school health procedures are carried on in a routine and regulatory fashion without regard to the feelings, the wants, the comfort, and the understanding of both parents and children, much negative learning is likely to take place. Therefore, one of the contributions of the physician and the nurse to health education is to make sure that all their procedures and methods result in positive rather than negative learning on the part of their clientele.

Discussion Questions

1. What is one contribution the physician and nurse could make in terms of their client's health education needs according to Derryberry?

2. What is the likely consequence of poor physician or nurse communication in the context of a school health service?

References

Adams, R. W. (1953). Notes on the application of anthropology. *Human Relations, 12,* 10–14.

Allport, G. W. (1953). The teaching-learning situation. *Public Health Reports, 68,* 857–879.

Anderson, E. J. (1950). Ideological barriers to effective teaching by health workers. *Public Health Reports, 65,* 661–669.

Foster, G. M. (1953). Relationships between theoretical and applied anthropology: A public health program analysis. *Human Organization, 2,* 5–16.

Koose, E. L. (1954). *Health of Regionville—What the people thought and did about it.* New York: Columbia University Press.

Mead, M. (1953). *Cultural patterns and technical change.* Paris: United Nations Education, Scientific, and Cultural Organization.

Preventive Medicine in Medical Schools—Report of Colorado Springs Conference. (1953). Baltimore: Waverly Press.

Saunders, L. (1954). *Cultural difference and medical care: The case of the Spanish-speaking people of the southwest.* New York: Russell Sage Foundation.

Schottstaedt, W. W., & Wolfe, S. (1955). Collaboration of the medical school and the health department in teaching medical students. *American Journal of Public Health, 45,* 1097–1100.

Shapiro, I. (1951). Doctor means teacher. *Journal of Medical Education, 26.*

Skinner, M. L., & Derryberry, M. (1954). Health education for outpatients. *Public Health Reports, 69,* 1107–1114.

World Health Organization, Technical Report Series No. 89. (1954). *Expert committee on health education of the public—first report.* Geneva: World Health Organization.

6

A New Technic of Health Education for Use in Baby Stations

Interest in the use of tests as a technic for motivating the general public to acquire information has recently been stimulated by the use of quiz games as teaching devices in health education and other fields.[1] In Newark, New Jersey, the Baby-Keep-Well Stations have adapted with considerable success the popular quiz session to an educational purpose, through the employment of "true or false" contest methods with groups of mothers who attend conferences.

As originally planned, using true-false statements as an educational device had as its primary objective instructing mothers in proper procedures in infant care. When the plan was put into operation, however, it developed that it was equally valuable for other purposes. It pointed out to the physicians those facts about baby care that were relatively or completely unknown to many of the mothers, and it also uncovered a number of wrong ideas that the mothers had. By concentrating on facts that were unknown and on the correction of wrong impressions, the physicians were able to make the instruction much more profitably. Furthermore, if he had previously taught some point now being tested, a physician could judge how effective his instruction had been.

Coauthored by Julius Levy, Mayhew Derryberry, and Ivan Mensch. Originally published in the *American Journal of Public Health*, July 1942, 32(7), 727–731. Reprinted with permission.

The test questions constructed for initial trial dealt with the following phases of maternal and child hygiene:

Feeding
  Artificial or bottle feeding
  Breast-feeding
  Cod liver oil
  Orange juice
Development
  Habit training
  Sleep
  Teething
Common infant disorders
  Constipation
  Cradle cap
  Crying
  Diarrhea
  Vomiting
  Care of diaper and skin
Clothing
Fresh air

The questions were prepared by the physicians and were, in general, based on actual experiences at baby stations.[2] Many of them were intended to present mistaken or commonly held ideas such as "Crying injures a baby's lungs," "Teething causes colds," and "Belly bands keep the back straight."

After the first contests in the fall of 1940, succeeding ones have been conducted at intervals ranging from 1 to 3 months, with from 5 to 15 participants at each. The physicians at the stations have, in each instance, announced the date of a contest several weeks in advance and reminded the mothers in the interval. In addition to the physician's reminder, the nurses during home visits have encouraged the mothers to attend.

Although in general the quiz sessions have been conducted as contests, a few physicians have preferred to omit the competitive feature and have, instead, a question-and-answer period. In each instance the physician introduced the session with a brief informal talk in which he explained the method that would be used and usually compared it with the radio quiz programs with which most people are familiar.

In conducting the contests, two distinct methods have been used. When the first method is followed, each member in turn is asked a question. About 25 questions are used, so that each participant has an opportunity to answer once or twice, to give reasons for her own answer, and to comment upon those given by others. According to the second method, the group is divided into competing teams. The division may be arbitrary, based on seating arrangement, for example, or on some characteristic such as the number of children a mother has. In the team arrangement the usual method of scoring has been to give one point for each correct answer and an additional one or two points credit for a correct explanation or reason for the answer. If the individual who gives the correct answer (true or false) cannot also furnish a correct explanation, the other side is given a chance to do so. The physician who conducts the contest also briefly summarizes the information after each question has been discussed.

In the time allotted to a contest with its attendant discussion (usually less than an hour) the physicians find that they can use 18 to 25 questions, selecting those pertinent to the problems most commonly found in their particular stations. Since there are available 160 questions from which to select, the physician has considerable latitude with respect to the topics he may wish to have discussed. By conducting the contest before the child health conference, it has been found that in general attendance has been improved.

Since the true-false contest was a new technic in health education, there was need for some evaluation of its effectiveness, when used by several physicians, before its real value could be determined. In order to find out more exactly how the method operated, stenographic transcripts of contests conducted by 7 physicians, each in a different health station, were taken between November 1940 and April 1941.

Five of the physicians used about 25 questions each, but the other 2 used 146 and 62, respectively. In the latter two contests, the percentage of questions about which there was no comment, discussion, or explanation was 60 in the first case and 90 in the other. The doctor sometimes said, "Yes, that's right," or "No, that's wrong," but gave no further interpretation. It would appear that at least two contests achieved only a very limited amount of teaching, since there is nothing in the record to indicate that the physicians even made certain that correct answers were not the result of guess work.

Contrasted with the type of contest that is little more than a recital of questions are the other 5 of the 7 analyzed. There was discussion and explanation in over 90 percent of all instances, and in no case was a question passed by without some comment. In two of the contests there was not a single question to which the answer was not discussed.

In the type of situation when there is secured not merely information in the form of discrete items of fact but an understanding of related facts and an explanation of reasons, it is surely fair to say that real teaching has been achieved. The physician, therefore, has opportunity to find out what the participants know or do not know and also to present new or unfamiliar information, correct wrong impressions, and make sure that reasons are properly related to practice. That can only be done, however, if the physician observes certain cautions in using the contest technic in his child health station. As one observer remarked after screening a true-false contest: "The success of the contest depends almost entirely upon the person who runs it and how he does it." The manner in which the physician conducts the quiz is most important to the effectiveness of this method of teaching mothers. This implies active participation by the physician, not a mere recital of a series of items.

The first two contests discussed above illustrate test situations in which the educational value was reduced and definitely limited by the use of large numbers of questions. Mere recital of questions consumed a major part of available time and allowed little or no explanation. The "all right," "yes," "that is correct" type of comment by the physician serves as praise for the one participant to whom it is directed and is a source of satisfaction only to her. However, others present can derive no educational benefit from noninformative comment; hence a valuable opportunity for teaching is lost when there is not additional explanation of the answer. Such discussions need not be long or very detailed. The following transcripts emphasize the importance of the physician's position as educator:

1. Always shake a lot of powder on the buttocks when the baby wets. True or false?

DOCTOR A

MOTHER: False.

DR.: Why is that wrong?

M.: It's not necessary. It sticks and cakes. You can oil the baby, use olive oil. For one thing, I have heard you can give the baby pneumonia from the dust.

DR.: This mother has thought about this. It will cake around the creases. Dust the powder on a puff and put it on. But the baby cannot get pneumonia from putting powder on the buttocks.

DOCTOR B

M.: False.

DR.: Correct.

2. Never use table sugar in the formula—there is not enough nutrition in it. True or false?

DOCTOR A

MOTHER: False.

DR.: Why?

M.: Because I never heard of any other kind of sugar to use for a baby.

DR.: Table sugar is just as good for a small baby as any other kind of sugar. Only in special cases do we use other sugars.

DOCTOR B

M.: That is false.

DR.: You are right.

3. Teething causes colds in babies. True or false?

DOCTOR A

MOTHER: False

DR.: Why?

M.: Teething does not cause any kind of illness. Baby may not have been dressed properly. It may have been in a draft.

DR.: That is what we are trying to bring out. Teething only causes teeth.

DOCTOR B

M.: False.

DR.: That's right.

In any evaluation of the quiz technic in health education, it is necessary to consider, in addition to its effectiveness in terms of

learning, the attitude that it produces in participants. The following transcripts are indicative:

> PHYSICIAN: I should like to ask you mothers what you think of
> these contests. Do you like this method?
> PARTICIPANT: Very much.
> PHYSICIAN: Do you think it makes much difference if you know
> *why* things are done?
> PARTICIPANT: I think if you know *why* you do these things, you
> are more apt to do them, and do them *right*.
> PHYSICIAN: Do you like this session, mothers?
> PARTICIPANT: Yes. Very much.
> PHYSICIAN: All of you?
> PARTICIPANT: Yes. You learn something. Have questions on older
> children next time.

The physicians conducting the contests have also expressed
their opinions of the technic in such ways as:

> DR. A: I think it's the best means of getting discussion. It's the
> best way the Baby Station can get all the mothers to take part.
> DR. B: The contests are nice, but I think the information you
> want to get across is better delivered by the five or ten minute
> talks we give all the mothers before each conference. The con-
> tests are popular, though; the mothers make mistakes and all
> laugh, and we have a lot of fun.
> DR. C: The best plan is to have the contest before the con-
> ference. In that way you have better interest and more moth-
> ers stay.
> DR. D: About forty to forty-five minutes is the optimum length
> of time for the contest. It doesn't work well if you take much
> more time than this. And each station should space them at
> least 3 months apart. You can't have the quizzes more often than
> that if you want to keep the mothers interested in the game. But

3 months is just about the right time to repeat the contest with the same mother.

The discussion and the quoted comments and criticisms above, taken together, highlight the characteristics of a good contest. Briefly stated, these may be considered the following:

1. Participation by all who attend.
2. Informality and the "game" spirit.
3. Emphasis on subjects of current interest and also on subjects unknown or relatively unknown to the participants.
4. Adequate discussion and explanation of the reasons for the answer.
5. A coordination and summary (on the part of the physician) of the information brought out during the discussion.
6. Length not to exceed 40 to 45 minutes for maximum interest to the participants.

Through the use of the true-false contest in baby stations, one of the primary interests motivating mothers to attend child health conferences is satisfied. The mother's desire for service and information brings her to the station. Physical examination of the baby and the physician's recommendations constitute the service, but the mother also receives information on maternal and baby care during the conference.

The health education technic described here can increase the amount of information about maternal and child hygiene that the mothers get and can also aid physicians to determine where teaching is most needed and how it will be most effective.

Summary

1. An adaptation of the popular quiz program has been introduced in baby stations.

2. Quiz contests can assist a baby station physician in giving information about maternal and child hygiene and thus aid in educating mothers in adequate health procedures by a popular technic, new in the field of public health education.

3. By means of contests, both physicians and mothers learn. The physician finds what subjects of maternal and child hygiene require special emphasis because they are unknown or relatively unknown to mothers—information that can be utilized in improving subsequent child health conferences.

4. How the contest is conducted depends principally upon the physician who serves as moderator and educator in the test situation. The amount of teaching done is directly related to the way in which the quiz period is handled by the physician.

5. Characteristics of a good contest are:
   a. Participation by all the mothers.
   b. Informality and the "game" spirit.
   c. Emphasis upon subjects of current interest and other pertinent problems.
   d. Adequate discussion and explanation of reasons for answers.
   e. Coordination and summary by the physician of the information brought out during the discussion period.
   f. Length not to exceed 40 to 45 minutes for maximum interest.

6. Contests not having the characteristics above have little value in health education.

7. Although it has not been experimentally demonstrated, it is believed that variations of the quiz technic can be used in other types of public health clinics.

Discussion Questions

1. Discuss the role of tests and quiz games as techniques for motivating the general public to acquire health information.

2. What are the two distinct contest methods that were described in the chapter?

3. Who learns from the use of contests and health games, what do they learn, and why?

4. What are three characteristics of a good health education contest?

Notes

1. See, for example, Mayhew Derryberry and Arthur Hichsmann, "Using Tests as a Medium for Health Education," *Public Health Reports*, 55, March 22, 1940, p. 489, and "The Quiz Corner as a New Informational Technique," Bureau of Agricultural Economics, United States Department of Agriculture, July 1941.

2. The use of the quiz session in Baby-Keep-Well Stations and the original set of questions were suggested by Dr. Ralph N. Shapiro, a member of Dr. Levy's staff.

Part II

Education

A Challenge to All Health Professions

Overview

Mayhew Derryberry believed that education is a service to be given by all health professionals, not just by health educators. He played a key role in moving health education from telling and selling to providing opportunities for many people to learn through discussions of individual, family, school, and community health problems and programs. Dr. Derryberry often stated that the health educator on the public health team had the responsibility for sharing knowledge and research about how people learn so that other professionals could improve their educational efforts. The next seven chapters reflect this belief.

The opening chapter, Chapter Seven, presents Derryberry's major study on the educational efforts of public health nurses in home visits. Presented to the National Organization for Public Health Nursing, this study created tremendous interest, both negative and positive, when it was presented. In this study, teaching is examined as it exists in practice as well as in theory. The study focuses on the learning of the patient rather than the teaching by the nurse. The need for the teacher to adapt instruction to the interests, concerns, and limitations of the learner is a significant finding of the study. Derryberry dramatizes how learning theory can be used to improve practice and uses excerpts from verbatim transcripts to heighten reader interest.

Chapter Eight shows how the teaching of health professionals can become more vital and meaningful through the use of taped transcripts of what actually occurs in field situations. Coauthored with Margaret Arnstein, it demonstrates Derryberry's thesis that the educator functions as a partner with the learner, not as a sole authority in education.

The next two chapters give emphasis to patient education and are among the earliest references to appear in the literature. At this time, the focus of health education was almost entirely on the well person, with an emphasis toward conforming patient behavior to meet the perceived goals of the health professional. Derryberry offers a much larger consideration of human wants and desires, regardless of whether the person is sick or well. He translates psychological motivational theories into practical application for program development. Furthermore, satisfaction with the learner's performance as a motivating force is emphasized. Today we call this *feedback*. He discusses fear and anxiety in the context of understanding how feelings function in influencing behavior rather than suggesting an unrestrained use of these forces.

The last three chapters in Part Two show the growing sophistication of the public health education profession. Conflicts between public health educators and other groups, such as the physical education community and the school health education professionals, are examined. Derryberry tried to neutralize these intraprofessional tensions by stressing that the nature of the public health field itself, that is, the growing chronic disease and environmental issues of the day, demanded new problem-solving approaches. He encouraged the application of new findings from research in the social sciences, for example, Lionberger's work in diffusion theory, plus the sharing of the research conducted by the military in World War II.

During the period represented by these chapters, Dr. Derryberry's leadership in the field of public health was beginning to emerge. Likewise, through Derryberry's support for the development of a curriculum in public health education at the graduate level in schools of public health at various universities and for broadening the interest and commitment of the federal government in health education, his important role in improving the academic preparation of health educators and widening the scope of health education practice was being firmly established.

7

The Nurse as a Family Teacher

It is hardly necessary to summon arguments in support of the statement that the public health nurse should be a teacher as well as a nurse. To teach, according to the dictionary, is to make aware of. And the public health nurse who fails to make her families aware of health and the paths to health must surely be little more than an automaton who performs some services, to be sure, but leaves her charges none the wiser. It is not only the educators who put the nurses in the ranks of the teachers. The National Organization for Public Health Nursing in the reports of its survey of public health nursing conducted in 1931 and 1932 makes the point that departments of health, departments of education, and public health nursing associations emphasize the teaching aspect of the nurse's work.[1] Yet the same survey found that in actual practice the average home visit had little educational value. The nurses' performance appeared at its lowest level in what, ideally, should have been one of their most important services.

Accordingly, about a year ago, the Public Health Service undertook an analysis of the educational work of public health nurses, in the hope of discovering some way by which it might become more effective. The objects of the study were to determine, as far as pos-

---

Originally published in *Public Health Nursing*, June 1938, 30, 357–365. Reprinted with permission.

sible, the virtues and failings of the nurses' educational efforts and, on the basis of the findings, to make recommendations that might lead to higher achievement. The data are verbatim transcripts of nursing visits in the home. The stenographic notes were taken by experienced workers who accompanied nurses on their routine home visits.

The study has not yet progressed to the stage where definite results can be shown and conclusions presented. However, a preliminary study of the material now available, viewed in the light of our knowledge of the way in which learning takes place, indicates that certain general educational principles are readily applicable to the teaching of nurses.

Interest—A Factor in Learning

Probably the most important factor in a learning situation is the interest that the learner may have in the material to be learned. Thorndike found in his investigations that "learning without interest of some sort does not occur to any appreciable degree."[2] If the families whom a nurse is trying to teach are indifferent to what she tells them, it is not very likely that she will be able to alter their health behavior to any great extent.

But it may be argued that everyone is interested in health. This is only partially true. Few well people are willing to do anything out of the ordinary to conserve their health; the sick are the ones to whom health is of paramount interest. An individual who is ill invites the physician and nurse to visit him and asks for their advice and assistance. He is uncomfortable, and in his eagerness to feel well once more he will for the most part rely on their instructions. If he is told to submit to an unpleasant treatment or observe a rigid routine, he will follow the more or less dictatorial orders of the physician and nurse. He seldom demands an explanation for things he is told to do and even less frequently is given one. He does what he is advised because he is interested in the outcome—recovery of his health.

But the well individual, and frequently the ambulatory patient, feels that his state of being is satisfactory. He is seldom interested in inconveniencing himself in order to follow a health practice advocated by public health workers. The following reasons given by mothers for not attending child welfare clinics illustrate apathetic attitudes and will have a familiar ring to all public health nurses:

NURSE: You haven't had him in to the health station.
MOTHER: He's getting along all right, and we didn't think it necessary.
NURSE: You haven't had Barbara into the clinic since June, and June is such a long time.
MOTHER: Yes, it is, but she is getting along nicely.

Such conversations as these could be repeated many times from our data, not only with child welfare cases but also with school-children, venereal disease patients, and contacts to tuberculosis patients.

Because of this lack of interest in hygienic habits on the part of the individual who is not sick, the task of raising his standard of health conduct is a difficult one. We cannot say to him as we do to the sick man, "You must do this," or "You should do that." To be of value, our teaching must be motivated in such a way that it will induce an active rather than a passive response.

Frequently nurses whose work we studied assumed that the patient's interest in preventing diphtheria, stamping out syphilis, or controlling tuberculosis was as great as their own. It would be fine if this were true, but we all know that it is not. Note the following verbatim extract from a nursing visit to secure reexamination of tuberculosis contacts:

NURSE: Did George and Ruth go back to the clinic?
MOTHER: No, they didn't go.
NURSE: How about Ruth? Is she still working?

MOTHER: Yes. She said she doesn't want to go back to the clinic. She said she doesn't want to know how she is getting along.

NURSE: I know, but she would much rather find out in time. She could go on Thursday night at seven-thirty. She hasn't had an X-ray for some time.

And from a child hygiene visit:

NURSE: Has the baby had the needles for diphtheria?

MOTHER: No, she didn't get the needles.

NURSE: They should have these things done. As they get older and go out in the street and come in contact with other children, it's best that they should have these things. Do you give the baby cod-liver oil?

MOTHER: Yes.

NURSE: And her eggs?

MOTHER: I give her eggs, but not often. Spinach and carrots and baked potato. But I didn't change her milk.

NURSE: Then you should bring her in, because she should have that changed, and the baby weighed. When they give the needles, they will give you a card. You should keep that, because when she goes to school they will ask about it.

The mothers in these two cases have probably been animated by as lively an interest in correct health practices as the average ten-year-old boy has in compound fractions when his teacher tells him to learn about them because she tells him to.

This overemphasis on the accomplishment of a definite objective without consideration for the patient's interest, or without permitting him to feel that he has any initiative in the matter, too often approaches a kind of police work. Unquestionably, the objectives have their own importance, and the nurse properly considers them her job. But she has another job, too, and brusque insistence on administrative and technical details may rob her forever of opportunities to be of educational service. For example, the following conversation took place in a child hygiene visit:

> NURSE: Do you take the little boy in to the child hygiene clinic?
> MOTHER: Yes.
> NURSE: He was vaccinated and got his protection for diphtheria?
> MOTHER: No, he never got his vaccination.
> NURSE: You should take him up there, too. Of course, he has to have these things before he starts school, so it's much better that you get them now. Do you feed the baby regularly?
> MOTHER: Yes.
> NURSE: You take the little boy up so you can get him vaccinated and get his protection for diphtheria, and when he starts to school, all that will be done, and you won't have to bother with it. And you take this one up there regularly.
> MOTHER: All right.
> NURSE: How are you getting along with baby, all right? What about his formula? You make all the formula up at once?
> MOTHER: Yes.
> NURSE: All right, then you take the baby in and we won't bother you. If you don't take it in, we'll have to come back.

And on a tuberculosis follow-up visit, the conversation was:

> NURSE: How long has it been since your husband died?
> MRS. JONES: The end of May.
> NURSE: The clinic nurse told you for two years you would have to be checked up, and Phyllis, too.
> MRS. JONES: After the death?
> NURSE: Yes, two years after. So when they give you a date, you should come back.

In contrast note the following, where the objectives of the visits are almost identical with the examples above:

NURSE: She will soon be six months old, and you will soon be thinking about getting the toxoid for her. It is the treatment that is given to children to prevent them from getting diphtheria. Have you heard of toxoid?

MOTHER: Toxin-antitoxin shots? I had them when I was a child.

NURSE: We advise you to have that when the baby is nine months old. It is to prevent the baby from getting diphtheria. You know diphtheria is a serious disease for young children.

NURSE: Has Ellen had an examination since you knew you had tuberculosis?

MRS. SMITH: Oh, no. She's fat. She's healthy.

NURSE: But just the same she was exposed and really should be examined. Tuberculosis is a contagious disease; you catch it from being around people who have it. So any person who has been in contact with anybody who has had tuberculosis should be examined. The doctor will give her a tuberculin test. That is to show whether the tuberculosis germs have entered into her body, and if it shows positive, they take an X-ray to find out if there is any damage to her lungs. We often find children with positive tests, which shows that they have germs in their system. Then the doctor takes an X-ray to find out if these germs have done damage to the lungs. That is a very good thing for children, don't you think?

MRS. SMITH: Sure, it is good.

NURSE: Everyone who has been exposed to the disease should have an examination. They may look all right and feel all right. When the disease begins, she might not even know it. The way it starts sometimes, there is no cough, no pain, or any other way you can recognize it. Some people with it are overweight. Wouldn't you like for her to be examined, to be sure?

These latter visits, in addition to being less dictatorial, are excellent illustrations of the way in which health teaching may be motivated. They present information concerning the importance of diphtheria immunization and the reasons for examining those who are contacts of tuberculosis patients. By having the facts before them, the families are able to recognize the importance of the advised actions. This is by no means a novel idea, but in our study we found it a frequent failing of the nurse to insist dogmatically upon a specific course of action without offering the family any explanation of its value. Long ago we abandoned learning by rote in our schools; it is time we discard it in public health education as well.

Teaching by Example

Another factor that may handicap the nurses in presenting convincing arguments for the health behaviors they advocate is the negligence of public health personnel in following these practices themselves. Recently we made a survey of the health practices of about 800 public health workers, among whom were 234 nurses.[3] It was found that a fourth of the children of public health workers were not protected by immunization against smallpox and diphtheria. Although the nurses scored considerably better than the other public health personnel, 10 percent of the nurses' children between the ages of 1 and 15 had not been given these two protective measures.

A fifth of the nurses had not had a Wassermann test; and of those who were married, a third had not persuaded their husbands to have this test. Still further, only 20 percent of the nurses who had had a Wassermann test had specifically requested it. They had the test because it was either routine or required in connection with their work. Is it surprising that we experience difficulty in convincing others of the need for specific health practices when we are so negligent ourselves? Is it possible that we are not really convinced of the value of the practices? If this is true, we should not urge them on others; if we are convinced, we should be the first to follow them.

I Would Like You to Do This

A method of motivation used extensively by many of the nurses is to ask the patient to cooperate with the nurse or health department in the achievement of some objective. It is illustrated in the following verbatim extracts:

> NURSE: The health department is very anxious that the mothers bring the babies to the child health center.

> NURSE: I would like for Carleton to be examined because I think he is run-down.

> NURSE: We would like for you to come to have the Schick test for Harry. Then the same day we could have the baby immunized, and then we ask you to come back with him in six months to have the Schick test. The Schick test is the only way we have of knowing whether the work we wish was done.

From these conversations, it would appear that the child is to be brought to the clinic to satisfy some vague aim of the nurse or health department and that the parent's interests are not involved. The nurse is imposing her own objectives upon the mother as sufficient motivation, disregarding the obvious and almost certain appeal to the mother's interest in the welfare of her baby.

There are, of course, many mothers who do not feel that they need any instructions from the nurse and consequently are not too receptive when a nurse calls and begins to outline the routines for taking care of the baby or the hygiene of pregnancy. Some nurses handle such a situation effectively by describing the services of the health department or public health nursing organization. It would be excellent if more would follow their example. Here is a case in point:

> NURSE: I'm from the _____ organization. May I come in?
> MRS. BROWN: Sit down.

NURSE: I am coming to tell you of the services we offer to those who are expecting babies. The names of all the patients that come to the hospital prenatal clinic are referred to us, and we make a home call to invite the mothers to mothers' club. We instruct the mothers in matters pertaining to the baby before and after it's born. We help the mothers with any problems they may have about clothing and diet and their own care, and all that. You see, at the hospital clinic they don't have time to teach the mothers care of themselves. Any little problem whatever that comes up that you don't understand—you come to mothers' club and bring it up, and they will try to explain it to you to the best of their ability. They will show you how to make the baby's clothes if you are interested in making the clothes.

MRS. BROWN: That's very nice.

Another means of arousing people's interest in health practices and securing their cooperation is the rendering of real service in time of need. This method is most successful in organizations that maintain a bedside nursing service. Unfortunately, in many official agencies it is a policy not to render bedside care. Note the following situation where the nurse making a visit to a tuberculosis patient found her in bed:

NURSE: Have *you* been able to get back to the clinic?

MRS. GREEN: No, I was planning to go today but I feel too sick.

NURSE: Did you call a doctor in?

MRS. GREEN: Yes. He told me to stay in bed.

NURSE: Well, I am so sorry. I am not going to talk to you much this morning, so I won't advise you about going into the clinic since he has ordered you to stay in bed. I will report you in bed. Has a visiting nurse been in to see you?

MRS. GREEN: No.

NURSE: If you do think you need a nurse, be sure to get in touch with the visiting nurse.

What attitudes are created in patients by such a restriction on the activities of a nurse? It is easy to imagine the patient recounting the incident to her family and neighbors, concluding with a sniff and some variation on the "Them-that-can-does, them-that-can't-talks" theme. The prestige of the nurse is reduced along with her chances for successful health teaching. Under the best circumstances, the patient is likely to feel that the nurse offers to help only when there is nothing to do, or possibly, that she is not capable of giving any real service. The nurse has no choice but to follow instructions when the policy of the local health department does not permit her to give care to the sick. Nevertheless, it is often found to be a real handicap to her in her relationship with her patients.

Misuse of Record Keeping

We find, too, a strange fixation among public health workers in connection with record keeping, which frequently gives rise to unnecessary difficulties. Sometimes it is the fault of the administration, sometimes of the nurse. Too often, securing information for a record card becomes an end in itself and is forgotten as a means to a desirable end. Undoubtedly records have their uses, but a patient must be puzzled and resentful when he is ordered to tell the health department about his citizenship, his parents, where he has lived, what he does, and how much money he makes in order to learn that he should drink milk and eat vegetables, see a doctor, or go to a clinic where he will probably be asked the same set of questions again. It would be interesting to know how much of this information is ever referred to for any reason whatever. In a case such as the following, the patient can't fail to feel that he, as an individual, is of little moment as compared to the nurse's interest in the purely mechanical processes of her job.

NURSE: [bluntly] Are you married or single?
MR. GRAY: Married.
NURSE: Where were you born, Mr. Gray?

MR. GRAY: Scotland.

NURSE: How long have you been in the United States?

MR. GRAY: Twelve years.

NURSE: Have you citizenship papers?

MR. GRAY: Yes. Oh, I have answered those questions a thousand times.

NURSE: Well, every organization has its own set of questions to ask.

Or, on a first visit to a tuberculosis family:

NURSE: How old is Walter? Is he thirty years old?

MRS. PENN: He is thirty.

NURSE: He is single, isn't he?

MRS. PENN: Yes.

NURSE: Where was he born—In the United States?

MRS. PENN: No. He was born in Austria.

NURSE: Is he a citizen?

MRS. PENN: Yes.

NURSE: What is his occupation? [Answers to the next several questions are omitted] How many rooms do you have? How many living in the household? Your first name? The father's name? How old are you? And the father? You are a housewife?

MRS. PENN: Yes. Is this catching?

NURSE: Yes, if you come in contact with it, yes.

MRS. PENN: Well, what can we do?

NURSE: What does the father do?

MRS. PENN: Basket maker. So what can we do?

NURSE: Just a minute. I will tell you all about that. Your address before this?

This conversation is not only an illustration of placing too much emphasis on records but also of the failure to take advantage of an expressed interest of the patient.

Adapting to Needs of Learner

One principle of teaching that is particularly important to the nurse as a family teacher is: Instruction should be adapted to the individual's symbolic level. In other words, instruction must be given in language easily understood by the patient and, wherever possible, delivered piecemeal, in bits adapted to his ability to retain it. This is a more exacting requirement than is generally recognized. The educational and mental equipment of different people varies widely. Ordinarily opportunities for frequent repetitions are limited, and consequently information must be given in a form readily comprehensible.

Our study has indicated that nurses do attempt to adapt their vocabulary to the patient's mental level. In developing a short method of determining the relative time a nurse devotes to teaching during a visit, we found that on an average, her conversation was conducted in four-letter words.

Nevertheless, it is difficult not to slip occasionally into familiar technical language that is meaningless to the patient. Observe these cases:

NURSE: [Asking about two children in a tuberculosis sanitarium] Are they active cases?
MRS. FIELDS: What does that mean? Does that mean whether they are getting worse or better?
NURSE: It means are they positive?
MRS. FIELDS: I don't know. They have spots.

The nurse's next statement was: "You have no other children?"

NURSE: [On a tuberculosis follow-up visit] We wouldn't be coming if he were an arrested case. When he is an arrested case, we won't come at all.
MRS. NEAL: Restification—what is that?

During a follow-up visit for syphilis, this was the conversation:

> MRS. FOX: The nurse claims the dose was too strong. She came out to see why. I stopped treatment, but I never went back. My arm would swell.
>
> NURSE: She was explaining to you that the doctor has to have the reactionary measure to show the physiological effect on your body, and the next dosage he would give you accordingly.
>
> MRS. FOX: My husband told me I would get along all right now, and I don't want to take any more.
>
> NURSE: Well, I think with a history like yours the doctor would advise you if it was at all imperative that you have that dosage according to the degree of involvement. If it were necessary to give the same dosage, then it would be necessary for you to have bedside treatment until that wore off. Even then that would be better than neglecting so serious an affair as that.

If you have ever asked an economist about the monetary situation and had him reply in a swift flow of technical financial terms or even had your automobile mechanic explain in detail what was wrong with your transmission or carburetor, you know how confusing the jargon of another field can be. Our own terminology is so familiar to us that it is often difficult to recognize it as meaningless to others.

Apparently failure to adapt advice to the patient's background occurred most commonly in giving general instructions such as, "Eat lots of nourishing food," or "Take plenty of rest," or "You must observe the precautions," when the patient did not know what is the "nourishing food," how much is "plenty of rest," or what are the "precautions" for a tuberculosis patient to follow. So long as the patient remains in ignorance of the implied details of such terms, he cannot change his behavior to comply with the instructions.

In contrast, some of the nurses planned menus with their patients and cooperatively worked out with them schedules of rest,

sleep, exercise, and eating. It is recognized that good nursing practice has prescribed this method of teaching for some time; yet many
of the nurses in our study gave very general advice that was totally
inadequate as a guide for the patients. Although our study will not
permit an evaluation of how much instruction at any one period of
teaching a patient can remember, we question whether a patient is
able to recall all that a nurse teaches her when the period of teaching covers as much as an hour or more. Some of the nurses spent as
much as an hour and a half on prenatal and infant hygiene visits.
During that time they covered almost all the material on the
hygiene of pregnancy or the care of the infant.

For example, on one visit the nurse taught rather fully concerning the following items: the desirability of medical care during pregnancy, how it could be obtained, and what the doctor would do
for the patient; the value of immunization for the three children;
the meaning of urinalysis, including an explanation of each step
in the process; the arrangements for home delivery, including discussion of supplies, methods of securing certain items, making of
pads, set-up of toilet tray, and calling a physician for delivery; diet
of the patient and family, including a discussion of the values of
canned milk and the ways to use it; dental care; clothing for the
mother and baby—their type and how to utilize substitutes; exercise, rest, elimination, drinking of water, symptoms of toxemia, and
adjustment of expenditures to budget allowance. One wonders how
many of the details the patient was able to recall and put into effect.

Summarizing the Visit

The possibility of the patient not remembering instructions suggests
another teaching aid that was used very frequently by the nurses.
Since repetition is one of the factors that bring about learning, the
practice of summarizing at the close of the visit the important items
taught the patient helps to fix them firmly in his mind. This technique is essential when the nurse has been obliged to teach many

things during the same visit. Here is a sample summary of a visit that was made by one of the nurses:

> Nurse: All right, Mrs. Hill, I think that about finishes our message to you today about little Sally and the baby. Let's go over what we have had. Little Sally, between now and the next time I see her: We're going to take care of those lovely teeth and try some recipes for liver. And our little baby: We're going to come up and see about three-hour feedings instead of the four-hour feedings because you think your milk supply is decreasing. And in the meantime you're going to try to get more milk for yourself and ask the doctor about the cereals. Is there any question you want to ask me?

In addition to a verbal summary of the visit, we venture to suggest a written summary, which would be given to the patient. This procedure was not found in any of the visits we have studied thus far. Yet those of us who attend classes practically always take notes of one kind or another. Of course, the patient seldom makes the notes, even though it might be desirable for her to do so; consequently it becomes the job of the nurse. The only written material that any of the nurses left with the patient was information about a physician, clinic, or social agency to which the patient could apply.

A written summary, properly executed, would serve two important purposes. It would remind the patient of the things that the nurse had taught and keep him aware of the things he was supposed to do. It would also help the nurse to check for herself the material she had taught. If the nurse used carbon paper and the summary were made out in duplicate, it could serve as the nurse's record of a visit to the family, thus permitting the nurse at subsequent visits to review what she had previously taught and continue her teaching at the point where she had left off. By revising present methods of recording in the home so that these carbon copies could serve as a nurse's report of the visit, the job of record keeping would be automatically solved. Whether or not such a procedure would be effective cannot be stated without experimental trial. We hope that some of you will evaluate it.

Finally, there are certain administrative procedures that limit the effectiveness of the nurse as a family teacher. All these are factors over which she has no direct control. Two of them are mentioned here in the hope that administrators may make such changes as are necessary to remove these handicaps to good teaching.

The first of these factors is the lack of coordination between clinics and field service. In a well-organized service the nurse presumably coordinates her teaching in the home with the findings in the clinic. To do this there must be some administrative machinery by which the field nurse is informed of the findings in the clinic. Consider the following example:

NURSE: Have you been in the clinic lately? [The nurse should have been notified so she wouldn't have had to ask.]

MRS. WOOD: I went a week ago yesterday.

NURSE: A week ago yesterday. Did you take a specimen of your urine?

MRS. WOOD: Oh yes.

NURSE: Did he think you were getting along all right?

MRS. WOOD: Yes.

NURSE: We would like for you to drink eight glasses of water a day. It shouldn't be so hard to do that, now that it is hot.

MRS. WOOD: The doctor told me to stop drinking so much water because my feet swell.

The nurse's standing orders for instruction were contradicted when the patient was examined at the prenatal clinic. Yet the nurse had no means of knowing what the physician had found. Such situations tear down the patient's confidence in the advice given her either by the doctor or by the nurse and sometimes both. Unfortunately, such lack of coordination exists all too frequently.

A second way in which the effectiveness of the nurse's teaching is hindered by factors outside her control is the failure of the clinics to deliver the type of service she describes. When patients attend clinics at the suggestion of the nurse and find it to be an unpleasant experience, they are less inclined to listen to the nurse's advice on other problems. Consider the following in an infant hygiene visit:

MRS. BROOKS: The only thing I am worried about is that his navel extends out a little. You see, I thought it was a navel rupture, so I went over to the doctor as you told me to do. He didn't say anything at all about the child's navel, so I asked him about the baby's navel. So he said, "I think it's a little ruptured." I said, "Well! Will you tell me for sure." And he said, "I think it is; don't worry about it," but he never examined the baby's navel at all. *That's one reason why I didn't go back.*

Another mother of an infant with excoriated buttocks stated:

I went to all the trouble of taking her to the clinic. That woman doctor just said "hello" and "goodbye." She didn't say a word about the baby's buttocks or anything.

There are other administrative procedures that interfere with the effectiveness of the nurse as a family teacher. These are, however, sufficient to illustrate that field nursing cannot succeed without adequate coordination with all the other efforts of public health workers.

Summary

Teaching is like selling. Just as one cannot say that he has made a sale until someone has bought, neither can we say we have taught until someone has learned. Interest in the thing being taught is a prerequisite of learning. Therefore, all health teaching of the nurse must consider the patient's interest and build on that. Some of the methods of stimulating interest as revealed by our study are:

1. Informing the patient concerning the reasons for the health practices he should follow rather than telling him the things he must do;

2. Describing the services that the patient is entitled to if he wishes to use them;

3. Rendering to the patient a service that he actually needs. Some of the procedures that tend to antagonize are:

   a. Ordering the patient to perform a health practice because he has to do it anyway since it is the health department regulation.
   b. Failing to render a service when such is needed.
   c. Asking many questions to fill out a record.
   d. Failing to make the objective of the teaching something the patient wants to do for his own satisfaction.

To be successful in our teaching, we must practice what we preach. Or, stated medically, we must not prescribe medicine we would not take under similar circumstances.

Another essential factor of effective teaching is the adaptation of the material to the limitations of the learner. This includes teaching in terms familiar to the public, not giving more material than can be remembered, summarizing at the close of the teaching period, and perhaps giving to the patient a written summary of the teaching.

None of these suggestions will yield maximum results if they are followed without consideration of the human side of the job. In our work we must remember that the attitudes instilled in the patient through all of his contacts with public health workers determine whether or not our teaching will be effective.

Discussion Questions

1. Although public health nurses could be effective educators about health, what factors were thought to handicap nurses in arguing for health behavior changes according to Derryberry?

2. How could some of these shortcomings be rectified?

3. What else is needed to yield maximum results from patient education?

Notes

1. National Organization for Public Health Nursing, *Survey of Public Health Nursing* (New York: The Commonwealth Fund, 1934).

2. E. L. Thorndike, *Adult Interests* (New York: Macmillan, 1936), p. 47.

3. Unpublished material gathered by the U.S. Public Health Service.

8

Nursing Visit Transcripts as Training Material

In all professional training, modern educational institutions bring theory and practice together whenever possible. If the student is training for any profession that involves human relationships, his knowledge of actual situations, their complexity and emotional content, is of utmost importance. Thus, schools of social work use case studies and verbatim interview reports; medical schools bring patients to the classroom and clinic; teachers' colleges employ lesson plans and stenographic reports of classroom work as teaching devices. All these methods have as one of their primary purposes the imparting to the student of a knowledge of the intricate human relationships with which he will have to deal in his professional career. In each instance such illustrative material supplements the practice work in social agency, hospital, or model school classroom, as the case may be.[1]

In the professional training of public health nurses, similar procedures are followed. Case studies, field record forms, and sometimes copies of actual field records of cases are made available to the student. But up to the present, no verbatim reports of actual home visits have been available for instructors of public health nursing to

Coauthored by Mayhew Derryberry and Margaret G. Arnstein. Originally published in *Public Health Reports*, December 20, 1940, 55(51), 2351–2355. Reprinted with permission.

use with their students. The teaching value of such material has been felt so strongly that many instructors have written imaginary visits based upon their past experience. Although such fabricated visits have been used with considerable success, they often sound artificial, and students are likely to question whether the situation described actually arises. Naturally, such resistance interferes with the learning process.

It is with a distinct sense of satisfaction therefore that the Division of Public Health Methods, National Institute of Health, is able to announce that transcripts of 23 public health nursing visits are now available to nursing instructors upon request.[2] The transcripts reproduced were selected from reports of 1,200 visits collected during a study of educational activities of public health nurses.[3]

The presentation of complete conversations, of both the nurse and the family, clearly demonstrates not only the nurse's teaching technique in a specific situation but also the response of the family to this teaching. Each visit is placed in its proper setting by supplementing the transcript with a copy of the record of all nursing and clinic visits prior to the time of the transcribed visit and of the services for a 2-month period after the visit.

Uses of Transcripts in Public Health Nursing Courses of Study

Perhaps the most important use of transcripts in teaching public health nursing lies in the fact that in this way a whole class may, so to speak, witness a given home visit and discuss it as it proceeds—a procedure obviously impossible in the actual home situation. Not only detailed analysis but also general discussion, if desired, is thus possible, with the added distinct advantage that no one need rely on memory alone to keep in mind precise points of procedure to be evaluated or commented on. In other words, the content may be kept before a group indefinitely; or, conversely, routine material may be quickly passed over without waste of time. Since neither simultaneous discussion nor the "slow-motion" effect is practical with a real home visit, these possibilities give the transcript a unique value as a method for introducing nurses to the theory and practice of home visiting.[4]

With no attempt to list all possible ways in which these materials may be used, it may be well to examine a few teaching situations in which the transcripts have been found to be effective. The list of such situations and methods of use could, no doubt, be amplified indefinitely. It is hoped that through the ingenuity of other instructors in the field, many other methods may be developed.

With beginning students, who are not sufficiently familiar with public health nursing procedures to be able to analyze a visit as a whole, it has proved most useful to choose excerpts illustrating points under discussion.

For example, in discussing the desirability of appealing to the family's interest in the welfare of its members, such excerpts as the following might be used to contrast teaching techniques.

Patient's Interest in Her Own Welfare Considered

NURSE: The baby has to have calcium to make bones, and if you don't give it in the form of milk, he'll take it from your teeth.
MRS. C.: Oh, I don't want to lose any of my teeth.
NURSE: Well, that's why you should drink milk.

Patient's Interest Ignored

NURSE: How about those calcium tablets?
MRS. B.: No ma'am, I haven't got them yet.
NURSE: But now is the time to take them. The doctor will be provoked that you haven't.

Or, as an illustration of the fact that a statement or direction may be substantially correct but, because it is not sufficiently explicit, a lay person may not know exactly what to do, the following contrasts might serve:

Insufficient Advice

NURSE: Don't nurse the baby every time she cries. She isn't always hungry.

Specific Instruction

NURSE: You should nurse her every 4 hours by the clock. You have a clock here so you can see it, and you should wake her up when it's time to nurse. What time did you nurse the baby this morning? The last time?

MRS. A.: Ten o'clock.

NURSE: At ten. Then nurse her again at two, then at six and ten at night, and once in the middle of the night, and start at six in the morning.

Aside from such elementary techniques as those illustrated here, the transcripts contain examples of almost all the common teaching and psychological principles. Comparison and contrast help to give concrete meaning to a principle and facilitate understanding of its application.

Students with public health nursing experience may profitably study entire visits. Such students are first asked to note the purpose of the visit and observe the extent to which it was achieved. They then analyze both good and bad points in the visit according to the principles of family health teaching. This exercise may be made equally constructive if students will indicate how the family's questions, comments, and responses might have been handled in each situation in which the nurse's teaching is adversely criticized. Positive emphasis is given to the good teaching or mental hygiene techniques illustrated in the visit.

When any such assignment is made, it is highly important to make certain that students understand fully the limitations of verbatim records, which can present only the bare words of a call but little or no evidence as to attitudes—the nods, smiles, frowns, and gestures that are as expressive as words and sometimes take the place of them. Furthermore, a transcript cannot record the pace of the visit. What may appear as a long uninterrupted series of instructions may, in the actual visit, have been broken by the nurse's moving about the room giving care or pausing for the patient's nod or other gesture. Students may need to be cautioned against an overcritical attitude toward colloquial speech, grammatical errors, or poor sentence structure in transcripts. The transcripts are not edited or polished to appear as written documents; they are conversational and therefore informal.

Transcripts are valuable in teaching students how to keep records. After reading a transcript, students make narrative notes of the visit and plans for the next visit. This procedure is particularly advantageous for beginners, inasmuch as they can give full attention to selecting facts that are important to record without being confused by the field situation in which they must but remember and hurriedly record the content amidst the confusion that is so often found in a home. After the students have completed their records, plans for the next visit are discussed in relation to the records they have made and also in relation to the transcript. Thus, when the student goes to a field agency, she is better prepared by having had some practice in recording.

For advanced students, transcripts and records provide material for special studies. For example, one may study the adequacy and completeness with which field nurses record their visits by comparing the content of the transcript with the nurse's notations.

Through study of the transcripts, students in supervision may escape the common educational pitfall of learning abstract theory and principles but not their application to practical situations. Such a student should read each transcript and indicate what steps she would take to supervise the nurse who made the visit. This may involve simply outlining the supervisory conference with the nurse, or it may go so far as to include plans for the nurse's further education if the student feels that the nurse needs more complete and accurate knowledge. A whole class can discuss the supervisory techniques that would be called into use in supervising a nurse who made such a visit; group discussion often throws much light on the student supervisor's problems. The relationship between supervisor and staff nurse is the key to all the supervisor's functions; transcripts afford excellent additional opportunities to discuss all phases of this key relationship, starting with the characteristics of the nurse as shown in the visit. Since the transcribed visits were made by a variety of staff nurses, many different personal assets and liabilities may be studied in the light of supervisory procedures that might be used in dealing with them.

Transcripts of actual visits have already proved an invaluable aid in teaching public health nursing to students, not only because they closely approach actual observations of field visits but also because, as is not possible in real visits, a whole class may discuss identical situations with the instructor. It is felt that this advantage of transcripts should open a wide field for further experimentation in their use.

Discussion Questions

1. How can transcripts be used profitably in public health nursing?

2. What is the documented value of transcripts and records in public health practice?

3. What is the role of public health education in nursing in the twenty-first century, and what are the competencies necessary for effective practice?

Notes

1. From the Division of Public Health Methods, National Institute of Health, Washington, D.C.

2. The supply of copies is limited; distribution is therefore restricted to instructors in public health nursing schools and to educational directors of health departments and other health organizations.

3. Papers describing the study and presenting some of its findings are: "The Nurse as a Family Teacher," *Public Health Nursing, 30,* 357–365 (June 1938); "How May the Nurse Become a Better Teacher," *Health Officer, 3,* 253–268 (January 1939); "Administrative Procedures That Interfere with Effective Public Health Nursing," *Health Officer, 6,* 13–23 (May 1939); "The Nurse as a Teacher of Tuberculosis to the Family," *Transactions of the 35th Annual Meeting of the National Tuberculosis Association,* 1939; and "Evaluation of Health Education Content and Materials," read at the Health Education Institute, Pittsburgh, Pa., October 16, 1939.

4. Transcripts are not to be considered a substitute for the observation of actual home visits, but the latter are likely to be much more meaningful if the student has analyzed transcripts previously.

9

How to Influence Health
Behavior of Adults

Public health educators have developed through past years a
body of health information, standards, and rules for healthful
behavior. This approved hygienic etiquette is now presented to
the public, which finds itself in much the same position as poor
Alice in Wonderland when confronted by a bottle so beautifully—
if dogmatically—labeled "Drink Me." The chief difference is that
the educators often have not bothered to label their product very
attractively. And, too, Alice was a child whose life was uncompli-
cated by the memory of past experiences or conflicting commands.
The chief motivation of her acts had been to please her elders by
doing as she was told, so she drank from the bottle. But the health
educators are dealing with adults who believe in acting to please
themselves. Whether directly or indirectly, this is almost invari-
ably the basis for their behavior. Here, then, is the fundamental
principle that should guide all our efforts to induce the public to follow hygienic habits. Will the public find pleasure in following
health practices because they satisfy some basic desire or prevent
some annoying situation from occurring?

The indignant reply may be, "Well, of course, everyone wants
to be healthy and therefore will want to follow good advice on

Originally published in *The Health Officer*, July–August 1939, 4(4), 114–117.
Reprinted with permission.

health behavior." But does this statement, which is so frequently and glibly made, accurately describe the attitude of the general public whom health educators are trying to reach? It is undoubtedly true of those who are ill. A sick person so desires health that he will endure all sorts of inconveniences, suffer humiliation, and accept dogmatic orders without question in the hope of recovery. He is anxious to avoid further discomfort such as he is now enduring, and this urge is a strong motivating force toward better hygienic practices in the future. Information and advice given in these circumstances are likely to be accepted. But the well person, in an environment comparatively free from such apparent dangers, can see no reason why he should change any of his present habits since they are not interfering with his sense of well-being. Furthermore, it is difficult to imagine himself in pain. Sickness strikes other people but not him. He'll not cross any bridges until he comes to them.

Perhaps public health educators have not recognized the distinction between the basic interests and desires of those who are well and those who are sick or partially so. Certainly many of them have not utilized the heightened interest of the sick as a means of motivating health behavior as much as they might, because they have maintained that it was their task to prevent illness rather than cure it. Consequently they have focused on the well individual almost to the exclusion of rendering guidance to the sick. By so doing they have frequently closed the door of opportunity for motivating preventive health practices. Though there may be serious administrative problems connected with the health supervision and instruction of the sick and convalescent, especially by official agencies, the chance for maximum educational results is much greater among the sick than among those who are not immediately concerned about their own hygienic habits.

In addition to the sick who are willing to follow health practices, the educator is afforded another interested group whenever some imminent threat of illness, such as an epidemic or some other environmental hazard, occurs. At such times many individuals have an urge to follow hygienic practices because they fear the loss of their existing state of well-being. The extent to which fear and consequent urge become widespread was shown by an analysis of a sampling of inquiries to the Public Health Service for 1933–35. It was found that during the encephalitis outbreak in St. Louis, the volume of correspondence on that subject was far greater than that relating to other subjects, and unusual interest continued during the following year. An organization ready to handle such inquiries adequately is reasonably assured of an interested audience that will react favorably to any instruction or advice that may be given. Yet I once heard a health educator declare he was so busy preparing radio scripts, bulletins, and popular health pamphlets that he never had time to give more than the most perfunctory attention to letters asking for advice on specific health problems. Thus he turned his back on an interested audience already in a receptive mood in favor of an indifferent one.

Health departments anxious to do a worthwhile educational job should give careful attention to mail requests, although they are generally considered the chief headache in the office. It is true that there are many cranks writing letters to public officials, but they can generally be recognized, and the sincere requests deserve the most careful advice possible. For it is man's way to value advice he has sought and be annoyed by that which is thrust upon him.

This latter principle of human nature applies to a number of other public health procedures whose objective is influencing health behavior. Since one is not inclined to follow advice that isn't sought, it would seem to be far better to offer health advice and guidance to the general public only where it is requested than to give advice or urge health practices where we feel they are needed. This is particularly true of nursing service. The individual who has invited the nurse in and is expecting her will reap the full benefit of the instruction given, whereas the individual visited because the nurse thought the instruction was needed may be concerned about other things and learn little from the experience. Although I recognize the danger of using the interest of the client as the sole criterion for selecting cases for home calls, it is nevertheless an extremely valuable criterion to use where the service is limited and certain cases must be omitted from attention.

Fear as a method of motivating health behavior has already been mentioned in relation to epidemics. Many health educators feel that it should be applied on a much wider scale. As evidence for their contention, they point to the way in which the manufacturers of patent drugs have exploited the fear motive in developing markets for their products through advertisements, most of which use the appeal "Don't let this happen to you." A glance at the sums of money spent annually for almost worthless drugs indicates the success achieved by such appeals. Other health educators, while admitting the potency of fear as a motivating force, point out that its exploitation in connection with the prevention of disease might have the highly undesirable effect of turning us into a nation of hypochondriacs. The use of fear, however, in situations for which a specific behavior removes the reason for fear would seem to obviate the above danger and present a legitimate use of such motivation. For example, developing a fear of smallpox and diphtheria as a means of inducing parents to vaccinate and immunize their children might be a valuable method of promoting these two preventive measures because, once protected, there is no further cause to fear. On the other hand, developing a fear of cancer or tuberculosis as a means of inducing medical attention for those two diseases is of doubtful value, for seeing the physician will not prevent the disease even though it does increase the chance of cure.

In seeking motivation for sound health practices we should not overlook the tremendous potency of group attitude. It has been said that acceptance within the social group to which one belongs is the mainspring of human behavior. Therefore, in urging any specific health behavior we should bend our efforts toward changing the attitudes of the group rather than concentrating on attempts at influencing individuals within the group. To accomplish this last purpose,

effort may be focused on certain leaders of thought in the community rather than on the individual needing the specific service.

A health officer in a large city had been unsuccessful in promoting immunizations of preschool children in a particular section
of the city. Intensive drives, house-to-house visiting, newspaper publicity, and distribution of pamphlets had all been tried to no avail.
He studied the community and learned that the priest was the
leader of thought. As soon as the situation was laid before the priest,
he promised to see that there would be no more resistance. The
next week the immunization clinics were crowded to overflowing.
Other health workers use local individuals to motivate health conduct by having them lead health discussion groups and promote
interest in health attitudes and behaviors. This is a legitimate use
of the Mrs.-Jones-over-the-back-fence type of instruction.

But the motivation of health behavior cannot be assured
because of the initial interest, urge, or stimulation of an individual.
If the practices are to be continued, the individual must derive satisfaction from the outcome. If, on the other hand, the resulting
behavior is annoying, the individual will not repeat the practice.
This principle has a direct bearing on many of the behaviors and
attitudes public health educators are trying to teach. For example,
if a contact of a tuberculosis case, convinced of the possibility of
infection and desiring to keep free from the disease, visits a tuberculosis clinic, is cordially greeted, is given prompt and efficient
attention, has his privacy preserved, and is carefully instructed on
all the questions about which he is concerned, his experience will
have been satisfying and he will likely return at the appointed time.
But if, as so frequently happens in public clinics, his experience is
unpleasant, the examination is seemingly cursory without any
explanation of the findings, and he is ordered to return in six
months, his dissatisfaction will strongly motivate him to avoid the
clinic in the future. If he continues in good health, he is likely to
feel a contempt for the health organization as well as its representative who asked him to go to the clinic; on the other hand, if he

does contract the disease, he will blame them for not helping him when they had the chance.

In such situations there frequently results that phenomenon known to psychologists as "associative shifting," whereby an individual who has had an unpleasant or unsatisfactory experience at the hands of a particular group or organization is likely to be negatively inclined toward all other efforts of that group. He may even be driven for the solution of his health problems to quacks, whose ethics do not limit them in the extreme methods that they use to motivate behavior that is profitable to them. But associative shifting also operates positively. One seeks help and advice from those who have previously helped him and won his confidence. Therefore, if an individual has been satisfied by one contact with a health organization, he is more likely to follow their advice on other matters.

The importance of being satisfied with the outcome as a motivating force for health practices is perhaps best illustrated by the lack of success that has followed the educational efforts for periodic examinations. Although many media of health instruction have been used to encourage annual health examinations, the practice is confined to relatively few individuals. Even many of those who are entitled to free examinations as a benefit from an insurance policy do not take advantage of the offer. Evidently they do not feel that the benefits obtained are sufficient to justify the effort. And this thought suggests the necessity of urging only that health behavior which is strictly essential. If we try to induce people to form a number of health habits, some of which are known to be valuable in preventing disease but others of which are actually unimportant, we should realize that when the latter are discovered to be worthless, the public may conclude that none of our advice is worth considering.

In promoting many health practices, public health organizations have resorted to coercion through legal restrictions. Milk control, water sanitation, sewage and refuse disposal, and many procedures for the control of communicable disease are now regulated by law in most localities. Proponents of syphilis control have recently incorporated certain preventive practices into law. There are also advocates for further extension of legal coercion for immunization against diphtheria, vaccination against smallpox for the infant, compulsory X-ray examination of all contacts of tuberculosis cases, and so on. However, the success of legal coercion really depends upon the effectiveness of the health educator. He must convince the public of the importance of the measure or, in other words, motivate the particular activity through some other means. Otherwise its enforcement is possible only through police methods, and this may be disastrous, for it combines in one organization the functions of leader or teacher with those of a militant enforcement officer. Frequently where leadership is difficult, enforcement is resorted to with a resultant development of an unfavorable attitude in the individual to whom the enforcement is applied.

This discussion has not attempted to cover all the appeals or the human wants that might be used in motivating health behavior. It has limited itself primarily to a discussion of the initial interest of the individual as being fundamental to bringing about any behavior and the equal importance of satisfaction resulting from the performance of the act. Whenever interest in some form or other is absent, and when satisfaction, either immediate or remote, does not accrue to the individual as the result of any act, there is little chance that the act will be repeated. It has been shown that the nature of the drives and motivating forces with which we are dealing is specific. A universal interest in health behavior cannot be assumed, else the practice of hygienic habits would be much more widespread, but wherever it is found, every effort should be made to satisfy it. Neither can fear nor group attitude be used with all individuals. Knowledge of the general factors that induce people to behave as they do is essential, but if our effort to influence health practices is to be effective, we must individualize the methods in terms of the factors that guide the behavior of the specific person or groups being reached. Such factors as age of the individual, the social group in which he moves, the prejudices he has, the ambitions to which he aspires, and the health problems with which he is faced will influence the motivation we use to induce him to practice hygienic habits.

In pointing out the limitations of various motivating forces there has been no intention to exhibit a defeatist attitude. Instead it is believed that a recognition of the limitation in the procedures we use may cause a better selection of methods and increase the success of our health education efforts.

Discussion Questions

1. How does Derryberry view the role of group attitude in seeking motivation for sound health practices?

2. What are some factors that increase the likelihood of adherence to health recommendations?

3. To what extent do "fear appeals" influence motivation to practice positive health behaviors?

4. What has research revealed about the use of fear appeals in health education since this article appeared in 1939?

10

Health Education for Outpatients

Workers in hospital outpatient clinics have an unusual opportunity for health education. People who come to the clinic do so because they have a health problem. It is of real concern to them. And the clinic is where they expect to get help. What takes place in the clinic can be more meaningful educationally than academic discussions or lectures about healthful practices at times when people are not actively concerned about their health.

There is an analogy between health education and medicine. Medicine is the art of applying the basic biological sciences for the benefit of the physical health of the individual. Health education is the art of applying an equally basic body of knowledge about the ways in which people acquire information, develop attitudes, and change their behavior about health. Health education requires diagnosis of the particular situation before methods are chosen, just as medicine requires diagnosis before treatment is prescribed. However, there is a tendency for some to choose an educational method that has proved successful in a particular situation for which it was designed, on the assumption that it is generally effective in all situations. This same tendency is sometimes observed in medicine. A dietitian tells this story:

Coauthored by Mayhew Derryberry and Mary Lou Skinner. Originally published in *Public Health Reports*, November 1954, 69(11), 1107–1114. Reprinted with permission.

One of the older physicians on the staff had ordered an extremely high-fat diet for a diabetic patient. A week or so later, diet orders with a very high fat content came down to the diet kitchen for two other diabetic patients. Thinking there must be some good reason for this deviation from the hospital's usual practice, the dietitian went up to the ward to inquire. The new intern said in surprise, "Oh, are those diets unusual? Why, I just ordered what old Dr. Brown had prescribed for the last diabetic patient he had here." As it turned out, Dr. Brown had put his patient on a ketogenic diet during the hospitalization period for a special reason. In routinely following the other physician's prescription, the intern had unknowingly prescribed diets that were not appropriate for his patient's needs. Such a procedure would, of course, be condemned by the experienced physician who thinks about the whole when a patient complains about a single symptom. In good education, too, the whole range of educational principles must be examined in order to select the best methods for a particular purpose.

How People Learn

It may be beneficial to take a look at some of the basic knowledge about how people learn before exploring ways of educating patients in clinics. Part of it will be familiar—some ideas have been recently documented by research, others are "educated hunches"—but application of the following five points is well worth all the emphasis that can be given.

First, all learning is motivated within the person, not by exterior force. Education in the real sense begins only with a problem of immediate interest to a person. The patient in the clinic has some problem of present concern to him, or he wouldn't be there. Thus, a condition favorable to learning already exists in the patient.

Is maximum use made of this opportunity? Beyond that immediate interest, people are truly motivated to do only those things that they think help achieve something they want or help cope with their own special personal problems. These goals may not be clear to the individual or to the person working with him. As a matter of fact, they are likely to be unrecognized by either. Nevertheless, they are the determining factors in what is learned in a given situation. Learning takes place more effectively when the experience has meaning for the learner and he is able to see the full implications of the experience.

Second, learning is an active process. It occurs only through the person's own efforts. So long as he is passive toward a situation, he will learn little. Yet, how often are people told what to do, lectured about tuberculosis or cancer, handed leaflets about health subjects? How often does the patient's "Yes, Doctor," or "Yes, Miss," response to the information given him delude the clinician into thinking the patient is learning? Sometimes there has been real interchange of ideas, but at other times the patient's assent is simply to free himself from an undesirable situation or to prevent exposing his lack of understanding.

Third, a person selects what he sees, hears, or feels largely because of both his past and present interests or motivations, and this selection determines what he learns. Furthermore, what is learned and how it is learned differ from one person to another because each comes into a given situation with a unique background of experience and point of view. For example, three people walk down the street past a poster announcing a chest X-ray schedule. The man who wants an X-ray will see the poster and go to the clinic. The man who thinks he has no need for an X-ray may not see the poster at all. The third person may see the poster all right but will avoid the clinic because of negative feelings about all clinics, because he is afraid of negative feelings about tuberculosis, because he has had a recent X-ray, or for other reasons. The response to a simple poster arises out of complex feelings. Consider then, the tangled skein of past experiences. These enhance or hinder his ability to utilize the educational opportunities in the clinic.

Fourth, behavior is seldom changed because a person has been told to do something different. He will change his behavior in a prescribed manner only when he understands what to do and when he sees the action as leading to the satisfaction of a felt need. He must want to learn the new action. He must also know clearly what action he is to take. Finally, he must see that the action will help him achieve a goal that is important to him. This characteristic of the learning process is particularly important in the clinic. How often information is given in medical terms that mean nothing to the patient! Besides that, the patient may not readily understand that the behavior advocated by the nurse or physician is related to the solution of his own health problem. He may then remain unconvinced that the procedure will cure his ailment. It is important for the clinic staff to remember that the patient is not likely to carry out any suggested action to meet his health need which to him appears to be in conflict with his way of life. The fact that the advice is acceptable to the person giving it often blinds that person to the ways in which the information may conflict with some deeply held value of the patient. This failure to consider the personal element sometimes defeats the clinician's goal.

Fifth, the attitudes of the groups to which the patient belongs are a significant force. Most people tend to conform to the accepted standards and sanctions of family and friends. These may determine whether information is accepted or rejected and whether the person takes any action. It is often difficult to recognize many of these group influences because they may be unrealized by the patient himself. The factors that appear on the top layer often camouflage the real values held tenaciously underneath. One expression of the way group pressures operate is through the cultural patterns of the people. These patterns are not readily discernible, and the assistance of educators and social scientists will be needed to discover the cultural medium in which a patient lives if it is to be used with insight in his education.

Current experiments with new research methods are providing additional perceptions about cultural reactions and their relation to learning. Although the full meaning of these studies is not quickly understood, and the facts are apt to be forgotten since they do not agree with prevailing concepts, it is desirable to look at some of the recent developments in the field because their significance has often been overlooked.

Stratified Attitudes

Studies on class stratification in the United States show a society made up of fairly well defined classes.[1] These studies agree, too, that: (1) each class has different values in which it believes and which it preserves, and each has different attitudes toward education; (2) each class tends to reject people who are in another class; and (3) members of each class have different ways of managing their own lives.

The class system of this country is not like that of the European countries. It is distinctly our own. Most professional people in medicine and the allied fields are drawn from the middle and upper-middle classes. Most middle-class people think that what they believe is the common belief of all right-minded, intelligent people. This attitude trips up many educational efforts. It results in annoyance and leads to the comment that people are uncooperative, stupid, hostile.

Not everyone in the United States regards infant health, life, or death the way this middle class does. Nor will everyone learn easily to change behaviors regarding health and medical care unless these changes are behaviors valued by the group to which he belongs. People who are in one social class do not accept easily the teaching given them by a person from a higher social class. More respect must be accorded the varying resistances of the different cultures in our society.

Most of our observations of the expressions of cultural values are empirical and tinged with unconscious prejudgments. Only a few studies that get at this kind of fact have been done in the health field. One that deserves thought was done recently at the Veterans Administration Hospital (West Kingsbridge Road) in New York City.[2] This study attempted to pin down the effect of cultural differences in patients' responses to pain. Among the groups selected for intensive study, the Italians and Jews were described as tending to "exaggerate" their pain. Free expression of words, sounds, and gestures is expected, accepted, and approved in both Jewish and Italian cultures. A patient from an Italian culture is more apt to be concerned with the present. If his pain is eased, he will relax and forget his sufferings and manifest a happy and joyful disposition. The Jewish patient, however, is often reluctant to accept the analgesic drug. He explains this in terms of concern about the effects of the drug on his health. He is apprehensive about the habit-forming aspects. After being relieved from pain, many Jewish patients continued to display depressed and worried behavior. The conclusions of this phase of the study were:

1. Similar reactions to pain manifested by members of different ethnocultural groups do not necessarily reflect similar attitudes to pain;

2. Reactive patterns similar in terms of their manifestations may have different functions and serve different purposes in various cultures.

From this, there would seem to be practical implications for education. First, there is not a public of patients but many groups within the total patient clientele. Also, there is no quick way to bring about changes in behavior within these different groups.

Many of the symptoms that bring people to clinics are life crises—social and emotional as well as physical. A mother concerned about a new baby, a breadwinner recovering from a heart attack, a family adjusting to the diagnosis of cancer in a member—these are real-life situations. At such times, barriers to learning are lowered. However, life crises produce many anxieties, and the patient may raise barriers to learning if the approach appears to be too great a threat to his goals of personal security.

The fact of having to admit illness, for the most part, threatens the familiar image of the patient's own successful ways of meeting life. Illness calls into play unaccustomed responses. The patient is more apt to worry about the unfamiliar. He has to ask for help, and these feelings about seeking help can be charged with guilt. Staff members may share emotionally charged feelings about seeking help or dealing with illness. Their inner judgments affect the inflection of voice and physical gestures. These become cues to which the patient reacts favorably or unfavorably, raising or lowering his defenses accordingly. In fact, what the patient perceives is just as potent a force in his education as the planned instruction during a lecture or individual conference.

For an educational program to make the most of its opportunities, the clinic staff must seek more knowledge about, and be willing to accept the worth of, patients' values and knowledge. There are two kinds of educational opportunities in a clinic that may be considered against the background of educational principles—the ones you plan for and the ones you don't, or opportunities for indirect and direct educational programs.

Indirect Education Programs

A thoughtful, objective look at what goes on in the clinic will indicate some of the instances and situations in which unplanned education occurs. What does the patient see? What is he made to feel?

What the patient learns depends on the clinic atmosphere—its climate. An inquiry into its physical makeup is a good starting point. For example: to what extent has the staff impersonalized the hospital-clinic routine? Must the patient sit in brown and dingy corridors? Does someone explain to him what he is to expect and why; and is he prepared to spend the time required? Is the unit aware of what the wait means to the patient; and is the patient uncertain while he waits?

Uncertainty creates fear, and fear is apt to produce anger, which, though it may be expressed in many ways, often appears as resentment or apathy. When there is vagueness about the details of therapy, it is perfectly normal for the patient to imagine the worst. He will cooperate more readily when he knows about routine matters.

A public health nurse tells about the time she was suddenly taken ill while on her vacation. The hospital physician she called urged her to come to the outpatient clinic. There she had to wait a long time, feeling more and more miserable. Finally, she was vaguely aware of a stiffly starched nurse advancing toward her and carrying a hypodermic needle. The strange nurse told her to get up on the table in the cubicle "over there." It was only because of her hospital training that the public health nurse questioned this command. As it turned out, the physician had had an emergency call. He had been sure from the patient's description of her symptoms that penicillin was indicated and had left an order for it to be given.

In this instance, it was particularly fortunate the patient spoke up—she knew she was sensitive to penicillin. But what might some other patient, not a nurse, have learned about medical practice from such a vague experience, so unrelated to his own understanding of cause and effect and expectations of medical service? And what kinds of feelings would such a patient transfer to the next situation? Simple thoughtfulness will reassure a patient, make him less demanding and more ready to hear the advice of the staff. It will make a positive health education experience the more likely.

The Physician's Role

The medical director can set the stage in which real education occurs, or he can defeat the opportunity for education. Among other studies bearing this out, the Denver study of tuberculosis hospitals[3] shows that the organization of a hospital often does not encourage sufficiently free exchange of information between various professional services. When the barriers are down, so that there is a pooling of information concerning patients, all benefit. It is the medical director who creates the climate in which this can happen.

The position that the physician holds in the patient's regard is the rock upon which treatment succeeds or fails. If the patient is given the feeling that the physician is interested in him personally, he is able to utilize other aspects of the medical care much more adequately. This was seen in Boston in the diabetes education program sponsored by the Diabetes Field Research and Training Unit of the Public Health Service. How the physician referred the patients to the group classes made a difference in the patients' willingness to come to the classes and to accept the information given by the nurse and nutritionist throughout the eight-week session.

The staff's perception of how it feels to be a patient will be increased by each member's participation in situations that parallel those experienced by the patient. There is a growing trend to plan situations for the staff in terms of the conditions in which patients find themselves so that they can better understand how it feels to be a patient. Many a hospital routine has been changed by wise physicians or nurses after they themselves have been real-life patients. It is not possible to, nor would one wish that every person could, have the experience of being a patient. Accumulated knowledge, however, attests the contribution to patient care and education of contrived experiences that develop insight. At Boston Psychopathic Hospital, staff members are offered an opportunity to take a drug which can create in well people for approximately 24 hours the feelings that a schizophrenic patient experiences. This sensitizing experience is not possible or necessary for all of the hospital staff. But it illustrates the idea of devices by which one may become more sensitive to a patient's feelings.

Staff members have also tried role-playing of "how it feels to be a patient" and are enthusiastic about the usefulness of this technique. There was a health department, too, that changed its entire procedure for handling telephone reports of communicable disease after the role-playing of "what happened on a call about a suspected diphtheria case." Another technique might be to have young medical students get the "feel" of clinic processes by going through a clinic identified only as patients.

The Patient's Response

It saves time and makes for effective education to know the patient's opinion. After all, the patient acts on his own opinion whether it is correct or not. A simple, well-planned interview with the patient usually will obtain the necessary information. When patient opinion is known, it is possible to plan an educational program that will hit the target more accurately.

Most patients realize that they are not competent to judge medical care, but they become impatient when their wishes and ideas are ignored. Their progress toward recovery and in education can be delayed by rules and procedures they do not understand and by indifferent personnel. Positive education is not apt to occur in a discontented person. Many people lose their dissatisfaction when they realize that the clinic is sufficiently interested in them to find out what their opinion is. One study of patient opinion found that most dissatisfied patients complained about not having the hospital schedule explained.[4] Is this worth exploring in outpatient clinics? The interviewers in this same poll were startled by one complaint that may have significance for outpatient clinics. Patients who were generally well satisfied did not feel that they had received enough information about how to care for themselves at home. The poll-takers concluded that "it was evidence of the failure of nurses and doctors to seize opportunities for health teaching, as well as showing a lack of interest in the patient as a person who will continue to exist and have health problems related to his illness even after he leaves the hospital. It could show, too, a lack of integrated planning with allied health agencies for follow-up care."

Direct Education Programs

The "diagnostic" process[5] of telling people things is not the most successful or satisfying way of working educationally with them—it is often dangerous, and its effect cannot be foreseen. It would seem preferable to adopt the "therapeutic" process of helping people to recognize things for themselves. However, since many shared attitudes are derived from the teacher-pupil experience of academic life, the attitude that one educates people by doing things to them is carried over into, and dominates, the educational relationships to patients. The difference in the diagnostic and therapeutic processes is between doing things "to" or "for" people and doing things "with" them. These ways of thinking affect the indirect and direct education that is done.

Printed literature, exhibits, and information racks are useful tools in an educational program, but the extent of their effectiveness depends on thoughtful planning for their use. The Veterans Administration Hospital in Rutland Heights, Massachusetts, used to give packets of pamphlets on tuberculosis to every new tuberculosis patient admitted. They lay untouched on the bedstands. However, when racks were put in the wards where the men could make their own selections, pamphlets began to disappear, in considerable variety and number.

Another and even more significant use of health literature is that reported by Schwartz.[6] The Cornell University Medical Center Outpatient Department in New York City started using pamphlet racks with a wide range of subject matter. Some of the staff were cynical.

Why child guidance leaflets in an adult clinic? they asked. Who on those benches requires prenatal care? A glance would show that the average age is 60. But patients waiting on outpatient benches, like people everywhere, have families. They did not discard family problems or interests at the clinic door, and the pamphlets disappeared.

The educator was still not satisfied, and another approach was tried. This time only one copy of each leaflet was made accessible.

It was clearly marked "Please do not remove this booklet from the clinic. If you think a copy will help you, talk with the nurse about obtaining one." These pamphlets were mixed with copies of the *Saturday Evening Post* and other magazines. To the surprise of the clinic staff, there were 136 requests for the leaflets in the first four weeks. Pamphlets in hand, the patients came and asked for information. The conferences that followed brought to light all manner of problems not directly related to the patient's reason for coming to the clinic. Transfer to physicians of information important to the treatment of the individual patients was a valuable result.

Advising and planning with patients and their families on what to expect in connection with medical therapy can produce favorable educational results. The study on hospitalization of children for tonsillectomies[7] conducted by the Albany (New York) Medical College Department of Pediatrics is an example of such anticipatory planning. Among other things, this study showed that young children resented a jab with a hypodermic needle. The child was told that the only jab he had to take was the finger prick for a hemoglobin reading. The staff found that if young Philip knew in advance that his finger would receive a slight prick, such as he gets dozens of times playing, followed by the appearance of a round bead of his own beautiful red blood, he was likely to watch without anxiety while the bead of blood rose in a little glass tube, just as he had been told it would. Mother might stand by trying to keep from shuddering, but Philip was fascinated. This is health education of real significance.

Any number of people, given the opportunity, will welcome the chance to help with the clinic's education program. It is not at all necessary for the clinic to do it alone. If mimeographed maps or guides to the clinic routine are needed, volunteers can solve the problem. If the staff is too busy to take time to talk with foreign-born folks who struggle with English, the local adult education center may be able to supply volunteers from its foreign classes.

If time will permit in-service education of staff, a plan used in Boston may be the solution. There, 9 hospitals and 11 official and voluntary agencies set up a committee on outpatient education to plan ways for improving educational practices. Educators are members and suggest improvements for the staffs to try. Other services for which the hospital clinics do not have time to recruit independently are provided in other ways.

Volunteers provided the Lubbock Memorial Hospital in Lubbock, Texas, with pamphlet racks and kept them filled; they also provided transportation for the indigent. While doing this, they learned about another need and have helped the hospital develop an African American prenatal clinic. Now they are working on community understanding of welfare problems that affect the hospital. Thus a double educational goal is being served. Not only are the patients in the hospital learning, but the volunteers have discovered many opportunities for effective action.

Group activities are one of the more significant methods that can be used by clinics to provide learning opportunities. This method is being tried in a wide variety of situations. Group discussions with parents in child health conferences at the Lillian Wald Health Station in New York City,[8] group discussion with parents and families of premature babies and of children with rheumatic fever at Gracie–New Haven Community Hospital, New Haven, Connecticut,[9] the group work with diabetic patients carried on in Boston by the City Hospital and the Diabetes Field Research and Training Unit of the Public Health Service, and the group work with obese patients at Herrick Hospital in Berkeley, California, indicate some of the experiments. Group work with patients who have had coronary attacks has been proposed. Alcoholics Anonymous is working closely with some hospital clinics in group discussions with alcoholic patients. Group methods of education can be used to help

parents of handicapped children learn how to work more successfully with their own children.[10]

"Group activities" in this context does not mean classes in the
traditional lecture form; it means, instead, ways of bringing people
together to create situations in which they feel free to discuss their
own reactions about the problems in question. They learn from
each other and give support to each other. The classic study[11] with
mothers of young infants on feeding orange and cod liver oil, done
at the University of Iowa Hospital, brought out clearly the advantage of decision-discussion methods. In such group discussions,
incorrect ideas are likely to be rejected by the group; people are
strengthened by group attitudes of their peers and supported in
changing or in tentative new convictions.

Leadership for this kind of group discussion is a skill. Only
recently has it been taught in school. Moreover, new studies in
group discussion methods are going on all the time. The clinic staff
that is interested in exploring this method would be well advised to
consult with local resources for help in adapting these skills to their
special needs.

Another Challenge

Not many in public health or hospital administration are specialists in education methods or have the skills of social scientists. As
in the medical field where general practitioners sometimes fail to
recognize a symptom that a specialist would spot at once, so in the
education field it is easy to miss significant opportunities for education. Social scientists can be called on for help on problems in these
fields. More and more hospitals are asking educators or sociologists
to observe their practices and to suggest more effective ways of
working. The demand is growing for consultation and service from
anthropologists, health educators, and adult educators.

These different professional groups will not provide a common
body of accumulated knowledge with ready-made answers. The

professions are advancing together into new, experimental, and more profound ways of working with people. Although these newer methods are not so well formed or definitive as the older academic ways of teaching, they can, when wisely used, offer greater satisfaction. Imaginative people in a clinic, who take their responsibilities thoughtfully, will be challenged to find out from day to day what the patients are learning and to enhance that knowledge positively.

It is important for everyone to become more familiar with the nature of the cultures and the ways of life of others: their goals in life and their values, beliefs, traditions, customs, and taboos with respect to health and illness. More must be known about the objectives for which people are to strive, and, conversely, more must be understood about the aspects of life that mean very little to them. These understandings are not easy to acquire. Since understanding is limited or not always possible, perhaps respect for differences is an attitude to nurture.

The only people who are really going to do anything for the patient are the persons who work with him. Not everyone is equally ready to learn about health at all times. But there are times in a lifetime when an individual is ready. One such time is when he comes to the outpatient clinic for service.

Discussion Questions

1. What is the role of individual values and attitudes in health education programs as described in this chapter section?

2. What does the term *indirect education program* denote?

3. According to the text, what is the role of culture, belief, and customs in learning and teaching about health?

4. How is what Derryberry has to say about motivation and how people learn consistent or different from what Bandura has to say in social learning theory?

Notes

1. D. B. Nyswander, "The Implications of New Educational Concepts for the Prevention of Prematurity," *California's Health, 10,* 1–7, July 15, 1952.

2. M. Zborowski, "Cultural Components in Responses to Pain," *Journal of Social Issues,* 8(4), 16–31, 1952.

3. National Tuberculosis Association, *Report of the Denver Hospital Study,* New York, 1952, 30 pages.

4. M. Randall, "Polling Patient Opinion," *University of Minnesota Hospital Staff Meeting Bulletin, 19,* 9, December 5, 1947.

5. A.T.M. Wilson, "Implications of Medical Practice and Social Case Work for Action Research," *Journal of Social Issues, 3,* 11–28, Spring 1947.

6. D. Schwartz, "Health Promotional Literature for Clinic Patients: An Experiment by the Nursing Service of the New York Hospital, Cornell Medical Center Outpatient Department," *American Journal of Public Health, 43,* 1318–1323, 1953.

7. R. Winkley, "When a Child Must Go to the Hospital," *Child, 17,* 34–36, November 1952.

8. S. M. Wishik, "Parents' Group Discussions in a Child Health Conference," *American Journal of Public Health, 43,* 888–895, 1953.

9. A. Kirchner, "Parents' Classes in a Maternity Program," *American Journal of Public Health, 43,* 896–899, 1953.

10. S. Milliken, "Group Discussion of Parents of Handicapped Children from the Health Education Standpoint," *American Journal of Public Health, 43,* 900–903, 1953.

11. M. Radke and D. Misurich, "Experiments in Changing Food Habits," *Journal of the American Dietetic Association, 23,* 403–409, 1947.

11

Today's Health Problems
and Health Education

The health problems of greatest significance today are the chronic diseases and accidents—in the home, at work, and on the highway. Large-scale epidemics, their investigation, and their control no longer demand the major attention of public health workers.

The extent of chronic diseases, various disabling conditions, and the economic burden that they impose have been thoroughly documented by the Committee on Interstate and Foreign Commerce of the United States House of Representatives.[1] Health education and health educators will be expected to contribute to the reduction of the negative impact of such major health problems as heart disease, cancer, dental disease, mental illness and other neurological disturbances, obesity, accidents, and the adjustments necessary to a productive old age.

The new and unique role of health education in helping to meet these problems can perhaps be clarified through a review of some of the differences between procedures that have been successful in solving the problems of the acute communicable diseases and those that are available for coping with today's problems.

Originally published in *Public Health Reports*, December 1954, 69(12), 1224–1228. Reprinted with permission.

Disease Prevention

The tools for dealing with the health conditions of today are not as specific and precise as those that have been available for the contagious diseases. The medical and sanitary sciences have provided public health workers with specific measures for prevention of these diseases—vaccination, immunization, safe water and milk supplies, sanitary sewage disposal, and insect vector control. When properly utilized, these measures have protected people from the several communicable diseases. But even in situations in which individuals do not avail themselves of these protective measures and contract a given disease, there are antibiotics and other chemotherapy agents that are specific and effective. No such specifics exist for preventing the chronic diseases, the degenerative conditions of old age, or accidents.

Medical science has, however, made possible the prevention of the more serious consequences of many of the chronic diseases. Seegal and his co-workers[2] listed 16 chronic diseases that medicine can now control by early diagnosis and treatment and 35 chronic conditions that are subject to partial control. No specific preventive is available for accidents or obesity other than changes in behavioral patterns.

Closely related to the lack of specific and precise methods of dealing with the chronic diseases is the difference in the manner in which these diseases occur. The onset of the chronic conditions is much more insidious than was the onset of the acute conditions, such as the contagious diseases, from which the patient became seriously ill in a very short time and either recovered quickly or died. Therefore, the motivation to act with reference to the slowly developing problems of chronic disease is not nearly so great as was the motivation to act in preventing the contagious diseases.

Because the onset of a chronic condition is gradual, education regarding the accompanying physical changes is difficult. Early detection of the disease means that the individual must either take routine examinations or tests when he feels perfectly well, or else he must become skilled in detecting in himself slight deviations in functioning and seek attention before the disease or condition has progressed too far.

Obstacles to Health Education

For many reasons, the task of health education, which is normally difficult enough, is made much more difficult by the lack of specific procedures for preventing today's ills, as well as by the absence of completely effective curative measures. Because control procedures are vague, the actions that health educators try to teach individuals to take to prevent or to cure disease are less well defined than were the actions necessary to control the contagious diseases. The relationship between the desirable actions and the effective control of chronic disease is, by the same token, much less obvious to the public eye.

There are additional difficulties in stimulating appropriate individual action to prevent or control the chronic diseases. A single action, such as being vaccinated or immunized, protects a person for a period of time—often for a long period of time—whereas the actions that must be taken to prevent further disability from a chronic disease often require a complete change in the pattern of one's daily living. Changing one's diet and changing the kinds and amounts of physical and mental activity permitted require radical readjustment in an individual's life. Because it is not possible to define adequately the actions persons should take, because these actions do not seem to relate directly to prevention of a condition, and because these actions may require radical changes in life, it is extremely difficult to effect desirable changes in behavior.

Present-day health problems differ from those with which public health traditionally has been concerned in the amount of individual understanding necessary to prevent and cure the diseases or to avoid accidents. Avoiding disability and death from these causes depends a great deal more on individual understanding and action than did the prevention of the infectious diseases.

Not every person needs to know about or take specific preventive action to be protected from a communicable disease. For example, if a community, through the action of a few of its citizens and its government, installs a safe water supply and sanitary sewage disposal, all members of the community will benefit. The immunization of even a few children in a community affords some protection to the others, for each immune child in a population reduces the chance of transmission of the disease. Godfrey[3] in his epidemiologic study of diphtheria, reported that "in only two instances known to the writer has a community that had attained 30 percent immunization of its under-five age group suffered even a moderate epidemic."

Such community protection is not possible with the chronic diseases or accidents. Each individual is responsible for taking whatever action is necessary if he is to benefit from the various measures that medical science has provided for preventing or controlling today's diseases. Furthermore, not only must the individual take the action, but he must do it at an early stage of the disease, at a time when the findings of medical science will still benefit him. So far as accidents are concerned, however, even though he tries to avoid hazards and to take all prescribed precautions, he is not always safe unless other people also know what to do and then do it.

The Health Educator's Job

The differences between the methods for prevention of acute and of chronic diseases greatly increase the scope and difficulty of the health educator's job. Each person must be reached with the educational message in a way that will ensure his response, or else the efforts of health workers accomplish nothing. It is not enough to produce positive results with a few persons or even with the majority. Even approximating the achievement of such an all-inclusive goal will challenge every resource and all the imagination health educators can muster.

The problems of greatest community health significance today affect adults and older persons much more than did the contagious diseases. To be sure, many children suffer from rheumatic fever, diabetes, and some of the other chronic conditions, but the majority of the persons affected by chronic diseases are adults. As a rule, it is much easier to convince parents to take action for the health of their children than it is to convince them to do anything about their own health. Furthermore, the fact that health education for today's problems must be an attempt to effect change in the behavior of older adults adds to the complexity of the task ahead.

Integration of Services

Coping with today's problems effectively requires much more integration of health and related services than was necessary in making the progress of the past half-century, when control of the communicable diseases was primarily a medical problem and when the entire responsibility was often assigned to the public health department. In the more successful health programs, the cooperation of the private physician was enlisted and the educational resources of the community were employed, but public health authorities have usually retained sole responsibility for preventing the spread of disease.

On the other hand, controlling the chronic diseases and solving the problems they bring to a family require the integrated efforts of many groups. All the medical resources of the community must be tapped—its health department, private physicians, and hospitals—as well as the facilities and services of many other social and welfare agencies if individuals with chronic disease are to be brought back to their maximum treatment, but the social, economic, and emotional factors arising out of a longtime illness must be considered. Home care, rehabilitation, retraining, and opportunity for employment of the handicapped are among the services needed. These are provided by a variety of agencies, all of which have shared responsibilities and must work together if they are to reduce the chronic disease problem. To accomplish the integration of these services in the control of the chronic diseases requires that workers in the various agencies become more efficient in collaborative thinking and in carrying out a cooperative program.

Integration of health and welfare services poses two distinct but equally difficult educational problems. The first of these concerns interagency planning and program operation. How can the working policies and practices of agencies that historically have functioned almost independently be modified to coordinate with other agencies for maximum service without duplication or conflict? Solving this problem means education of not only the executives and workers of the agencies but also of members of their boards. Furthermore, the emphasis today on clear-cut lines of administration and responsibility, the difficulties involved in joint planning, and the disapproval of joint program operation by specialists in administration make this problem even more difficult. Nevertheless, all who are interested in attacking successfully today's problems must contribute toward finding more effective ways of integrating the necessary skills and services. The second educational problem that this complex of agency services poses is the likelihood that conflicting advice will be given to the public from the several agencies, and the increased possibility that an individual may become dissatisfied with one or more of the groups with which he must deal. Such experiences make the task of stimulating continued positive health action on the part of the individual extremely difficult. To the extent that the individual imparts his feelings of dissatisfaction to his associates, they will be resistant to taking the desirable action suggested by the health educator.

In this connection, educators have a special responsibility to sensitize the personnel of health and welfare agencies to the educational effects of the service experience of an individual and particularly to the potent influence of an unpleasant or unsatisfactory experience.

Health Education Content Today

The preceding discussion of educational difficulties in coping with today's health problems emphasizes the challenge with which health educators are faced. Let us look at a few implications of this challenge for educational content and method, and for the appropriate places to concentrate our effort.

If the challenge is to be met, most of the educational efforts must be concentrated upon adults outside the classroom where the problems may arise. It will not suffice to give students in grade school or even in college a body of the latest scientific information and expect them to use the information when they reach the age when chronic diseases are most prevalent. Such an expectation overlooks an important research finding in psychology—we forget rapidly information that is not functional in our daily lives.

But even if people did remember everything they learned in grade school or college, would the latest scientific information of today serve as guides to the behavior of students when they become older? Certainly everyone would hope not, for with the dynamic nature of medical research today, there is every indication that many of the tools for dealing with the diseases of today will become much more precise. If the limited information now available were remembered and used by students in later life, it might serve as a deterrent to the real action the students should take. To illustrate this point, here is an exact quotation from one of the textbooks of about 40 years ago: "A life out of doors all day long, summer and winter, has cured many cases [tuberculosis]. It is now considered the only cure for the disease."[4] Certainly no one would want people to act in terms of that information today.

What, then, should be the educational focus? Rather than concentrating on imparting an organized series of health facts, should the major emphasis not be on developing among students skill in solving health problems when they occur? In every school or college, some health situation is constantly arising in which individuals or groups must take action for their health. All too often, instructors decide upon the action to be taken without giving students the opportunity to gather information regarding the problem, to evaluate it, to develop their own solution, and to put these solutions into operation.

If, however, students have the experience of making the decisions, they will learn how to assemble pertinent facts from a variety of sources—a far more important achievement than that of having acquired an extensive body of knowledge about health. They will also have an opportunity to develop the ability to discriminate between reliable and unreliable information. This latter skill is particularly important at this time, for with the rapid advance of scientific discovery, it is often not easy to distinguish research achievement from the exorbitant claims of quacks or the overzealous desire for publicity on the part of a pseudoinvestigator.

One other aspect of the educational content of today's health problems that should be considered is that the action which must be taken to deal with the present problems frequently conflicts with some of our traditional value systems. We have been a pioneering people, more concerned with advancing our economic welfare and that of the country than with the health and other hazards encountered in the pioneering effort. As a result, we tend to look with a certain amount of disdain upon the person who is concerned with avoiding danger, or who exercises reasonable caution in avoiding crippling injuries or disabling disease. Could it be that this value system accounts in part for lack of concern about the rules of health, dangerous conditions around the home, or for the tendency to take unnecessary risks in order to get somewhere in under-record time? Now that we are no longer pioneers in the sense that we do not need to take undue physical risks in order to progress, should we not consider a change in implied approval, if not outright praise, that our culture places on those who disregard the rules for health and safety? If society frowned upon taking unreasonable and unnecessary chances, it might be a real stimulus to positive action for controlling the ravages of chronic diseases and accidents.

Aging presents another type of cultural problem. To provide financial security for individuals as they grow old, fairly rigid retirement systems have been developed. When these systems were being established, they were considered a real social advance in that an individual's support was assured as he reached old age. Coupled with these insurance systems there gradually disappeared the long-cherished cultural pattern of families looking after their older members and fitting them into the family structure. Consequently, there has arisen a tendency to set older people aside as they retire. They are left without activity and usefulness—literally placed on the shelf. We are now coming to realize that much of what is popularly called senility is really confusion, moodiness, forgetfulness, depression, and irritability brought on by social isolation and lack of mental stimulation—with little or no organic deterioration. A Norristown, Pennsylvania, physician[5] has been successfully treating patients with seeming senility through individual and group psychotherapy, creative crafts, and recreation, because he is convinced that mental decline can be postponed.

It would seem, then, that our educational task in retarding the physiological and mental deterioration of older persons is to help reorient our cultural patterns with respect to them before and after retirement and to provide these senior members of our society with educational opportunities for developing some of their latent talents or realizing some of their avocational desires.

Summary

Almost unbelievable progress in reducing death from the communicable diseases has been made in our lifetime. Health education has had some small part in helping to bring about this achievement.

Today, we are faced with a host of health problems that require individual action if people are to benefit from the findings of scientific investigators. Bringing about that action requires education. The task is made unusually difficult because of the insidious nature of the chronic diseases, the lack of any action individuals may take, the age-group that must be influenced, the large number of agencies that are involved, and the need for modification of some of our cultural patterns and value systems. This is the challenge to the profession of health education.

Discussion Questions

1. What were the health problems of most significance during the 1950s?

2. How do these problems compare to today's health problems?

3. What changes in the environment might make changes in health behavior easier to initiate and maintain?

4. What were some problems noted in chronic versus acute health problems and their prevention as discussed in this chapter?

5. What approaches have been used today to prevent accidents or injury, apart from changing individual behavior?

Notes

1. U.S. Congress, House of Representatives, Committee on Interstate and Foreign Commerce, *Health Inquiry on the Toll of Our Major Diseases—Their Prevention and Control*, Preliminary Report No. 1338, 83rd Congress (Washington, D.C.: U.S. Government Printing Office, 1954).

2. D. Seegal, H. Cocher, K. B. Duane, Jr., and A. D. Wertheim, "Progress in the Control of Chronic Illness," *Hygeia*, *27*, 48–50, 52, 1949.

3. E. S. Godfrey, "Study in the Epidemiology of Diphtheria in Relation to the Active Immunization of Certain Age Groups," *American Journal of Public Health*, 22, 237–256, 1932.

4. H. W. Conn, *Physiology and Health* (Boston: Silver, Burdett, and Company, 1916), p. 189.

5. M. E. Linden, "The Miracle in Building," *Currents*, January 1954. Reprinted by Pennsylvania Citizens Association, Philadelphia.

12

Health Education in Transition

To be invited to give the first Dorothy B. Nyswander lecture is a single honor and one of which I am deeply appreciative. It is all the more pleasing to me because I count Dr. Nyswander as one of my close friends. I have chosen "Health Education in Transition" as the subject for this lecture, partly because so much change in health education has occurred since Dr. Nyswander first entered public health and partly because of the dynamic changes now in progress.

Many forces are importantly related to the process of health education—the health level of the people, the disease problems causing disability and death, the health resources available, the physical location of the people, the communication media, the economic and cultural resources, the kinds of action people must take to improve their health, and the facts known about behavior and its change. A review of the changes in these elements should help to focus today's health education efforts and may point toward possible future developments.

What were the conditions existing roughly a quarter of a century ago? When Dr. Nyswander began her pioneer work in public

Originally published in the *American Journal of Public Health*, November 1957, 47(11), 1357–1366. Reprinted with permission.

health, how adequate was the information that could be given about the health problems of that time? What were some of the educational and sociological situations that influenced the health education efforts? What was known about learning and behavior change that could be applied to health education tasks?

One-fourth of the deaths were from acute infectious diseases. Diphtheria, scarlet fever, pneumonia, septicemia, whooping cough, infant diarrhea and enteritis, tuberculosis, malaria, dysentery, and syphilis were the diseases that held the forefront of attention. They were the concern of both the professional health worker and the public. Why these diseases demanded so much attention and interest is quite understandable when one considers that in the early twenties, the number of reported annual deaths for most of the more fatal infectious diseases exceeded the number of cases now reported annually. Actually, the average annual deaths from all infectious diseases for the three-year period 1924–1926 was 305,000; whereas for the period 1954–1956 the average was 82,000.[1]

The significance of these figures becomes all the more evident when it is recalled that the population in which they occurred was less than two-thirds of its present size and also that reporting of vital events was much less complete then than it is today.

These were the problems toward which public health and health education were directing attention in the late twenties. To be sure, chronic diseases and other disabling conditions were among us, but by and large, they were looked upon by the people as the natural result of growing old. It was the acute illnesses that aroused the people's concern. When disease struck, usually many members of the community were involved, onset was fairly sudden, and the end result was often tragic.

The widespread interest of people in avoiding the infectious diseases was a real asset to health education. People responded to education about the need for health departments, and many were organized about that time. What is more, the departments were given unusual authority to enforce regulations and carry out sanitary measures to reduce communicable disease hazards. This community action may have somewhat obscured to workers of that day, and even of this, the motivational factors in the situation, as I shall attempt to point out later.

But other elements in the situation at that time were not so favorable for effective education on how to avoid these diseases or reduce their impact, if one was stricken. There was not always clear, specific information that could be given on what to do. To be sure, vaccination against smallpox had been a preventive since 1798 (1800 in this country),[2] but this protective action often was not readily taken because the aftereffects of vaccination were frequently painful and disfiguring. Mass immunization against diphtheria became available in the early twenties, but for most other conditions no specific individual action could be advised, either to prevent the disease or to cure it.[3]

Such information and advice as was given was on general cleanliness—thought of as next to godliness—and rules of hygiene. The exact relation that taking baths and observing such other rules bore to specific disease prevention was not scientifically determined and hence was often impossible to explain to the public.

From the standpoint of education, approximately 6 percent of our population 10 years of age and over were illiterate, and the median number of school years completed was only about eight years.[4] Among groups with such limited educational experience, it was difficult to interpret scientific findings of medicine into meaningful terms for behavior change.

Nearly one-half of the people lived in rural areas, where opportunities for communicating information were infrequent.[5] Health workers had little chance to study the existing health ideas and practices of these rural folk as a basis for planning meaningful education.

Even where there was specific health information to communicate to the people, there was not the extensive mass communication network of today. Radios did not become available commercially until 1926,[6] and, of course, television was mentioned only in science fiction.

The average weekly earnings of all wage earners were under
$27 per week.[7] The extremely low income of many people, which this
average reflects, may not have reduced their concern about health,
but in the struggle for the other necessities of living, they often
could not afford the health action that might have been indicated.

Individuals engaged in health education (there were a very few
pioneering health educators) were not only hampered by a lack of
scientific medical knowledge, by limitations in communication,
and by educational and economic considerations but were just as
seriously hindered by the lack of understanding of how people—
especially adults—learn and change their behavior. Much research
had been done by psychologists, sociologists, and anthropologists,
and was being done at this time, but their findings had not yet been
made available in forms that health workers found usable.

Much of the effort of the psychologists was being devoted to psychologic testing of intelligence and personality traits, together with
statistical manipulations or interrelations, in the search for causal
factors. In general, psychologists were not too interested in practical
problems. Social psychology, as such, had not yet been accepted as
an experimental social science. Group behavior was explained using
such vague concepts as "instinctive social forces," "the mob spirit,"
or "the group mind." The public health worker found little practical advantage in understanding these concepts.

The sociologists' contributions were, primarily, systematic
descriptions of society and the inner workings of the social components of a community. Health workers, in general, felt more at
home with the methodology involved in such descriptions, for it
more nearly approached the type of data collection and treatment
they were accustomed to using in their epidemiologic investigations.

Insofar as anthropology was concerned, it was just beginning to
focus on modern culture. Much of the investigative effort up to this
time had been spent in intensive field work, recording in detail the
customs of the primitive peoples of the earth. In general, social scientists had little to offer public health in the way of practical knowl-

edge, primarily because they were not too interested in communicating what information they had uncovered. At the same time, public health workers were scarcely aware of social science as a rich source of help for their problems. Even had they been aware, the communication problem probably would have been a barrier.

Lacking systematic and scientifically established knowledge about ways of educating the public and of changing their habit patterns, health workers often borrowed methods from fields of endeavor whose goals seemed analogous to those of public health. The methods of the advertiser were borrowed and widely used as health education technics. For example, one health department developed the slogan "Health Is Purchasable" as a means of getting appropriations. If these methods were questioned, they were justified by statements such as: "The businessman uses these advertising procedures to sell his product. If they didn't pay in terms of more sales, you can be sure he wouldn't use them. Why shouldn't we use his methods to sell health?"

In an effort to interest schoolchildren, the health message was sugar-coated. Health songs, poems, dramatizations, fairy stories, and the like were used extensively without any follow-up or measurement of their value.

Such was the situation when our honored guest first accepted a research position in a health agency. Now let us look at some of the developments that have taken place during the period of her service in public health. These are the changes to which she has been constantly adjusting to provide up-to-the-minute leadership in health education.

First, in the medical and health area itself, the clinical and natural science laboratories, together with field experiments, have concentrated on determining the specific cause, as well as the most effective control agent, for each of the major infectious diseases. With such specifics as mass protection through sanitation, immunizing agents, sulfa drugs, penicillin, and other antibiotics, most of the infectious diseases have been brought under control.

Second, means of communication have increased at an almost miraculous rate. It would be difficult to find a household without at least one radio. In August of last year the Bureau of the Census reported that 76 percent of our households had one or more television sets. The circulation of periodicals has almost doubled, and the distribution of newspapers has increased, though at a much slower rate. Thus, there are few people in the United States who are physically cut off from new information that might have value to them in improving their health.

Third, discoveries in the field of atomic energy no longer astound us. We have come to expect them. However, one that may have real significance for health improvement was signalized early this year. A complete luncheon of appetizer, entree, vegetables, salad, and dessert—prepared from food that had been preserved over a considerable period of time by radiation—was served to a large public group in Washington, D.C. The guests were most enthusiastic about the natural flavor of the food. Consider what this can mean for nutrition and nutrition education, not only in this country but all over the world.

Fourth, there are many other material developments in electronics, chemistry, physics, and the like that have contributed to our way of living. They all make possible the realization of some of our goals, so that time and energy are available for other pursuits. They are considerations that will enter into health education planning now and in the future.

Fifth, many economic and sociologic changes have taken place. Practically all of our population can now read. The median years of school completed by persons 14 years and older is more than 10, and a fourth of our total population is in school. We are rapidly reaching the stage where most of the complexities of health problems can be communicated and understood by all of our people who have a desire to know and understand. The total national income of almost $400 billion is the highest in the history of the country. In terms of individual income, the median for urban and rural nonfarm families surpasses $4,000, and farm income, though somewhat below 1952, has improved much in the last quarter-century. This greater purchasing power makes vastly improved and increased health services a possibility. But we must be realistic and recognize that other desires come into play when people consider how to spend their income.

There is one other sociologic change that I would like to mention. Rural living is becoming less and less attractive. Earlier, half of our people lived in rural areas; now the proportion is barely a third and is constantly decreasing. At the same time there is a movement away from cities to the suburbs. The real sociological and educational significance of this trend is only beginning to be investigated. There is some evidence that there is greater community spirit in suburbia than at the center of the city. At the same time there is competition between community loyalty to activities at the place of work and those at the place of living. Here is a problem that health education will need to study both for programs today and in the future.

While not as spectacular as the technological applications of the physical and biological research findings of the past 25 years, nor as apparent as the economic and sociologic changes just mentioned, progress in understanding the "how" and "why" of human behavior has been equally significant. Until World War II the psychologists, sociologists, and anthropologists, each with their own unique methodology, probed human behavior in terms of their own frame of reference. For example, the Freudians focused their investigations on the inner dynamics of the person. Others, like the behaviorists, concentrated their study on variables external to the individual. Still others of the Lewinian school stressed in their investigations such concepts as goals, objects, or activities sought by people. They studied extensively the decision-making process, particularly as it relates to actions a person or group will take voluntarily.

World War II created a new setting for social science study and investigation. It brought together researchers from the various groups or schools of thought, forced them to communicate with one another and to apply their theories and ideas to specific problems concerned with the war effort. Out of the joint work on such problems as recruiting and selecting persons for specific war tasks, selling war bonds, reducing absenteeism, increasing production, and raising morale, a more general kind of orientation in the behavioral sciences emerged. As a result of the practical outcomes from these combined efforts, both government and industry made available large sums of money for theoretical and practical research on human behavioral problems. Yet, with all the advances they have made, no unified theory of human behavior acceptable to all the scientists has been developed that health educators can apply to their work. However, some broad concepts are available for our use.

Behavior is now seen as the function of a great many variables—motivational, perceptual, social, and cultural. How an individual acts and thinks in specific situations seems to depend on inner drives arising from his personal goals and needs, his perception of the situation, and his past experiences, plus the influence of external factors of the situation, including the cultural patterns and social structures in the society to which he belongs. Common goals and experiences of people result in the observed similarities in the behavior of groups, while the individual's own peculiar experiences and motivations produce ways of acting, thinking, perceiving, and believing that are unique to him. This formulation emphasizes the need for health workers to obtain far more specific information about the goal, personality needs, perceptions, and value patterns of individuals as essential data for planning educational programs for health improvement.

It has been shown that people everywhere organize themselves in certain ways that divide them into different cultural, class, or status groups, with a resultant limitation on full communication between groups. What better illustration of this concept and its operation do we need than the cultural and status differentials between doctors and laymen and the problems in communication that result? Improving the communication between such groups, and especially doctors and the public, is a task that will demand much ingenuity on the part of health educators.

In the health work in other countries, as well as among some of the minority groups in this country, the importance of existing cultural patterns and concepts has been shown by social scientists. They have also analyzed the way in which cultural patterns may be brought about or resisted and how these have meaning to our health planning.

A complete catalogue of social science concepts useful to health educators is beyond the scope of this chapter. Enough has been given, however, to suggest that the progress behavioral scientists have made over the years provides a rich storehouse for educators and practitioners in the public health field. In addition to the scientific findings on behavior, there is the development of new methods for uncovering meaningful information about individual and group behavior. Methods of sampling, interviewing, open-ended questioning, projective technics, and other such procedures have been improved and developed. In health education we need to become acquainted with ways of adapting these research tools and making use of them in our day-to-day practical work.

One other encouraging development is the trend toward behavioral research in the content area of public health. The work of Paul, Simmons, Saunders, and Koos, as well as the work of Knutson and his staff in the United States Public Health Service, is merely the beginning of what will be a tremendous expansion of the theoretical and the practical research in this area.

In this rapidly changing social and technologic milieu, what are some of the problems facing health education? The major specific health problems are those of chronic diseases, accidents, alcoholism, and mental illness. As we contemplate the job to be done in connection with these problems, I should like to emphasize some essential differences between them and the problems on which so much progress has been made in the past. For many of the infectious diseases, responsibility for control rested with the health authorities.

The health department, through some measure such as water treatment or enforcement of sanitary regulations, provided protection for all the people, regardless of their own personal actions. Even where prevention depended on the people taking some action, it usually was a single act, such as immunization or vaccination, which was relatively inexpensive and not too inconvenient. Very often the action was taken on behalf of a child and not for the health of the individual who took the action.

But prevention or control of the conditions facing us today demands quite a different set of behavior patterns. Self-initiated action is required of the person whose health is involved. The indicated action may often lead to considerable expense, may be grossly inconvenient, and may require major readjustment of the individual's habit patterns.

For each of the diseases that have been "conquered," science discovered a single direct cause in a bacterium, virus, or other invading organism and provided a specific preventive or control measure. The direct cause-and-effect relationship between actions taken by the people and the results achieved were easy to demonstrate. If children are immunized for diphtheria, pertussis, and tetanus, they do not develop the diseases. Penicillin quickly conquers streptococcal infections, and DDT demonstrably reduces the mosquito population. In such situations, education is relatively easy, for the effects of the advised action are readily apparent to the individual.

Over the years the success of scientists in finding the single cause for each of so many diseases and in developing a specific for either its prevention or control has led the public to expect a continuation of miraculous discoveries of fairly simple, easy-to-use remedies. Witness the rapid acceptance of the polio vaccine when it was released. It is doubtful that any other medical discovery has been accepted by the public with such alacrity. And this has taken place in spite of some of the unfavorable circumstances that arose. This public expectation of a single causation of disease entities and ready acceptance of new discoveries, particularly when they are simple and easy to take, is a real handicap to health education in today's problems.

So far as we know, the chronic diseases and other health problems of today are caused by a multiplicity of physiologic, psychologic, and sociologic factors. It is not likely that a single causative organism or chemical will be found. Neither does it seem likely that a single preventive or control method will become available. Of course, I realize that tomorrow some laboratory may discover a formula for the Fountain of Youth that will outdate this information, but from the evidence now at hand, we are forced to assume that such control as can be accomplished will probably depend on a series or combinations of actions, some, if not all, of which will demand changes in habits of a lifetime. Furthermore, even if the actions for prevention or control are effective, the cause-and-effect relationship is not likely to be so readily apparent to the people. When people expect a single causation for a given disease and a single action to bring about control, it will not be easy to stimulate a series of actions the effect of which cannot be easily demonstrated. May I say, also, that this problem exists no less with the profession than with the public. It is difficult for the professional person also to identify clearly the role of education in dealing with problems that are ambiguous as to cause and complex in their solution.

This widespread expectation that a single disease has a single cause and a simple cure plays directly into the hands of quacks. Recently, Postmaster General Summerfield reported that "sure-cure" medical quackery by mail had "reached the highest level in history." During the past year, "postal inspectors have prepared cases representing an annual loss to the public of fifty million dollars."[8] To develop ways to combat quacks in their exploitation of this advantage is a challenge to us in health education. Many lives could be saved that are lost because of dependence on quacks.

The task of effecting an understanding of multiple causation is made even more difficult by the lack of scientific evidence and resultant lack of medical agreement on the combination of causes, the relative importance of each cause, and the combination of steps that one needs to take to avoid the conditions. Even in diabetes, where the disease process is better understood than in most chronic disorders, there are purists insisting on strict diet or chemical control; the free dieters prescribing symptom control; and the middle-of-the-roaders that combine chemical and symptom control.

In less well defined areas the differences in treatment are even more varied. Imagine the confusion of patients who may get conflicting advice on what to do about their illness from differing house officers or residents, even in the same teaching hospital. Recently, we have had a health educator working in the chronic disease ward of a general hospital. One of her important findings was the diversity of medical opinion on what kind of adjustments—diet, work patterns, drug therapy—the same patient should make. What kinds of learning experiences can the educator create for constructive behavior change when the change needed is not well established? I recounted this dilemma to a leading medical educator. His answer, though scientific, in no way provided a solution for the problem. He said, "Well, the evidence shows that widely divergent methods seem to have approximately the same degree of effectiveness."

Until medical research has proof of causes of our present conditions and effectiveness of combinations of habit patterns in controlling or curing each condition, health education is going to be seriously hampered in making its potential contribution to the reduction of the disabling conditions occurring today. In addition to the difficulties health education faces with respect to the health problems and to the educational work that can be done, there are two other realities in our society that have a bearing on the future of health education. The first concerns the degree to which health operates as a motivating force in determining behavior.

Earlier I indicated that the public's and the health worker's common concern about the acute infectious diseases might have obscured to the public health worker the importance of motivation in the public's behavior. We tended to assume that the interest of the public in health, as a goal in life, was equivalent to ours. We are now beginning to discover that health, per se, is not always the important goal that motivates people's actions. Stouffer, in his study of the concerns of a cross-sectional sampling of Americans, showed that health, either their own or that of someone in the family, was mentioned by only 24 percent of the people.[9] Rosenstock, in his pretest sample for a study on perceived needs of people, found a similar figure. He was able to identify one group that always mentioned health; this comprised the parents of small children. Their concern was not about their own health but about that of their offspring. Here is a health concern that has remained relatively constant over the years.[10]

But the large majority of the population have concerns other than health. Their present physical condition seemingly is no deterrent to the achievement of personal goals, such as professional, economic, social, or political success. Witness the long, strenuous hours put in by our physicians and the resultant high rate of heart disease in that occupational group. Certainly, no health adviser would prescribe the rigors of campaigning to which our politicians subject themselves, nor the all-too-frequent banquets that the successful ones must attend. It may be disconcerting to us as health workers to accept the existence of this low level of concern about health. This is particularly so, since the social scientists have demonstrated that people do not act unless they are motivated or otherwise see their action as satisfying some goal they have.

Another reality that health education must face is that many of the social problems of today require action on a broader front than the present operating definition of health embraces. Problems of the aged, juvenile delinquency, civil rights, slums (city and rural), and unplanned suburbia—all have health aspects, but sometimes health plays a minor role.

Full solution of the problems requires the skills and talents of many professional groups and organizations working together. For example, meeting the problems of the older person demands the skills of individuals who can help on income maintenance, recreation, vocational rehabilitation, education, housing, and health—to mention only the most obvious ones.

These last two facts, namely, that the primary concern of many people is with goals other than health and that the scope of social problems in communities embraces many more facets than health, pose real difficulties for health education in the future. Are we, as health educators, going to manipulate the people or otherwise pressure them into doing something about health and neglect the other aspects of the broad problems confronting them? Are we going to work with them to achieve some aspects of their goal, so that they will reward us by working on the health problems of our concern? Or are we going to help people, individuals and groups, to achieve the constructive goals they have regardless of their relation to health? And if we do concentrate our effort outside the health area, how is our health administrator going to perceive us, even though our efforts may contribute ultimately to long-term health improvement? These questions pose a real dilemma for us in health education.

Surely, there are a number of ways in which the problem can be met. One possible direction might be the broadening of the health educator's role so that he might be able to help individuals and communities cope with the problems of their concern. In such a role he would do the same things that good health educators do, except that the content area in which he works would not be limited to health. Specifically, the task would be to assist people to obtain the best technical resources available and also help them to comprehend the "pros" and "cons" of the alternative actions they might take. Once they reach a decision he would help them in planning the step-by-step action they need to take in order to reach their goal. To be effective, he would need to know the sources of technical competence on a wide range of problems but not necessarily be the source of information himself.

Actually, what is being suggested is a type of professional community worker who will do for human betterment everywhere what the county agent or extension worker has started to do for the betterment of farmers in selected demonstration areas. The type of work may be signified by some such title as "Extension Worker for Conservation of Human Resources." Of course this title is much too long, but it suggests the breadth of educational responsibility involved. Think of the rapid, practical translation of scientific findings into improved human living if in every community of this country there were available a community worker who was effective in giving such educational service.

Perhaps some of you are thinking, "What would this mean for health education and health educators?" Would it not mean broadened scope of activities, greater freedom to work in all phases of human improvement, and opportunity to utilize to the maximum the findings of the behavioral sciences concerning individual and group behavior change? Ultimately, we might be joining hands with agricultural extension workers, rural development workers, and adult educators, each of whom would likewise broaden his scope and horizons as well as become more qualified in the fields in which he is not now working.

There are many unanswered questions about this concept. To whom should the worker report? How would the community worker keep up on all new developments? Who should pay for such a person? Would health, recreation, housing, rehabilitation, and other social program administrators be willing to permit communities to decide the problem on which they would work if the vested interests of the social agencies were not served?

These are only some of the many valid questions that need to be answered concerning this one proposal. Doubtless there are other suggestions for the kinds of constructive change that health education should be making to fit into the realities of today's society. As a young profession, we should be constantly seeking effective ways to improve human living and make it more satisfying. In so doing we shall need to be constantly alert to the problems of concern to the people and to utilize all that is known about the way people react, think, and work. If the new ways of working encounter administrative and organizational barriers, we should seek satisfactory ways of overcoming them. After all, administration and organization are creatures of our own development. They, too, are subject to change.

In honoring our guest tonight, we have reminded her of the vast changes she has experienced since she first started contributing to public health. To many of these changes she has made tremendous contributions. One last one, unmentioned until now, is the development of a professional corps of health educators. Her students, and the work they are doing, attest to the extensive contribution she has made to this development. As we in health education now look to the future and the possible expansion of the scope of problems on which we can work, I feel certain that we will accept the challenge and pioneer, as Dr. Nyswander has done—always thinking ahead, testing, revising, improving, and contributing to make the lives of all of those with whom we work much more satisfying.

Discussion Questions

1. What does the concept of multiple causation denote and what is the implication for public health education?

2. Given the complexity of chronic diseases, what ideas embedded in this chapter are likely to be useful today?

3. What were Dorothy Nyswander's main contributions to health education?

Notes

1. U.S. Public Health Service, National Office of Vital Statistics, Morbidity Analysis Section, Washington, D.C.

2. Milton J. Rosenau, *Preventive Medicine and Hygiene*, 6th ed. (New York: Appleton-Century, 1935), p. 4.

3. W. H. Park, *Public Health and Hygiene*, 2nd ed. (Philadelphia: Lea and Febiger, 1928), p. 84.

4. U.S. Office of Education, Research and Statistical Services Branch, Washington, D.C.

5. U.S. Department of Commerce, Bureau of the Census, *U.S. Census of Population*, 1950, Vol. 11, Part 1, Washington, D.C.

6. *Electronics Industry Fact Book* (Radio-Electronics Television Manufacturers Association, Marketing Data Department, Washington, D.C., 1957), p. 5.

7. U.S. Executive Office of the President, Council of Economic Advisers, *Economic Indicators* (Department of Labor Data, Washington, D.C.)

8. "Sure-Cure, Quackery Reaches Peak in Mails," *Washington Post*, May 12, 1957.

9. Samuel A. Stouffer, "Report of the American People," *Look*, 19, 25–27, March 22, 1962, and April 5, 1955.

10. Irwin M. Rosenstock, unpublished data.

13

Health Educator

Partner in Health Education

The theme, "Partners in Health," chosen for your annual meeting is certainly appropriate and timely. So far as I am able to ascertain, all the major health problems facing us today require for their solution cooperative effort by different categories of professional workers, and often these come from a number of organizations— private, voluntary, or official. To achieve a smooth working relationship among these many individuals and groups is a task for which few of us have the necessary skills. Hence the more we focus on understanding one another—and on how to work as "partners"—the more effective we can become in our health endeavors. Therefore, I salute you on your program theme. As a health educator, I am delighted to be listed as a partner with the doctor, nurse, social worker, engineer, sanitarian, nutritionist, and other workers. For all of us have an important part in health education. My purpose will be to attempt a clarification of the unique role of the health educator and perhaps suggest a few ways he works with his partners.

As a first step in clarification, let us make sure we are all talking about the same thing when we mention health education. To some

Originally presented at a Joint Session of the Health Officers' Section and the Health Education Section at the annual meeting of the Texas Public Health Association, March 7, 1961, Fort Worth.

health workers, health education means the various methods designed to induce people to guard their health. Looking at it this way, health education means pamphlets, news releases, television and radio shows, movies, and so on. In short, health education comprises these kinds of activities—regardless of the effect on people we are trying to influence.

To others, it means the entire process—the end result of which is the change that takes place in people rather than the actions we health workers take.

When we regard health education as changing or improving people's health practices, it becomes obvious that we are dealing with a complicated phenomenon. In fact, I should like to submit that it is equally, if not more, complicated than improving their physical condition. The steps in effecting health behavior improvement are closely analogous to those the physician uses to better his patient's physical condition. Let us review the steps.

Symptoms

The doctor begins to function when he is confronted with a patient who reports a series of symptoms—headache, nausea and vomiting, lower back pains, diarrhea, and the like.

The symptoms that health educators see are: a population in which large segments are not vaccinated against polio, many people disregarding the potential for lung cancer by excessive cigarette smoking, few cars with seat belts and many occupants of cars with belts not using this safety measure, many communities without sodium fluoride in their water and some communities that have dropped this cavity-avoidance measure.

The physician, in treating such symptoms, can immediately administer or prescribe symptomatic treatment. (Sometimes we call it "shotgun" prescribing.) For emergency conditions and the more common complaints, this is frequently the preferable treatment, and today, with wide-spectrum antibiotics, it often is successful.

In health education, we too can use symptomatic treatment and sometimes do. We can assume that the reason people are not protected from polio, do not adjust the fluoride content of their water, and so on is because they do not know what they should do. We can further assume that if we use a wide enough spectrum of information (television, newspapers, pamphlets, and so on) people will be informed and then act. In other words, we can use a shotgun of information beamed toward the public. Sometimes this will work.

Diagnosis

In most cases doctors are not satisfied to give symptomatic treatment; rather, they prefer to take enough time to make a diagnosis. In doing so, they gather evidence about the cause of the symptoms. This may include a history, blood analysis, electrocardiogram, X-rays, and whatever else is indicated. They may even call in consultants before deciding on the diagnosis. The two main parts of the diagnosis are: (1) What is causing the symptoms? and (2) How will this patient respond to the various types of treatment that can be administered? Is it necessary to give preparatory treatment, such as building up the patient, before initiating the medicine or surgery? The physician carefully considers many such questions.

Similarly, in health education we seek an educational diagnosis. Why are certain people not immunized against polio? Is it because of the cost? Are they afraid of its safety? Do they think it is ineffective? Do they object to interference with nature? Have their past experiences with the health department, hospitals, or private physicians been so unsatisfactory and distressing, they hesitate to return?

Or why do so many people smoke cigarettes when excessive smoking increases the chances of lung cancer tenfold? Have they read the data? Do they disbelieve it? More specifically, why do so many public health workers continue to smoke cigarettes? Are they slaves to a habit? Does smoking satisfy a goal? Can it be satisfied in another way?

Like the doctor, the health educator may call in consultants to provide additional information. These consultants generally come from the field of behavioral science.

Again, as in medicine, we must learn not only why people are not following good health practices, we must learn what methods and influences are likely to bring about a change in their behavior. For example, what kinds of influence will induce polio immunization among the low-income, low-educational groups in our society? Do they follow advice from the television and radio, or do they listen to individuals of their own status? Plainly, we in health education must seek such answers before proceeding to the next step.

Parenthetically, I should like to point out in this analogy that the tools and tests available for a diagnosis in health education are not as specific nor as well developed as some of those available to the physician. For that reason the educational diagnosis is likely to be much less precise. Nevertheless, the lack of precision should not be used as an argument that an educational diagnosis cannot be undertaken.

Treatment

Once the diagnosis has been made, the physician prescribes the treatment. Generally, it consists of two parts: (1) What should be done? and (2) Who shall do it? We all know that frequently the physician himself does not give the treatment. Rather he orders physiotherapy by a therapist, nursing procedures to be undertaken by the nurse, or gives directions to be carried out by the family or the patient himself.

In health education the prescription also breaks down into what should be done and who shall do it. Again, the health educator himself may not be the one to carry out the prescribed methods. Rather, it will be the person or groups most effective in bringing about the desired change. In some instances this is the health officer, in others the nurse, or it can be a person unconnected with the health department—such as a minister, priest, or political leader.

The physician has at his disposal a pharmacopoeia of drugs and other aids to use separately or in various combinations in treating his patients, or he can have the pharmacist make up prescriptions. He is thoroughly acquainted with the properties of the various drugs and the reactions they generally produce in patients.

So, too, there is a pharmacopoeia of procedures and aids in health education. For example, there are such techniques as individual instruction, the interview, group discussion, lectures, community organization. There is also a myriad of audio and visual aids, such as radio and television, movies, printed materials, and news releases. All of these can be drawn upon in our efforts to improve health practices. Each has its own value and limitations.

Just as the doctor can have the pharmacist make up a specific prescription, so the health educator can, within limits, develop his own particular aids. At this point, however, he generally calls in the producer of films—or whatever type aid he is considering.

The health educator is familiar with the various techniques and knows how to use them singly or in combination. He also recognizes that research has proved interpersonal or face-to-face communication the most effective method of education for behavior change. Discussing this fact, a professor of mass communication media recently said:

> If we break down the process by which people put into practice a new research finding, we see five main steps:
>
> 1. Awareness of the information;
> 2. Interest in the practice;
> 3. Trial of the practice;
> 4. Evaluation of its effect;
> 5. Adoption of the practice.
>
> Mass media are effective only in the first two steps of creating awareness and interest. More intensive methods

are necessary to effect adoption of a new practice in the large majority of people.

May I digress long enough here to repeat, in terms of the analogy we are using, what I said in the first part of this paper. All too many people regard health education as a pharmacy of methods and materials when actually it is the compounding of these ingredients—the analytical process—that is most important.

Follow-Up or Evaluation

Now to return to the steps that physicians take in their treatment of patients. They follow up on the effectiveness of their diagnosis and prescription to see how the patients react. If patients do not improve, the physicians reexamine their diagnoses and may change treatments.

Similarly, in health education we should evaluate the impact our efforts are having both immediately and in the long pull. If no results can be discerned, we need to reexamine our diagnosis and try another method. It may prove necessary to intensify our efforts in limited areas or completely change our approach. I am sure you recognize that this description of the health education process is an ideal one. In virtually no operating programs will you find such constant, meticulous analysis. But, I ask, is there any reason we should not try, where practical, this analytical approach to human behavior change? The scientific method has certainly served us well in our attempts to control both our physical and bacteriological environments. Should we not be as precise as possible in our educational efforts, just as we have been in our health control efforts? These questions take on added significance when we look at the shape of things to come. It is an old story to you that as the communicable diseases recede (due to our public health discoveries and efforts), the chronic, degenerative, or long-term illnesses are coming to the fore. For almost all of these conditions, our only preventive or control measures depend upon early detection and treatment.

From the standpoint of education, this means that each individual, if he is to benefit, must act in order to take advantage of whatever examining or screening procedures are available, and then follow whatever regimen is prescribed. Thus, one of our major tasks is to inform each individual in such a way that he will do what he should for his own protection.

Superficial consideration of this educational problem might lead one to conclude that it is a simple and easy task. In this country we have the most extensive media for disseminating information that has ever existed. Newspapers, radio, and television almost blanket the entire country. No person need be ignorant of scientific findings that would benefit him. We know from experience, however, that use of these media alone is not sufficient to bring about the necessary actions to improve people's health. I have already mentioned some of these. I wish I had time to review with you other research by social scientists that gives us clues as to why people are so obstinate or apathetic—that is, "obstinate" or "apathetic" *from our point of view*. But that is not the purpose of our present discussion.

Up to this point, we have seen through analogy that health education is an analytical-action process. We have noted that numerous health safeguards hinge on individual action and that stimulating such action is the task of health education. Now let's turn more specifically to our title, "Health Educator—Partner in Health Education." The health educator's chief contribution to the partnership is in helping plan educational phases of a program. Elements in planning are indicated by such questions as: What groups in the community—doctors, educators, commissioners, socioeconomic groups—will be asked to take action? What specific action will be required, and what is the timing? What are the current attitudes? Which resources will be most helpful? Will individual contacts be necessary? What educational aids are recommended, and how will they be most effective? Planning the educational phase of a program requires thoroughness and precision, a fact often overlooked.

Recently I read the preparations for an experiment to give live-virus polio vaccine to the total population of a community. The methods of giving the vaccine were detailed to the last minutiae, stating the number of plastic spoons required, how the handles should be turned, and how the nurse would make sure each person swallowed his vaccine. Epidemiologic plans for this community project were underway for seven months.

Two weeks before the vaccine was to be administered, health educators were called in to prepare and execute an educational program to induce people to be vaccinated. Would you agree with me *that it is* somewhat simpler to arrange plastic spoons and pour vaccine in them than it is to persuade people to participate? Yet we health educators frequently are denied our full partnership in the planning of programs. Our knowledge about people's behavior and possible ways to get response cannot be useful to the partnership unless our participation starts in the planning stage.

The job of the health education partner is an exacting one. He must be prepared for the task. If we may use the analogy to medicine again, the physician is a practitioner of the physiological sciences. He studies physiology, anatomy, pathology, chemistry, and bacteriology as major subjects. He may study to a limited degree the behavioral sciences. He then learns how to apply these sciences in the clinical situation. I like to think of the health educator as a practitioner of the behavioral sciences in the field of health. As such, he should be thoroughly grounded in the sciences of psychology, sociology, and anthropology, with some minor studies in the health field. These give him an understanding of human behavior. Then he should learn to apply these in the practical community situation. What I have described as educational qualifications are the ideal. Few of our health educators are as well prepared as they would like to be. But part of this lack of preparation stems from a lack of appreciation by many administrators of the complexity of educating adults about health, and the analytical work required. If health educators are not included in program planning, the necessity for their training does not become apparent.

Finally, the health educator is one of the youngest members of the partnership. His role is not altogether understood by other partners, and sometimes not even by himself. However, it is my conviction, as we go forward in public health through the years ahead, that the health educator will mature professionally and will contribute far more to the health partnership than he has been able, or permitted, to thus far.

Summary

1. Education of the public about health is an activity in which all members of the health partnership participate together. The physician, nurse, sanitarian, and health educator all have a role in the educational task.

2. Health education is an analytical as well as action process. Diagnosis of why people are following unhealthy practices, and then determining the best channels or means to help them improve their behavior, is essential to effective education.

3. Health safeguards of the future often will require individual action that can only be stimulated through health education.

4. The health educator as a partner in health brings his unique background in the behavioral sciences to assist in program planning.

5. The health educator can be most effective when his assistance is sought at the time that programs are being planned, not after decisions have been made.

6. For health educators to make their maximum contribution to the health partnership, they must be thoroughly qualified through professional preparation in the behavioral sciences

and have grown through experience in practical situations and in-service training.

To be accepted as a full partner in the health professions is gratifying to us as health educators. With your confidence and assistance, we will measure up by doing our part for the improvement of the public's health.

Discussion Questions

1. How is the importance of partnerships in public health portrayed by Derryberry in this section?

2. How can the health educator maximize his or her effectiveness according to Derryberry?

3. Do you have any ideas about how to further improve the professional status of the health educator today, an idea that Derryberry strongly advocated?

4. How do you react to Derryberry's definition of health education for today's health practice?

Part III

Establishing the Parameters
of Health Education

Overview

The chapters in Parts One and Two have documented meticulous efforts to quantify and organize data in an educational context so as to produce change in how the public health community perceives education and learning. One function of leadership is articulating what a professional field encompasses and what it does not. Accordingly, the chapters in Part Three chronicle the leadership position that Mayhew Derryberry took in order to establish the parameters of health education and to give continuous attention to the research base needed to improve the quality of educational effort.

In Chapter Fourteen, an essay delivered more than fifty years ago, Dr. Derryberry challenges the then popular belief that learning has taken place simply because teaching has occurred. He not only confronts this presumed correlation, he also attacks the notion that people are passive, pointing out that learning is occurring at all times, whether the professional is "teaching" or not. This chapter introduces logic, language, and experience, the components of comprehension, into the context of public health program development. It was at this time that the psychological principles for health education and their application for program development were gaining attention through efforts like that of the American Public Health Association Health Education Institute, formed in 1937. Derryberry brought behavioral scientists into the Public Health Service approximately ten years after writing this early essay.

In this era different viewpoints about health education and public relations were widely discussed and sometimes heatedly debated. The second chapter in this part points out that the fundamental difference between the two fields of endeavor is found in the objectives of each. Health education deals with problem solving and action, whereas public relations focuses on winning good will for an organization. Both approaches struggled for and succeeded in gaining support and a constituency.

A noticeable sense that the public health education profession was maturing emerges in Chapter Sixteen. Dr. Derryberry practiced his belief that knowledge must be translated into the terms most familiar to people, in this case health officers, medical administrators, and policymakers. The principles upon which health education operates are described in the terms most familiar to these audiences. In this chapter the relationship between the health educator as a practitioner and the behavioral scientist as a specialist is described for the first time. Derryberry employs diagrams and charts to show program relationships that previously had been confusing. He stresses the need for health educators to keep up with behavioral science findings. This is one of the first references in the literature to continuing education for health educators.

Chapter Seventeen provides an interpretation of relevant research from rural sociology, communication arts, and anthropology, as well as social psychology. At this time *communications* was an important buzzword. The partnership role the professional was to play with the public (or patients) is easily seen as the modus operandi of the future.

The family becomes the center of attention in Chapter Eighteen. There is a perception today that focus on the family is a *new* approach. However, in the 1960s Derryberry reported on the enor-

mous potential for learning and behavioral change through education of the entire family unit. He refers to five problems to illustrate
communication barriers between patients and medical personnel,
and he describes ways to approach these situations.

The maturity and professionalism of the field of public health
education is evident in these five chapters. The responsibility of the
health educator to maintain a high level of quality of effort is under-
scored time and again.

14

Taking the Public with You

At a recent discussion on health education, many public health workers were startled by the following challenge of a newspaper reporter: "Why is it," he said, "that, in a majority of communities, reductions in the health department budget can be made without stirring up much comment either in the newspaper or by the public in general; but if the budget for the education department is cut, an immediate community objection is registered in newspaper editorials and in other community action?" According to this reporter, the educators have "sold" their program and objectives to the public and the health workers have not.

It is, of course, impossible to discuss here the many reasons for this condition, or to describe the means by which the situation might be corrected. However, in the past, discussions of the problem of winning enthusiastic public support for health movements have been confined principally to plans for special sporadic campaigns, exhibits, or routine techniques in preparing pamphlets. All of these undeniably have their place in the health education program, but in concentrating energies on the machinery for publicity and propaganda, equally potent forces in the building up of favorable public attitudes are frequently overlooked. One of these, so

Originally published in *The Health Officer*, April 1938, 2(12), 615–621. Reprinted with permission.

obvious that it is almost entirely disregarded, is the matter of the contact made by various members of the health department with the public it intends to serve. Almost all of the work of the public health nurse and most of the functions of the health officer and sanitarian are alleged to be for the purpose of health education. Can it be that these efforts of public health workers are not actually educating the public?

By studying this problem primarily from the standpoint of the learner (who in the aggregate constitutes the public) and the way in which he acquires information, changes his attitude, or modifies his behavior, a number of considerations that should guide procedures in health education have been precipitated. The first of these is the distinction between learning and teaching. This difference is not a quibble about whether or not there is teaching if there is no learning, but certainly it cannot be assumed that learning has taken place simply because there has been teaching. This seems an obvious distinction; yet all too frequently it has been neglected. Many health departments are proud of the accomplishments of their health education program. They furnish as evidence of its effectiveness such items as the number of health talks delivered (sometimes without even considering the number present), the inches of newspaper space obtained, the number of pamphlets distributed, and the number of individual contacts made.

In the course of this impressive enumeration of activities, no mention is made of the effect on the public. Just because a number of motions supposedly directed at health education have been made, there is no assurance that the public has been educated. Neither can the assumption be made that the public is not learning when the health department is not teaching. As a matter of fact, learning is going on all of the time. It is not a faucet that can be turned on and off in the same way as can be done in the teaching procedures. Every contact that an individual experiences with a health department representative is a learning situation. The patient who comes to a clinic, sits on a bench in a gloomy room for two hours, and is finally given a cursory examination and told to see the nurse is learning about public health. Learning is taking place despite the fact that no conscious attempt has been made to teach him anything about health education. This is merely illustrative of many procedures in public health that are built on the assumption that patients are passive or even inanimate objects of treatment. Actually, the reverse is true; clients are actively learning at all times, and instead of coming along with the health department, they frequently learn to avoid contact with it.

A few examples of errors in health education procedures that may cause the public to learn some things that are contrary to the intended teaching may suggest ways of preventing such negative learning.

A Staff Divided

One of the factors that will interfere with successful teaching of the public is the issuance of conflicting advice by different members of the health department. Unless the entire staff, from the health officer to the clerk, has been educated to work toward the same general objective and in the same way, the public is likely to conclude that the material taught is false or that the behavior urged is unnecessary.

Here is a concrete case. An alert young man, having read much of the recent publicity and educational material on the control of syphilis, decided to have a blood test. He went to a clinic operated by an organization that had been urging blood tests for everybody and asked if someone could take a blood specimen for a Wassermann. The physician in the clinic asked, "Who wants it?" Somewhat abashed, the young man said, "Well, I heard that it was a good thing to do, so I thought I would have it." He was then asked curtly, "Have you had your breakfast?" He replied, "Yes," and although it was ten-thirty in the morning and he had had his breakfast at seven o'clock, the physician remarked in a superior manner, "Well, no good doctor would take a blood specimen right after you have eaten." The publicity had made no mention of any such reservation, and though the young man had followed specifically the advice given, he had been made to feel very uncomfortable. As a result of this experience, he is not disposed ever to have a Wassermann test and is inclined to discount all the fine publicity issued by health organizations.

The publicity need not have given the detailed procedure of taking a blood Wassermann; its purpose was simply to bring people to the clinic. A cordial reception and a careful explanation of the test on the part of the physician could very well have resulted in the making and keeping of a definite appointment for another hour.

Cooperation with the Medical Profession

Another factor that may teach people not to go along with the health department is its failure to seek the cooperation of the medical profession. Before urging any type of behavior or teaching any health facts, it is essential to know that the medical group agrees with the educational material and that it will give the type of medical care advocated. What good does it do to educate the public about the value of periodic health examinations if the physicians in the community are not "sold" on the idea? What if the physicians in the community give only cursory examinations, saying, "Oh, there is nothing wrong with you; why do you bother?" and dismiss the applicant with the bland smile reserved for confirmed hypochondriacs? Or what value will accrue from a case-finding program in tuberculosis should some of the physicians in the community tell the families, "Tuberculin tests are all tommy-rot" or "It is not necessary for the adult contacts of tuberculosis to be examined"?

By such experiences the public learns to disregard the advice of the physician, of the health department, or of both. Most often it is the health department that loses standing. In any case, the result is undesirable. Unfortunately, these situations arise all too often. So the job of taking the public with you requires taking the physicians of the community with you first.

Practice What You Preach

It is not only necessary that the health advice given the public be consistently the same whether it comes from the health department or the physicians; it is also necessary that we follow our own advice. "Practice yourself what you preach" is older than Christianity, but do we do it? If not, the public can point to us and say, "You haven't done this; why should I?" That many public health workers do not follow their own teachings was brought out in a recent survey on the subject.[1] The survey covered about 800 individuals working in public health organizations. It was found that less than half of them had had a Wassermann test and even fewer of their spouses had been given a test; over a third of them had never had a tuberculin test or a chest X-ray, and two-thirds of their wives had had no examination for tuberculosis. Furthermore, a fourth of their children between the ages of 1 and 15 years had neither been immunized against diphtheria nor vaccinated against smallpox. Almost all of the public health workers had had a health examination at some time or another, but over half of them had had the examination merely as a prerequisite for their job or to secure insurance and did not have a definite plan of periodic examinations. As many as 15 percent went to the dentist only when they were aware of a carious tooth or when they had a toothache. What is your score?

Plain Speaking

Sometimes public health teaching has not been effective because the material has not been presented in a manner that could be easily understood. Too frequently technical jargon has been used to the complete confusion of those being taught. Recently a nurse was talking to the contact of a tuberculosis case who had been removed to the hospital. She was explaining that the individual could return from the hospital as soon as he had become an *arrested* case, whereupon the individual being visited said, "What did you say about restification?"

A health educator was talking to a third-grade class from a poor section about diet, and in her teaching said, "You children must *dispense* with tea and coffee for breakfast." Whereupon one youngster replied, "My mother won't let me have any more." Closely connected with this difficulty in teaching is the failure to make the instructions specific. To talk in general terms does little good. For example, a nurse who was visiting a tuberculosis child for the first time said to the mother, "You know you must take all of the precautions." Unfortunately, the mother did not know what was meant by "all of the precautions," and the nurse made no further explanation; therefore the advice was of little value.

How Do People Learn?

A few other important factors in determining what methods are likely to influence the public favorably come out of a study of the way in which people learn.

From his experiments in human learning, Thorndike has concluded, "Learning without interest of some sort does not occur in any appreciable degree." Therefore it is most ineffective to bombard the population continually with health facts or urge them to improve their practices if they have no interest in the facts or in changing their habits.

Peculiarly enough, few people are interested in health per se. "How then," someone asks, "can we make our teaching interesting?" Psychologists report that there are a few basic desires—"I-want's"— which man continually tries to satisfy. These are: hunger; a mate; comfort; power over nature, things, and people; and approval by his fellow man. It will be noted that health is not one of these basic wants. However, health teaching can satisfy the desire for comfort.

For that reason, it seems that health education should make more use of the salient appeal rather than of the health appeal. "You will feel better the next morning" is a much better argument for sleeping with windows open than to give as a reason, "It will make you healthy and strong." There is another consideration that should govern the way subject matter is presented. It might be stated dogmatically thus: A possible cause should never be related to an effect that the individual can refute from experience even though scientific experiment can demonstrate the cause-and-effect relationship.

It is difficult to convince the farmer who has secured all his water from an open, unprotected spring for the last 40 or 50 years that there is danger of contamination and disease if he does not protect his water supply. He thinks that he knows better. Forty years of experience has taught him that there is no danger. None of his family has been affected yet. And simply saying there is danger without explanation is not convincing. Take the case of the boy who went to school, and the teacher, who was trying to improve the dietary habits of the children, said to him, "Johnny, what did you have for breakfast this morning?" He said, "Pancakes," whereupon he was given a long tirade about the evils of pancakes and how they would influence his health in later life. The boy was unconvinced. He said, "My grandmother is eighty-five years old. She has been eating pancakes every morning and she's all right. I don't want to be any better than she is, so pancakes are okay for me." And the worst part about all this is that the public is likely to regard all of public health teaching as being inaccurate if their experience contradicts even a very small part of it.

Among the previously mentioned basic drives that cause individuals to behave in one manner rather than another was listed "approval by [our] fellow man." If teaching procedures interfere with the satisfaction of this basic drive, then the public is likely not to learn what is being taught. Consider the following experience. A nurse visited a recently arrested tuberculosis case and found the patient and a friend leaving the house. She was trying to impress upon him the advantages of continuous medical supervision. In the presence of his friend, she told him that the clinic could tell him whether he had the *terrible* disease any longer; if he did not have it, then he would be free from the *stigma* of the disease. Certainly this conversation was not such that the patient could feel he had gained the approval of his fellow man. Whether or not he learned the value of medical supervision and will seek it from that experience is questionable.

For Your Sake, Not Ours

Finally, in teaching it is important that the patient feel that the behavior being urged is for his own benefit, not to please the health worker or to satisfy some regulation. The following verbatim conversation between a tuberculosis contact and a nurse is illustrative:

MR. X: Did you want us to be injected?

NURSE: To be what?

MR. X: Injected.

NURSE: I don't want anybody to be injected. Do you mean examined?

MR. X: Yes.

NURSE: We do want that done, and when he [the tuberculosis son] comes home from the hospital, we want to see him and how he is feeling.

MR. X: He has had six or seven X-rays and they all came back negative. I am going up to see him this afternoon.

NURSE: I believe you expected to take the wife and the children to a private doctor?

MR. X: Yes, but it always slips my mind, but I will do it.

NURSE: All right—because we have to have the report.

MR. X: That is true.

NURSE: We cannot make the rules different for you than for anyone else.

If the individuals in this family are examined, they will likely feel that it was done for the benefit of the nurse rather than for their own benefit—if the preponderance of *we's*, *reports*, and *rules* in this nurse's teaching is any indication.

Summary

Taking the public with you in a health program requires much more than ordinary publicity and propaganda. Every act of every member of the department is a potential contributor to the goal. Whether the public comes along or is driven away depends on the degree to which there is recognition of the educational implications of all the procedures in the program. The following approaches are suggested as methods for making health education more effective:

1. Make certain that all members of the department focus on giving the same advice to the public, thus avoiding conflict of advice, which engenders distrust.

2. Be sure that the medical profession agrees with the educational work and that they will render the type of service promised to the public.

3. "Practice what you preach," or, medically stated, "Don't prescribe medicine you wouldn't take under similar circumstances."

4. Teach specifically in terms familiar to the public. Technical jargon is permissible only when the patient has learned its meaning and all its connotations.

5. Appeal to the basic interests of the public and thus motivate learning in terms of the fundamental drives of human nature. Be sure that in handling the public, they are not subjected to some experience that is annoying to them. This interferes with the satisfaction of a naturally basic drive.

6. Consider the public's educational level and former experiences and be sure that no effect is related to a cause that the patient believes from his experience not to be true, without complete explanation of the way in which the cause-and-effect relationship operates.

7. Urge the public to practice health behaviors not for the purpose of satisfying a regulation or a public health worker but to bring satisfaction to themselves.

These represent a few of the many considerations that should guide procedure in *taking the public with you*.

Discussion Questions

1. "Taking the public with you" in a health program requires much more than ordinary publicity and propaganda. What are some approaches for addressing this issue, as documented by Derryberry in this chapter?

2. What appeals can the health educator use to facilitate action, other than the appeal of improving health?

3. Give an example of a health education practice or approach that involves the patient or the public.

Note

1. Unpublished data assembled by the Division of Public Health Methods, U.S. Public Health Service, Washington, D.C.

15

Health Education and Public Relations

The terms "public relations" and "health education," as used in this statement, relate to objectives rather than to methods. In the field of public health, public relations refers to winning good will for an organization or for one of its programs; health education aims to facilitate learning about health and health problems and to motivate good individual and group health practices.

No organization can render maximum service without good public relations! If it is to serve most effectively, and be adequately financed, the people must know the functions of the organization, understand its problems, and appreciate its importance. Campaigns of mass information and publicity may improve an organization's public relations temporarily. But the continuation of good will for an organization, such as a health department, requires efficient, courteous service as well as publicity and mass information programs. Thus, every member of the health department in his intimate public contacts, while rendering a health service, exerts a marked influence on the level of public relations that the department enjoys. When a health department has good public relations, its opportunities for service increase. One of the

Originally published in the *American Journal of Public Health*, March 1950, 40(3), 251–252. Reprinted with permission.

services, health education, has as its goal a public that knows and practices good health behavior. In accordance with democratic principles of education, the service consists of a fourfold activity: it stimulates people to recognize health needs of which they were not aware; it helps them to obtain authentic and reliable information about their problems; it encourages them to plan for solving these problems; and it assists them to act on the plans they have made.

In acquainting people with health problems, all the media of mass information, as well as individual and group discussion, may be used. Also, the entire health department staff, through their individual home, clinic, and premise contacts, as well as group meetings, contribute to the health education objective. Thus, both health education and public relations are furthered through the activities of the entire health department staff, and both make use of mass media.

One fundamental difference, however, should be noted. The goal of health education is not fully realized until every individual understands good health behaviors, has a favorable attitude toward them, and habitually practices them. On the other hand, when an organization enjoys the support of its policy and program by a significant portion of the people, the major goal of public relations is achieved. In short, success in health education requires far more fundamental change in human behavior than is needed to achieve good public relations.

The public relations approach often differs from the health education approach. Usually, in public relations, approval and support of the health department's existing decisions are sought from the people; in health education, people are stimulated to make a careful study of their health needs and opportunities and to take an active part in making decisions that affect them. Public relations promotes a program for the people, while health education is a program of the people.

Discussion Questions

1. What is the difference between "public relations" and "health education"?

2. Why is public relations so important to any organization?

3. What common methods are used in both health education and public relations efforts?

16

Health Education

Its Objectives and Methods

In the documentation for the Twelfth World Health Assembly, it is stated that: "Health education embraces the sum of all those experiences of an individual that change or influence his attitudes or behavior with respect to health, and the processes and efforts of bringing these changes about."[1] This concept of health education recognizes that "many experiences of an individual have an impact on what he thinks, feels, and does about health" and that it is "more than mere information or propaganda."[2]

The particular significance of this concept for us is the emphasis placed on the individuals, groups, and communities toward whom the health education effort is directed. In other words, the primary concern is the degree to which health education is successful in helping the particular individuals or groups to acquire more information about health, to change and improve their health practices. The methods and materials used to achieve the desired results are a secondary consideration. In this sense, public health education is similar to what happens in our schools today. As parents, or others responsible for the younger generation, we are vitally interested in what our children learn. Our concern with the teachers, their methods, or the materials they

Originally published in *Health Education Monographs*, No. 8, 1960, pp. 3–9. Reprinted with permission.

use is important only as they contribute to the educational growth of our children.

Or let us use another analogy, that of selling merchandise. A merchant is concerned with the volume of sales when he talks about salesmanship. To be sure, he observes carefully how his advertisements in newspapers and magazines look and where they are placed on the page. Similarly, he listens and watches to hear and see his radio and television commercials. But his real concern with this phase of merchandising is that it produces an increase in the sales of his product.

And so it is with health education. Inches of news coverage, number of television programs, volume of printed materials distributed, and the like are secondary considerations to the question: *What changes have been brought about in the target audience?*

What, then, are some of the educational processes that go into bringing about increased health knowledge and improved health attitudes and practices? To me, the processes are almost completely analogous to those used by physicians in the practice of medicine. Let us examine more closely the similarities shown in graphic form on Table 16.1.

Those who practice medicine apply research findings from the basic biological and physiological sciences and to a lesser degree utilize the behavioral sciences. Those who attempt to improve people's health practices—those engaged in health education—apply research findings from the basic behavioral sciences—psychology,

Table 16.1. Similarities in Educational Processes Used by the Physician and the Health Education Worker.

The Physician	The Health Education Worker
The Underlying Sciences	
Physiology, Biology, Anatomy, Chemistry, Physics, to a lesser extent, Behavioral Science	Behavioral Sciences: Psychology, Sociology, Anthropology, to a lesser extent, Natural Science

The Problem	
Symptoms, such as: headaches, temperature, lower back pain, dizziness	Symptoms, such as: many children not immunized against polio; high mortality from coronary disease; failure to use cervical test for cancer; few people having periodic medical examinations

Possible Action	
Shotgun prescription	Intensive information program

Diagnosis Based On:	
History Pulse Blood pressure Blood tests Sugar & cell count Urinalysis	A person's or group's: history of past experiences; information or knowledge; culture and traditions; personal goals; perception of health practices, etc.

Treatment	
Who shall it be? Who shall give it?	Who shall it be? Who shall give it?

Pharmacopoeia	
Drugs, Rest, Diet Radiation therapy Physical therapy	Community organization; films, group discussions; individual instruction; lectures; news releases; pamphlets; TV

Follow-Up	
Periodic observation of: symptoms and progress	Periodic observation of: progress in change of attitudes and behavior

anthropology, and sociology—in their interpreting and stimulating practical use of the natural sciences.

The steps that these two groups of practitioners go through in applying their respective sciences are almost identical. The physician generally begins with one or more symptoms of disorder that the patient reports or that the physician extracts from him. The health education worker usually starts with "symptoms" also: evidence that an individual, a group, or a population is not practicing the findings of science that, if followed, would improve their health.

At this point, each can follow a similar course of action. The physician can treat the symptoms by giving the patient a "shotgun prescription." The health education worker can shower the people with information on the assumption that they are ignorant of the research that dictates certain desirable health practices. In certain limited and emergency situations this use of the shotgun type of action can be highly effective. However, these situations are relatively rare.

But in most situations, the physician will avoid, if at all possible, symptomatic treatment. He will proceed to make a diagnosis. Why does the patient have headaches, dizziness, a fever, or lower back pain? For this diagnosis he not only takes a history, but he may give the patient a number of tests. He may call in various technical experts, internists, radiologists, pathologists, and so on to the extent he considers it necessary to make a reasonably accurate diagnosis. Here he weighs complete accuracy and assurance against the time required, the expense involved, and other relevant considerations.

The skilled health educator, too, works on a diagnosis, an *educational* diagnosis. Is the failure of the people to follow sound health practices due to lack of information, or are they more interested in something else? Is some past experience with health services deterring the people from good health practices? Does the recommended health practice interfere with the achievement of some other goal they have? Do they see the practice of the health habit as lowering their status or bringing disapproval from members of their social group?

These are the types of questions to which the skilled health education worker needs answers in order to diagnose the cause of the poor health practices he has observed. In obtaining satisfactory answers, the health education worker may also call in experts—behavioral scientists—to assist in arriving at the educational diagnosis.

Just as the physician uses or adopts diagnostic tools from the sciences of which he is a practitioner, so the health education worker draws his diagnostic tools from the behavioral sciences. Admittedly, the tools of the health education worker have not yet been developed to the same degree of precision as those of the physician. Furthermore, they generally require more time to use and, in most cases, are more expensive to apply. Despite these drawbacks, using such measurements is far better than guessing at the diagnosis. And time is on the side of the health educator since it is seldom necessary that he reach his diagnosis in the same short period that is required in the case of a medical emergency.

Once the diagnosis has been made, the physician then prescribes a course of treatment and indicates who will give it. Sometimes he himself may be the principal person, as in surgery. Sometimes it is the nurse, physiotherapist, or members of the patient's family.

He may also prescribe certain medicines and procedures from his pharmacopeia as aids in the treatment.

Similarly, the health educator prescribes the educational treatment after he has reached his diagnosis. He, too, decides who should administer the treatment. It may be the doctor or the nurse, the priest, the family—or he himself may be the principal person to carry it out. The health educator also draws upon his pharmacopeia of educational aids and methods—community organization, exhibits, films, group discussions, individual instruction, lectures, news releases, pamphlets, posters, television programs, and so on.

The doctor constantly watches his patient. He notes how the patient is responding to treatment and, on the basis of his observation, refines his diagnosis and revises his treatment to make them more effective. He may, and usually does, accumulate evidence to evaluate his handling of the immediate and related future cases. The health educator also keeps checking the accuracy of his educational diagnosis and the efficacy of his prescribed treatment. During the course of it, he may suggest different people to carry out parts of the treatment or he may completely change the type of aids he has prescribed.

Finally, the health educator continuously evaluates his efforts in order to become more proficient in diagnosis, in prescribing educational experiences, and in improving the quality and effectiveness of his aids.

Our analogy to medicine is one way of viewing the processes involved in increasing people's health information, changing their health beliefs, and improving their practices. But there are other ways to look at this, and we in health education recognize the value of presenting the same concepts in a number of frameworks.

Let us look at the same phenomena from the physics analogy of lines of force. If I may repeat, the health education worker is concerned with changing the public's beliefs and practices about health and uses his efforts to bring about these changes. In its simplest form, this effort can be represented like this (see Figure 16.1):

The line of force between the health education worker and the public may be health education materials and methods of any kind—personal conferences, community organization, news releases, magazine articles, movies, radio, television, exhibits, pamphlets, and the like. In this simple physics representation, it would appear that the line, or lines, of force exerted by the health worker impinge

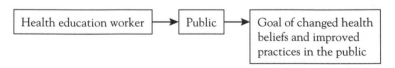

Figure 16.1. Simple Depiction of the Relationship of the Health Education Worker to Improved Health Practices.

upon the public without any interference, and the stronger the force, the greater the impact on the public—pushing them toward the goal of changed beliefs and improved health practices. Furthermore, this visual representation treats the public as an inert mass with no internal forces that influence its movement.

Certainly none of us subscribes to this simplified statement of changing health behavior, but is it fair to ask whether this visual representation does not closely correspond to the way we often carry on health education programs?

We still have the basic pattern—the health education worker is exercising force on the public to push it toward changed health beliefs and improved practices (in Figure 16.2 represented by a solid line). But instead of the line of force reaching the public unimpeded, we find a screen through which the lines of force must penetrate if they are to have any impact. This screen is made up of such factors as interests of the public, their motivations, their perception of our interests and concerns, their past experiences (particularly with following previous health advice), and a host of other influences that the health education worker needs to understand before he can find the ways for his line of force to penetrate this screen.

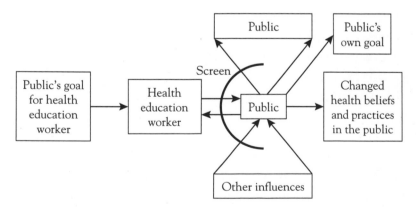

Figure 16.2. A More Dynamic Depiction of the Relationship of the Health Education Worker to Improved Health Practices.

Even so, the intensity of the line of force may be diminished as it finds its way through the screen. But the screen is not the only factor. There are other external influences exerting lines of force to push the public in other directions, toward other goals.

There are also *internal* forces operating from *within* the public, such as particular goals they may have set. It could be that the public is trying to exert force on us—to push us toward a goal they have in mind for us.

Let us look at a real problem in this framework. Some health education workers are concerned with the mounting death toll from lung cancer. On the basis of the evidence, they are exerting educational force on those who are smoking cigarettes to stop smoking or at least reduce the amount they smoke. The impact of the force of their educational effort on the smokers (the public in our chart) is diminished by lack of interest, the belief that lung cancer "can't happen to me," the fatalistic attitude of "I've got to die of something, so why not lung cancer," and other rationalizations that go into the smoker's screen. The tobacco companies, social pressures, and other cultural patterns encourage smoking (other influences). Sometimes I get the feeling that the smoker's goal for me (when I undertake to be a health education worker on this subject) is to shut me up. Despite this inadequate and incomplete analysis of the educational problem involved in cigarette smoking and lung cancer, I am sure all will agree that this analogy and analysis more nearly approaches reality than the simple exercise of force pushing to a predetermined goal. In developing these two ways of looking at health education, I have had three main purposes in mind:

1. *To draw attention to the many facets to be considered in improving the health practices of the public.* Frequently, the diagnostic phase—to determine the barriers or screen, the other external lines of forces and the internal forces that may be impeding the efforts of the health educator—is completely overlooked.

In other instances, there is failure to "prescribe" the person who will be the most effective teacher for the particular task. All too often health education is discussed only in terms of its pharmacopeia—that is, its methods and materials.

2. *To emphasize some of the complexities encountered in effecting health behavior change.* I submit that trying to diagnose why people do not follow desirable health practices and then to develop a treatment pattern to bring about improvement is as difficult (and perhaps more so) for the health educator as it is for the physician to diagnose and prescribe successful treatment for brain tumor or lower back pain!

3. *To indicate how important it is that our health education practitioners have a thorough understanding of the behavioral sciences.* The developments in these fields during the past two decades have been tremendous, so much so that many of the scientists themselves have difficulty in keeping up to date.

Summary

Health education is concerned with effecting improved health attitudes and behavior in the general public. Accomplishment of this goal requires careful and thorough consideration of the present knowledge, attitudes, goals, perceptions, social status, power structure, cultural traditions, and other aspects of whatever public is to be reached. Only in terms of these elements can a successful program be built.

Discussion Questions

1. What are some elements of the health education encounter that make it so complex?

2. What is the significance of this complexity for the health education worker?

3. How is the skilled health educator similar to the physician?

4. What other theories or models for health education practice does this chapter remind you of?

Notes

1. "Background Document Based on Summary Reports Received from Countries," used at technical discussions on health education of the public, Twelfth World Health Assembly, May 1969.

2. "Report of Technical Discussions on Health Education of the Public," Twelfth World Health Assembly, May 1969.

Better Communications

An Essential in Today's Public Health

A new phenomenon seems to have appeared on the horizon—at least it has assumed a new name, that of communications. Of course, people have been communicating with each other since the beginning of time, but only recently have we begun to dignify the process with the generic term.

In the past, when a person acted the way we told him to, we said, "*He understands.*" Or, conversely, "He *did not* understand"—if he did not carry out the request. Seldom did we say, "I did not make myself clear." Never did we designate the failure as a breakdown in *communications*.

Shift in Meaning

Today, the term has come to mean the *process of exchanging information that will lead to action*, and I believe this shift is due primarily to three factors:

1. Investigations into successful and unsuccessful transmission of information.
2. The necessity to make practical use of the ever-increasing amount of research findings.

Originally published in *Michigan's Health*, May–June 1961, pp. 43–46. Reprinted with permission.

3. The paradox of our enormous potential—mass media—that fails to reach large segments of our mass population.

Addressing the National Health Forum in New York, March 14–16, on the subject "Goals of Health Communication," Dr. Leona Baumgartner, Commissioner of Health for the City of New York, asked:

> Why is communication suddenly so important? The answer is that today we are dealing more and more with special situations, with an ever increasing load of research findings to translate into action, and special kinds of care that won't work unless we do communicate.
>
> We are passing from a medicine in which you do something to the patient into medicine in which we must do something with the patient, and in which the patient must do a lot more on his own. In speaking of "do-to" medicine, I am thinking of shots for tetanus and typhoid and diphtheria, of operations for appendicitis, of removing gall bladders.
>
> We can cure an estimated one-half of all cases of cancer today by finding them soon enough and doing for them what we already know how to do. If someone invented a drug that would cure half the present cases of cancer, the excitement would be beyond belief. We have such a drug—and I am completely serious: It is communication.

Much the same point can be made for glaucoma, venereal disease, tuberculosis, diabetes, and lung cancer; for the disabling effects of coronaries, strokes, and rheumatoid arthritis; and for avoiding the environmental hazards of air and water pollution, radiation exposure, and the like.

Improvement Needed

Other ideas voiced at the National Health Forum, which I would like to pass on, are three instances where communications should be improved:

1. *Among scientists*. More scientific findings have become available in the past two decades than in any two previous centuries. Scientists cannot keep up with the literature in their own specialty, let alone the research in allied fields.

2. *Among professional health workers themselves (that is, among the various categories, each of which has its own professional jargon)*. Without ready communication among the many disciplines, we cannot achieve the harmonious cooperation that is so imperative for good service to our clientele.

3. *Between professional health workers and various segments of the public*. It is this aspect which is perhaps of most concern to us and the one to which I shall devote the remainder of my remarks.

It has been well established that communication takes place only when the intended receiver has an interest in the message. We see, hear, and absorb only a few of the many pleas aimed at us. In fact, bombarded as we are—by radio, television, newspapers, billboards, pamphlets, and so on—with advice and urging on everything from hair tonic to Hi-Fi, we automatically sift out the few we will heed.

We recognize, too, that when we try to force communication with a person about a subject of no interest to him, or one that interferes with his own goals, he either does not hear or see the message, or he deliberately rejects it. Public health workers who are chain cigarette smokers illustrate this fact every day. It is, of course, plain that to communicate successfully with people, we must know their goals, interests, and requirements *as perceived by them*. We may realize that all classes of society, all ethnic groups, do not have our same aims and beliefs. Yet, as Dr. Baumgartner says: "We of the health professions are so overpoweringly and impossibly middle class, we assume that others think as we do and things important to us are also important to them. We talk to them in *our* language, and even if they speak English, they do not understand us."

Proper timing, as in most every field, is important in communication because people accept a message only when they are ready. We have long recognized that a young mother with her first baby is ready to learn facts about child health. We have not been so fortunate in finding the best timing for communication about other aspects of health.

I wonder how many more people would now be protected by Salk vaccine if we could have timed a vaccination program to capitalize on news of the successful field trials! Another basic fact we sometimes overlook is that people are much more likely to act if they can do it immediately upon receiving the message. Much of the success of the polio vaccination campaign in Columbus, Georgia, this spring hinged on this fact. In addition to spreading the word by every known method, portable vaccination stations were set up throughout the city, readily accessible to all comers.

All too often the classic advice to "See your family doctor" or "Go to the health department" falls flat when the recipient does not have a physician or does not know where his health department is.

Past Experience Plays a Part

The effect of past experience with a source of information affects our acceptance of messages from that source. None of us puts much stock in information from a source we have found unsatisfactory in the past. It pays us to consider the attitudes—right or wrong—that are held about health workers and their services by the people we are attempting to reach. The other side of the coin, of course, is that the more trustworthy and expert the recipient perceives the communicator to be, the more likely he is to take his advice. To quickly summarize the main factors that influence a person's acceptance and action on health messages, we find that:

1. People select the communications that fit their personal interests and motives.

2. People interpret communications in terms of their own needs and perceptions.

3. People's past experiences in health situations influence their selection and acceptance of a health message.

4. People are more apt to act when facilities for action are readily accessible and specifically designated.

5. People are more likely to act when they have high regard for the communicator.

As for the pattern or kind of health message, I suppose the most debatable one is the use of the scare technique to stimulate people to action. While a good deal of research on the role of anxiety in communications has been done, I know of only one study in the health area. In it the same message about dental care was communicated in three ways—to produce (1) minimal fear, (2) moderate fear, and (3) strong fear.

The success of the three statements of the message in changing dental hygiene practices was inversely related to the strength of the fear-producing messages. The general implication is that some anxiety arousal is necessary; otherwise the individual feels no reason to act. But producing extreme anxiety decreases the likelihood of action.

There is one other point about use of fear in our communications. To arouse fear without a clearly defined course of action to reduce the fear is a dangerous procedure. Psychiatrists tell us an individual cannot live with intense anxiety for any period of time. He will either deny the described danger as nonexistent or else he will take whatever action (or actions) he can think of that seems to reduce the danger. Regardless of which type of behavior the individual chooses—that is, denial of the danger or useless and ineffective action—he is not likely to respond to a subsequent communication urging a more effective type of action.

I must confess there is no direct field research confirming this theory, but laboratory experiments with anxiety-arousing stimuli attest to its validity. The possibility that the theory is true warrants caution in the use of scare techniques in our health messages.

Considerable research has been done on the arrangement of arguments in a communication. Without describing the data, let me outline a few of the findings. In situations where there are conflicting viewpoints, a two-sided presentation is more influential than a one-sided presentation if (1) the recipient is initially opposed, (2) he has relatively high intellectual ability, or (3) he will be subsequently exposed to opposing arguments. Perhaps these findings should be tested on the fluoridation controversy in communities not as enlightened as Grand Rapids!

Another type of research considers the person who issues the communication and its effect on the acceptance of the message. Two important findings are:

1. The more trustworthy and expert the recipient perceives the communicator to be, the more likely is his message to be accepted.

2. If a communicator's message has a definite intention of persuading others, then the chances are increased that he will be perceived as having something to gain if the message is accepted. Although he may still be considered an expert, he is judged to be less trustworthy as a source of information.

These are only a few of the findings I have culled from the research on the nature of communications. Abelson has put together in a summary volume entitled *Persuasion* many such findings stated in practical everyday language. I recommend that volume to you.

What's the Best Medium?

Often I am asked: "What is the most effective medium of communication for health messages? Is it movies, newspapers, posters, pamphlets, or exhibits?" In many respects this question is analogous to the question I might ask of a doctor: "What is the best medicine to use in illness?" In both cases the answer is that it depends on the situation and what result one is trying to produce.

However, there is some evidence on the effectiveness of various media. The National Association of Science News Writers made a random sampling survey of almost 2,000 individuals. They sought answers to such questions as: "Who gets what science news, where do they get it, and what do they think about it?" In the analysis they separate medical news from all other science news. They report that the percentages of people who use the various mass media to obtain medical science news are: newspapers, 60 percent; magazines, 20 percent; radio, 7 percent; and television, 25 percent.

However, when these percentages are broken down by sex and education, less than 20 percent of the men and 30 percent of the women with a grade school education or less ever read any medical science news. If our goal is to inform the better-educated people, newspapers doubtless are the best medium. Generally, however, we are attempting to communicate with people who have little education, not only to inform them but to move them to action. This study would indicate that for this purpose, mass media have serious limitations.

One other research finding on the effectiveness of mass media may be worth reporting. In 1941 David Goodman, in his New York University Ph.D. thesis, tested the relative effectiveness of sound movies, silent movies, sound film strips, and film strips with captions. Four comparable groups were given the same message, using one of these methods with each group. So far as information is concerned, the film strip was more effective than the movie, and the silent movie was more effective than the talking movie. This same type of study was performed in Czechoslovakia with almost identical results. All the research to date confirms one fundamental fact—that face-to-face communication in imparting information and stimulating action is superior to any other method.

All of you know the work of Radke on the value of group discussion-leading-to-decision as a method of changing food habits. Confirmation of this finding was reported by Betty Bond in her attempt to stimulate breast self-examination among women in Duluth.

Gladys Gallup of the Department of Agriculture states that mass media are most successful when (1) the message is simple, (2) the suggested action is close to present practices, and (3) the message is directed to the well-educated. Face-to-face communication is preferred when (1) the message is more complex, (2) the change in behavior is more extensive, and (3) the communication is for the lower educational and economic class.

Dr. Kumata, Professor of Mass Communications at Michigan State University, views the communication task of health workers in five steps: (1) interest—in the new message; (2) awareness—that a change could be made; (3) trial—give the change a try; (4) evaluation—do I like it? and (5) adoption—make it a habit. He further notes that for the first two steps, interest and awareness, mass media are quite effective, but for the last three—which seek action and habit formation—mass media are not particularly useful.

Discussing this matter at the National Health Forum, Leo Brown of the American Medical Association summed it up happily when he said:

> It takes two to tango, two to love, and two to communicate. But you have not danced until you have effected some motion. You have not loved until you have stimu-

lated emotions. And you have not communicated until you have caused some thought or action on the part of the receiver.

Communication is a two-way street. To get, you must give. To hear, you must listen. To see, you must first perceive. To read, you must comprehend. The wink of an eye, the shrug of a shoulder, the sway of the hips are often considered effective means of communicating. There are times when silence itself can have a tremendous impact.

Summary

Success in handling new public health demands of the second half of this century requires that we become much more precise and adept in an old technique—communications. We must improve communication from scientist to scientist, from scientist to practitioner, among practitioners who are working together, and from practitioners to those who benefit from our services.

We can begin by learning and putting into practice the existing research on the communication process. We can improve our skill by initiating research focused specifically on the communication of health information and improvement of health practices. If we concentrate on the recipient of health messages and his reactions, we will reap bigger dividends in future efficiency than by concentrating on various methods of communication. Finally, if we approach the matter of health communication with the same scientific methods that we apply in our attacks on disease, I am sure we will be equally successful.

Discussion Questions

1. What does the term *communication* mean?

2. Why did Derryberry believe communication was so important in health education?

3. Where were some of the communication improvements needed according to Derryberry?

4. What are factors that influence a person's acceptance of and action on health messages?

5. What is the best communication medium for health messages?

18

The Patient and His Family

A Focus for Health Education

Health education of patients and their families is receiving increased emphasis as a way of improving the health practices of people. It is also being recognized as part of the treatment regime of the patient. Health education in connection with hospital stays has long been advocated, though not frequently practiced. More recently, education about health has been emphasized in connection with all phases of medical care. In much of the discussion of health education in relation to medical care, the emphasis is limited to imparting information. In this chapter, the term *health education* will embrace *all* those experiences of patient and family with health personnel, organizations, and resources that affect their reactions to health situations. In other words, it refers to everything that influences the information people acquire, the way they feel about health conditions, and the health actions they take. What has aroused this mounting interest in the health education of the patient and his family? Let me mention just three of the many reasons:

1. It is well documented that motivation is essential to learning. Individuals who are sick are far more concerned about improving their health or taking action to prevent repetition of their

---

Originally presented at a meeting of the Western Branch of the American Public Health Association, May 28, 1963, Phoenix, Arizona.

illness than are those who are relatively healthful. Quite
often other members of the family of sick individuals become
more interested in health. At the time of an illness, there is
usually a greater motivation to learn, and health education is
likely to be more effective. (Some exceptions to this generalization will be examined later in this chapter.)

2. Concentration of educational effort on the family members of
   patients who seek medical advice will reach an increasingly
   large segment of the population. For example, 25 million hos-
   pitalizations are predicted for this year—one for every eight
   Americans. If we use the census figure of 3.6 persons per family, then it would be possible to reach 66.7 million people if
   every family were provided with some health education experience at the time of hospitalization of one member. If, in
   addition, health education opportunities were provided for
   the families of patients who go to private physicians, then
   more than half our population could be reached by concentrating on patients and their families.

3. For many, if not all, patients, education is a part of therapy.
   Patients and their family members are instructed about their
   illness and the actions to be taken to hasten the curative
   process. If sufficient attention is given to making available
   wanted information and providing a satisfying experience,
   the patient and family will learn much about what they can
   do to prevent future illnesses.

Health education centered on the patient and his family differs
in one important respect from health education focused on prevention. The former represents a crisis or at least a stressful circumstance. It involves anxiety and emotional reactions about which
we know far too little, and particularly how these anxiety feelings
influence the learning or health education that takes place. In a cri-

sis there is motivation, but one cannot be sure the learning that occurs will lead to future positive action.

In the general population, we are dealing with the normal individual or family, and with this group we often hear the wail, "How can I motivate them to learn and to act?" We sometimes take refuge in responding, "People will be motivated to learn and change when they are sick; therefore we should give more attention to health education in connection with medical care." Actually, we recognize that this generalization is not too accurate. Different people react differently depending on the illness they have or suspect. For example, Sullivan found that the families of rheumatic fever patients learned all there was to know (so far as they were concerned) about rheumatic fever within two or three weeks after the diagnosis. Their information may have come from the *Reader's Digest*, medical books, or friends. Nevertheless, they learned fast, and their opinions, even if erroneous, were not easily changed.

Various studies of people's attitudes and reactions to cancer give quite a different picture. People who know that their symptoms may be related to cancer delay longer in seeking medical care than patients with the same symptoms who are ignorant of the association. It is also reported that family members of cancer patients delay longer in seeking medical checkups than those in families who have had no cancer.

I mention these simply to illustrate that a family's experience with a disease does not assure that they have learned what to do about it.

Do we have evidence of people's reactions to other diseases or symptoms? Do we know what diagnoses people will refuse to accept as applying to them? A health educator recently told me that for a long time she could not accept the diagnosis of an ulcer in her own case. She also recalled a nurse acquaintance who felt the same way about her diagnosis of tuberculosis. The doctor said, "Well, come in tomorrow and we will treat your pneumonia." Because the reactions of patients and families may be highly specific, education based on a generality about people learning and changing when they are sick can lead us down very unproductive paths.

Turning to other obstacles, the literature is filled with anecdotes about the difficulty of communication between patients and medical personnel. First, there is the difference in vocabulary. All of you can recount examples, but a particularly pathetic one occurred on an Indian reservation. An Indian mother brought her baby, seriously dehydrated from diarrhea, to the doctor. He gave the mother a medicine and told her to go home and "push fluids" on the baby. The mother followed his instruction literally. She forced water into the baby until he strangled—and he died six hours later.

Second, there is the time factor. Does the doctor have time, or take time, to communicate? Just yesterday, while I was lunching with a general practitioner to discuss communications, he said, "I didn't take the necessary time to communicate with my last two patients because I was rushing to keep this appointment."

Third, the emotional stress often militates against clear and effective communication. In the past we have largely assumed that only the patient and his family were under stress. More recent data note that the doctor, as well as the nurse, may be unable to communicate clearly because of their own stressful feelings. The strain may be due to the immediate circumstance or to habit patterns established by past anxieties.

Fourth, too often the exposure to the communication is a single experience. There is no place to turn for reinforcement or confirmation. Nor have we built into the patient-family–health personnel relationship reinforcing or reassuring mechanisms.

Fifth, and perhaps most important, are the different perceptions of the doctor-patient, nurse-patient, and other relationships that vary almost as much as the individuals concerned. Well, what is being done to improve communications? Are we exploring and testing new methods or ideas? If we are, little of it has appeared in the literature. Some work has been reported in cross-cultures, primarily with Mexicans and Indians, but not much in the general population.

In a study to be conducted soon, Dr. Butterworth of our office plans to make tape recordings of doctor-patient conversations. Shortly thereafter, he will interview the doctor to ascertain exactly what he planned to get across to this patient. About two weeks later he will interview the patient to determine what the patient thought the physician told him about his illness and its treatment. He will also learn how the patient is carrying out instructions and what questions he still wants answered. If a breakdown in communication occurs, the recorded conversation of doctor and patient and the interview will be examined for clues. In subsequent cases, attempts will be made to overcome such difficulties, and this trial-and-error process will continue as long as it is productive. This is only one approach, but it illustrates the kind of exploration that can be done and a method of delving deeper into the matter, with built-in evaluation.

Another deterrent to effective education, closely allied to communication, is the number of sources of health information and the fact that so often they conflict. A further complication is our rapidly changing scientific scene. New medical discoveries seem almost miraculous. Patients and families are frequently confused when the doctor says the widely heralded method will not benefit their condition. Is it any wonder, then, that patients go shopping around for the popular diagnosis or miracle drug they want or, on the other hand, become such easy prey to quacks? Have we not, perhaps, been too content oriented or task oriented in our educational efforts? Have we not concentrated too much on "do this" or "do that," without adequate explanation and background for intelligent understanding and choice?

John Gardner, in his 1962 report to the Carnegie Corporation, strikes at the heart of a similar matter. In the following quotation he is talking about the education of youth to cope with rapid change, but his words seem to apply almost equally well to our education efforts with patients and families:

If we indoctrinate the young person in an elaborate set of fixed beliefs, we are ensuring his early obsolescence. The alternative is to develop skills, attitudes, habits of mind, and the kind of knowledge and understanding that will be the instruments of continuous change and growth on the part of the young person.

Even if such a goal for patients and families is too ideal, should we not at least move in this direction and experiment with ways of educating patients to accept change and to handle conflicting advice? You may ask me "How?" My answer is that it demands imaginative, creative exploration—a challenging activity for each one of us.

A third handicap to effective education of patients and their families is the complicated way we have organized health services. A family I know has a cerebral-palsied child. For two years, the family was referred to a variety of health agencies for different services. Each time they were asked a long list of questions, many identical to those previously asked. Yet no one agency put together the information about the child and how best to care for him. Fortunately, the father (a health educator) continued looking for resources until he found those that did fulfill the child's needs.

Hospitals can be as disjointed with their many specialty clinics. Aware of this, many hospitals are beginning to coordinate their services, but a large number have yet to start.

How are we counteracting the *negative* educational effects of this fragmentation of specialized services? Much is said about coordination, but is it the complete solution?

Marian Leach, working in the San Francisco Bay area, is approaching the problem in a different way. Starting with an index family from a health agency, she will trace their experiences in obtaining services from other agencies to which they are referred. If a breakdown in service or an unsatisfactory experience that can be remedied occurs, it will be discussed by the agencies concerned with an eye to correcting the situation and preventing a negative impact on the patient.

Throughout this presentation, I have been hammering at one essential point: our crying need to explore in depth ways of realizing the enormous potential for improving health attitudes and practices of families through more effective educational efforts by all concerned.

We cannot expect those whose primary task is direct service to the patient to make the meticulous type of exploration that is required. Just as research workers and their clinical associates explore ways to put a scientific finding into practice, those concerned with education and changed behavior must look for ways of utilizing the data we have accumulated in order to improve health attitudes and practices.

These explorations will not be cheap. They are complicated operations, touching on the reactions of professional personnel, the lay public, institutions, and practices with long traditions. However, unless we dare to venture, we can reap only partial benefits from the remarkable medical findings of past decades and those to come.

When we spend so much for medical research, should we not invest a small fraction of our creativity and funds in finding out how to make maximum use of all advances through health education?

Summary

Several reasons are presented to consider the patient and his family as a focus for health education. A few of the obstacles to successful health education in stressful situations are explored. Many more, only hinted at, are of equal significance. Finally, it is emphasized that we should not accept, as if it were an axiom, that all patient and family experiences are positive in their educational results. A plea is made for more creative and investigative effort by health professionals and institutions to make better use of their opportunities for health education with the patient and his family.

This is a complex matter, to be tackled by doctors, nurses, health educators, behavioral scientists—in fact, by all those interested in improved health behavior of the public. It is one to evoke our best efforts. I know we will respond.

Discussion Questions

1. How does health education centered on the patient and family (with defined health problems) differ from health education focused on prevention?

2. What are some obstacles to successful health education in stressful settings?

3. How can opportunities for health education of the patient and his or her family be improved?

Part IV

Community Health Education

Overview

I f one were to try to identify a particular, outstanding area in which Mayhew Derryberry continually mobilized his resources and efforts in the Public Health Service, it would be the area of community health education. Dedicated to the principle that only through the active participation of the people themselves can life patterns gradually be changed, Dr. Derryberry sought to demonstrate the viability of this principle.

Derryberry established the concept of community demonstration programs in health education and recruited a series of competent health educators to staff these projects, which were sponsored all over the country from Puerto Rico to California. He assumed leadership positions in organizations such as the American Public Health Association and encouraged his staff to exert leadership through organizing workshops, writing papers, and participating with other groups, such as the W. K. Kellogg Foundation and the National Training Laboratories, to improve the state of the art of community health education.

The first chapter in Part Four (Chapter Nineteen) emphasizes technique transfer between agriculture and public health, describing Derryberry's vision that problem solving approached in the style of the agricultural extension worker had merit in public health. He presents two community organization experiences: one starting with the recognized leaders in an area; the other with the people themselves. He felt that a "public health extension worker" could implement either approach for international health programs. These approaches later became the basis for training programs for community health educators. We now call the process *community networking*.

So far, the chapters have dealt with specific elements. In the chapters in Part Four, Dr. Derryberry puts the elements of program development together and offers a series of sequential steps to arrive at the desired goal. The result, illustrated in Chapter Twenty, is an early endorsement of training public health workers in the principles of community organization as well as in facilitating large citizen groups in thinking about and planning for improvement of their members' health.

In Chapter Twenty-One, coauthored with Nell McKeever, five insights present the implications for public health programs as the nation's priorities shift from the mass communicable disease control measures of the past to the individualized chronic disease control measures of the future. This chapter points out the tremendous consequences of this shift for health education practices. First published in 1956, it raises serious questions that still await concrete answers. It is up to today's public health educators to provide the momentum to effectively respond to these questions.

Finally, Chapter Twenty-Two, prepared for a World Health Organization Study Group, illustrates how the principles of health education can be applied as a practical matter to a given program area, namely, family planning.

19

Extension Experience in Public Health

Public health today has three great areas of interest: prevention of disease, control of disease, and promotion of positive health for all the people.

Within these areas are rich opportunities for cooperation between public health and agriculture, especially in working in war-torn areas. It has long been known that some diseases can be prevented or controlled effectively through the efforts of a relatively few people, thus promoting the positive health of a great number of people. Responsibility for resettlement sites, water supplies, and sewage disposal rests with experts trained to deal with these matters.

There is a second group of diseases, however, the prevention and control of which are possible only through active participation of practically all of the people. Experiments to find out how this participation on the part of the people could be enlisted in matters of health have been carried out by many groups, of which the Public Health Service and the W. K. Kellogg Foundation programs serve as examples of different approaches.

Coauthored by Mayhew Derryberry and J. O. Dean. Originally published in *The Contribution of Extension Methods and Techniques Toward the Rehabilitation of War-Torn Countries*, Report of the Conference on April 19–22, 1944, U.S. Department of Agriculture. Reprinted with permission.

The Public Health Service's experimental program in health education in war areas was an emergency measure at the outset. Trained health education consultants were lent by the Public Health Service to states and assigned by them to county health units in war-boom and extra-cantonment areas. After a careful survey of the health assets and needs of the county and interviews with key women in the communities, local women were stimulated to organize themselves (usually on the block plan) into study groups to learn about local health problems and what could be done about them. Through these study groups, many women were awakened for the first time to the fact that rats infested their town, that epidemics of intestinal upsets occurred because of unsanitary handling of food in local restaurants, and that prostitutes and "pickups" on their street corners were spreading venereal diseases to soldiers.

Women discussed these problems and, as a group, decided what they could do about them—and then did it. The professional worker acted at all times only as the catalyst who stimulated and expedited action but did not in any way take over the responsibilities of the local women. Though the program was initiated on an emergency basis, the foundations were laid for long-range programs to follow up.

A different approach to long-range community organization was carried out by the Kellogg Foundation in its seven-county demonstrations in Michigan. The problem was attacked by means of a widespread adult-education program designed to develop local leadership. Different approaches were formulated for the various professional and lay groups, both organized and unorganized. One group stimulated another to requesting guidance until, over a period of 12 years, scarcely a group remains in the seven counties that has not participated in some educational program contributing in some way to raising the health level of the area. The two experiments briefly described represent two different ways of using the problem-solving approach effectively. One starts with the recognized leaders in an area; the other, with the people themselves. Both have been successful because they have been fundamentally sound and executed in a democratic manner. They show, above all, that there is no one way to do health education, but the program must be adapted to local needs and follow to some extent the familiar pattern of the population.

These demonstrations of extension work with rural people perhaps point to one way in which problems in foreign countries could be approached in a realistic manner, not by handing out things free, but by stimulating local organization and lending a helping hand when requested, and by working through local leaders the people already recognize.

Through this problem-solving approach, which can be applied to any other field as well as to public health, the professional worker gives guidance and stimulus but lets the people develop their own solutions. Only through this active participation of the people themselves can patterns of life gradually be changed and better, more healthful habits be practiced.

Basic Principles

1. Community health education is an activity of the people, but well-qualified, trained personnel are needed to guide this work.

2. Personnel should not be spread too thin. Concentrate initial work in a small area and then expand to neighboring areas as leaders are found locally.

3. In going into an area, capitalize on existing community interests. Work on a problem in which the people are interested and gradually work around to those in which they should be interested.

4. Keep in mind and be guided by the standards, policies, practices, and mores of the group with which you are working.

5. Have a plan and frequently stop to evaluate progress. Let speed and method of procedure be determined by the people doing the traveling, not by the professional worker.

6. Better results are obtained if the people have a hand in the planning.

7. If policy is "demonstrate and withdraw," the training of local leaders or professional workers is essential to carry on the program after the demonstration personnel leave.

8. In emergencies, people experienced in the field of education can be given training on specific aspects of public health to carry on a program in their home communities. This type of personnel needs much counseling and close supervision.

9. A demand for services that cannot be obtained should not be created in the population. First, professional workers should be trained and provided with facilities so that they can "deliver" when the demand comes from the people.

Discussion Questions

1. What are the three great areas of interest in public health described by Derryberry?

2. Are these still relevant today? Why? Why not?

3. What are some basic principles of public health described in this chapter that remain globally relevant today?

4. What are some of the current global health issues in which health educators might be actively involved?

20

Health Is Everybody's Business

Not so long ago, one of the outstanding leaders of public health said, "You know, I used to think that the main purpose for bringing the community into the program was to get support for the activities we wanted to carry out." This statement typifies the public health thinking of a quarter of a century ago. Professional workers carefully studied the situation, developed a program that they considered good for the people, and then tried to obtain their support. Public health leaders were afraid to give citizens too much, if any, voice in the development of the program, for fear they might want to do something the experts didn't think right. Frequently, such statements as the following were made: "Laymen get too enthusiastic and move too fast." "They are uninformed and demand things we can't do." So long as the professional health workers could provide mass disease control through some activity of their own, like providing a clean and safe milk and water supply, or adequate sewage disposal, such an attitude did not detract from public health progress.

But today, the problems are changed, and the interests of citizens are becoming more intimately concerned with health. How to capitalize on this interest and bring about constructive group

Originally published in *Public Health Reports*, October 14, 1949, 64(41), 1293–1298. Reprinted with permission.

thinking and planning by the citizens is a major task for public health workers.

The problem has at least two important aspects: (1) how to involve large groups of people with varying backgrounds, interests, and experience in working harmoniously together, and (2) how to change the attitude of professional public health workers so that they will aid group thinking and planning by citizens for improvement of their own health. Some suggestions for working out these two problems may be gleaned from the experimental programs conducted by social psychologists, adult educators, industrial relations officers, and workers in community organization and social group work.

1. *The first and most important step in group planning by citizens is that the problem to be worked on should be selected by them and be one that a majority of the members of the group feel is important.* Too often in the past, the problem has been one selected by professional workers. But are the people always interested in the problems proposed by the public health professional? It is difficult to interest an individual in having a careful periodic medical examination for the protection of his health in the future when he has a throbbing toothache. Groups frequently can't be interested in preschool health programs when the filth around them is the problem that is disturbing them most. The immediate problem selected must be the one that the people recognize as important.

Sometimes the problem has been determined by a superficial annoyance of one citizen who is determined to dominate and have his problem solved, regardless of group concerns. This is not an easy situation to handle, but as groups become more skilled in working together, they will be able to avoid the pitfall of satisfying only a domineering citizen.

The most usual method of problem selection begins with a survey, sometimes conducted by experts but preferably conducted by the citizens themselves. All too often, however, the completion of the survey, making of recommendations, and printing of the report (to adorn library shelves) are accepted as the solution of the problem. A recommendation is made that somebody else do something, and through that method, those who should take action wash their hands of any further responsibility. If surveys are to be used, the people should make the survey or at least frame the recommendations for the action they will take.

The social psychologists suggest a problem census as the method for selecting a problem on which to work, that is, listing all the problems with which the various group members are concerned. Professional workers are always afraid that the laymen are not aware of the important problems. Actually, in any such compilation made by interested citizens, the entire gamut of health problems will always be covered. From the listed problems, priorities can be established through group decision.

2. *The goal to be achieved with reference to any problem must be realistic and not visionary and entirely idealistic.* In determining a realistic goal, it is necessary to appraise carefully the resources available to the group. Individuals and organizations must be given the opportunity to define their own level of participation. How many of us have seen Mr. and Mrs. Fix-It, who alienated many potential workers on a project by saying, "I have it all worked out: Mrs. Jones, you do this; Mr. Smith, your organization can do this." The hostile reactions to such a person need not be described. The only resources consistently available on any project are those that are volunteered. It is the job of the professional health worker to secure maximum volunteer participation.

Not only must the positive resources available be appraised, but there must also be a clear delineation of the factors in the situation that will interfere with achievement of the goal. For example, cultural and traditional food patterns need to be carefully considered in any program of improving nutrition. We learned this lesson in the war, and seldom now do we hear the comment in regard to immigrants' foodways, "I just can't get those people to eat an American diet." We learned then that the supplementation of the diets of various cultures was what was needed, rather than the standard (American) dietary pattern.

Another factor that must never be overlooked is organized opposition. Dr. Florence Sabin tells the story of her work in Colorado and how the people had worked for passage of a certain law. Because they had not foreseen that the law would be opposed by a particular group within the state, the law failed to pass. How to cope with pressure groups is a long story in itself, but as citizen groups gain more skill in democratic planning and action for the welfare of all the people, the influence of organized opposition will decline.

Still another consideration in the selection of a realistic goal is the need for some success early in the period of working together. It is far better to get a vacant lot cleaned up as a first step toward more vital citizen participation in health activities than to attempt to get every expectant mother under medical care when there are not sufficient doctors to give the care. The first success will give skill in working together so that more difficult problems can be attacked over longer periods of time.

Citizens can be aided in their selection of a realistic goal if they call in as technical advisers the professional experts in the field. The experts can give information, describe the limitations of various procedures, and perhaps even suggest other goals, but they do not tell the citizens what to select.

3. *The third step is the development of a workable plan.* When all the people have been involved in both the selection of the problem and the definition of the goal, they naturally will be in on the planning. Too often the first time all the people are brought in is after the plan has been developed by a professional worker, a voluntary agency, or a dynamic community "do-gooder." One of the reasons for not including everyone during the development of plans is the desire for credit by those who take over the planning function. Recently a national organization, which shall be designated by "X," developed a plan suggesting that the local chapters should get the cooperation of all other interested agencies in communities

in carrying out the plan, but also cautioning that the program must be kept an "X" organization project.

Perhaps we should take a hint from the Japanese Diet. It is said that each member of the Diet expresses his opinion as to how a given problem should be solved. Once having given his opinion, he no longer claims it as his own; it becomes the property of the group. From all the ideas proposed, a plan is eventually adopted that represents a universal group decision. If the plan should fail, the group and not any one individual is responsible for its failure. It is too dangerous for an individual to be responsible for the plan because a failure of the plan would require that the individual commit hara-kiri. In addition, the proposal is more likely to succeed because it has the backing of the entire group.

Ivah Deering, in her book *Let's Try Thinking*, says: "To think [a problem] through within and with the assistance of the group is to build under subsequent action a foundation which will stand greater storms and stresses, for it is made up of understanding, cooperation, and common effort." Therefore, if we want all the people to contribute more effectively to the total community health, we must find ways to let them do the planning.

4. *The fourth step is action.* Nothing is harder for a group to do than to get into action. Of course, if members of the group have been involved in the three enumerated steps above, they are much more likely to take action. Suggested aids for getting into gear are: (1) the group should commit itself both collectively and as individuals to do some specific thing; (2) there should be a time limit set; (3) the action to be taken should not require too long a time before the group reassembles to consider progress and further steps; and (4) if possible, every member should get some feeling of success.

5. *The results of the action must be objectively evaluated.* Quite often, and rightly so, at the completion of some project or community action there is a "success banquet." Such occasions serve a very valuable purpose, but should there not also be a much more soul-searching session? Perhaps the celebration is for publicity purposes.

But if citizens are to get more skill in solving health problems, should they not be willing to look back objectively on past performance and evaluate it, not so much in terms of the actual achievement as in terms of the process they followed? What were the steps they took that were most helpful in achieving the goal, and what did they do that could be improved? Did they have too many meetings or too few? Did they move into action without adequate plans? Did they have the best technical advice they could obtain? Did they use it in the best manner and at the right time? Were all the people aware of the problem, and did they have opportunity to participate in the planning as well as in the action? Only through such careful study (introspection, if you will) of the methods they used to work together, and the reactions of all the people toward the procedure and toward one another, can they learn to increase the quality and amount of improvement in health through participation.

Suggestions for Professional Health Workers

All the suggestions above have been directed primarily toward the ways in which citizens can effectively make health their business. Occasionally, reference has been made to the expert, or professional health worker, but only incidentally. Now let's turn our attention to those in that category and see what suggestions there are for them.

First, it may be said that the role professional workers play cannot be as clearly delineated. But there are some attitudes we should possess:

1. We must have faith, yes, even a conviction, that every citizen has a potential contribution to make for the betterment of his community. The quality and amount of the contribution may be great or small, but regardless of its magnitude or quality, every opportunity should be given for the contribution to be made. It is our job to help uncover any hidden resources that

may reside in people and to help them make their maximum contribution.

2. We must have faith in the democratic principle that the decisions of an informed majority are right. We must have that faith even though the decisions made by a group do not conform with our own opinions. If it is in our field of expertise, then we can only attribute the decision, which we may consider incorrect, as being our failure to provide adequate information, or, if we are truly objective and honest, perhaps we would face the possibility that we might be wrong. Sometimes professional persons overlook the fact that they are subject to human errors of judgment.

3. We must have faith that a group thinking together, and utilizing the contributions that all can make, can produce more and better results than can any one individual in the group working alone. Even though we repeat that we have profound faith in the group, we often act as if we did not believe our own words. A reason for this inconsistency may be that most groups have not developed skill in the mechanics of working together productively. Furthermore, most individuals with training in special fields know very little about how to guide a group toward the expression of its ideas. Because professional leaders become overprotective, they often fail to give the group a chance to practice independent thinking. Our job is not merely one of making special resources or information available to others. Our job is also to help the group to work effectively. This is a problem all its own.

4. We must be sufficiently patient to let a group take such time as is necessary to arrive at its conclusions. If information is given too quickly, the group may be pushed into indecision.

5. We must develop insight and an understanding of interpersonal and intergroup relations so that we can help individuals and groups get satisfaction from their participation and

increase their own feeling of worth among their fellow men. The studies of social psychologists are constantly enriching our knowledge of human motivation. Again and again, psychological research underlines the power of the need to be approved by one's associates.

6. We must coordinate our services and activities in order that we will not duplicate services or compete with one another in the field. Too few professional workers are available for us to waste their time and effort by using several persons to do what can be done by one with adequate planning. Certainly we should not tolerate duplication. Sharing responsibilities and services is one of the skills we must improve.

All over the country, citizens are becoming more and more concerned about the health of the nation. A few suggestions for making that concern more productive in terms of community action, using the skills and abilities of all people, lay and professional, have been discussed. It is hoped that putting the suggestions in organized form might stimulate wider and more intensive activity in the future.

Summary

Wider group participation in planning for health is contingent upon (1) developing group experience in cooperative action, and (2) educating professional public health workers in methods of securing such action from groups:

Members of the group should select their own problems.

The group's goal should be defined realistically and achieved by a program that is practical.

The methods employed in securing group action should be analyzed when the program is completed.

Professional health workers must have sincere faith, practiced as well as voiced, in the worth of methods of democratic action.

Further, they must increasingly strive to learn to deal with groups as an integral aspect of their own professional skills.

Discussion Questions

1. How does Derryberry view the role of the citizen in community-based health programs?

2. What are some problems related to groups of large people being involved in public health as described in this chapter?

3. How has this viewpoint changed over time, if at all, and what implications does this have for today's health educator and community-based participatory research in health promotion and disease prevention?

21

What Does the Changing Picture in Public Health Mean to Health Education in Programs and Practices?

Discussed here are five insights that need greatly to be sharpened if modern-day health education is to achieve scientific stature. The behavioral sciences are the means through which these insights may be sharpened. Incidentally, health educators are not the only health workers who need the help of these sciences.

Four years ago some of us had the pleasure of hearing C.E.A. Winslow discuss developments in public health education beginning with his appointment as director of a new division in the New York State Health Department called Publicity and Education. In his words, the publication entitled *Health News* "gradually developed in the light of the knowledge of the times." That was 1914, when the picture was changing from one in which technical staffs working alone or with a small segment of the population could design health programs and manipulate the environment for the benefit of the people to one in which people needed to be informed and to take some action if such diseases as diphtheria, smallpox, and malaria were to be controlled.

Coauthored by Mayhew Derryberry and Nell McKeever. Originally published in the *American Journal of Public Health*, January 1956, 46(1), 54–60. Address given at APHA 83rd Annual Meeting, Kansas City, Missouri, November 15, 1955. Reprinted with permission.

Fitting into the pattern of this 83rd Annual Meeting of the Association, the Public Health Education Section turns its attention to meeting the challenge of today's picture and attempts to project it into the future. Perhaps we should spend some time thinking about our heritage. Certainly, we would like to acknowledge our debt to the early leaders for their insight into change, for their vision into the future, and for their courage in exploring an untried area. We think, however, that these same leaders might be somewhat disappointed if we took too much time looking backward—our job is today and looking forward to tomorrow.

"In the light of the knowledge of the times," what do we see? We see our country no longer threatened by the dreaded epidemic diseases of a past generation. Through the extension of effective public health measures, the development of vaccines, serums, and antibiotics, and better medical care, the deadly communicable diseases of the past have been brought under control. But they have been replaced by other problems—heart disease, cancer, mental illness, arthritis, diabetes, accidents, and so on. These are the serious problems of today. They are the conditions to which we as public health workers must direct our attention if we are to fulfill our mission. As health educators, what is our place in this picture? What responsibilities are ours? Are we prepared to meet these responsibilities adequately? Or are we still hoping that the methods of 1914, which were effective in solving the problems of that day, will solve the very different problems of today?

We believe that we can document some changes, such as: a greater understanding that an effective educational program must provide people with opportunities to learn their responsibilities rather than depending entirely on the transmission of scientific facts; more concern with helping people and communities determine their health problems and use their own ways to solve them; a growing recognition that individuals and groups are unique in terms of goals, experience, aspirations, and ways of working; and more emphasis on the kind of planning in which community members join with technical staffs in developing health programs. However, we are in an era where, more than ever before, improvement in health depends upon constructive action of individuals and groups. How much understanding of human behavior and the process of education have we introduced into the public health field? If this is our primary responsibility, how can we strengthen our efforts? And, difficult as it is, how can we anticipate the future to be ready to meet the demands effectively?

Health education looks to two broad disciplines for its practices: the natural and developmental sciences for its content and the social sciences for its methods and technics.

At the present time, chronic diseases take a tremendous toll. Knowledge regarding ways of preventing the chronic and debilitating diseases is limited. The actions that must be taken to prevent further disability after the diseases are recognized are still somewhat vague and ill-defined, although medical science has made possible the prevention of the more serious consequences of many of the chronic diseases. To a very large extent, however, these preventive measures require changes in daily living, many of them unpleasant and some of them counter to social customs.

We may expect research in the natural sciences to provide data that will (1) lead to the prevention of the degenerative process, (2) reduce and curtail disability, and (3) improve tools for the early discovery of degenerative diseases.[1] As this progress is made, the behavior that people will need to practice in order to benefit from the discoveries will change, probably toward behaviors that are clearer and more specific than those we now know. For example, a short time ago there was a list of rules to follow to cut down the risk of polio. Informing people about these rules was difficult. Observance of the rules was even more difficult. The discovery of the vaccine provides not only a specific course of action, but the action and the results are clearly correlated.

We now have asparagine for epilepsy and reserpine and other drugs being used in the treatment of some mental disorders. We are told that even though all the factors associated with coronary occlusion may not be defined, it is certainly not out of the realm of possibility that a substance can be found that will prevent the thickening inside the vessel. Perhaps the day may come when we will be eating this substance in bread, drinking it in water, or taking it like a vitamin pill.

As scientific advances are made, they will be of benefit only if the findings of the laboratory can become meaningful to the people. Other "miracle" methods may be found, but now, and perhaps for some time to come, changes in daily living are going to be necessary to reduce disability. Through education, can we lead people from limited to broader understandings and practices? Can educators help people form desirable patterns of attitudes and behaviors in line with scientific facts? Studies of the resistance encountered in gaining acceptance of new health and medical discoveries, such as the study of the opposition to the effort to fluoridate the water supply in Northampton, Massachusetts, reported by Bernard and Judith Mausner,[2] can give us valuable clues as to what happens when it is taken for granted that people will act automatically on scientific evidence as presented.

Closely correlated with the increased importance of chronic disease, and yet a problem quite distinct, is adapting to growing old. As progress is made in preventing psychological and physiological deterioration, education must help to find a way to assist the senior members of society to make a satisfactory adjustment and an effective contribution while maintaining in society the kind of balance that will serve the best interests of all generations.

Accidents—home, industry, and vehicular—one of the most pressing problems of today, involve a myriad of factors, physical, psychological, and sociological. Much has been done in highway safety to improve road conditions, to standardize rules and regulations, and to provide adequate traffic controls. Automobile manufacturers are becoming more concerned and are advertising a multitude of safety devices, but little impact has been made because the real problem is the behavior of operators and pedestrians. Here is where the attack must be made, unless you are willing to say that the day will come when engineering science will provide the answer in electronically controlled highways and cars to be accelerated, steered, braked, stopped, and moved from one lane to another from highway towers.

In the area of mental health, it is doubtful that any one simple procedure will be found to develop full adjustment to one's environment. If we think of mental health in terms of a mature understanding of behavior, our own in relation to others, leading to a balance between ourselves and our environment, it seems unreasonable to expect any one miracle drug to attain and maintain that balance. We hope that medical and chemical research will provide answers to the serious mental disorders. We may also expect research to make more precise the steps involved in the development of personality patterns. In this age of reliance on outside resources to solve our problems and meet our needs, it seems of utmost importance to place emphasis on the need for people to develop their inner resources, have confidence in their own worth and the worth of others, and be able to work through their problems by drawing on their own skills and abilities. This too is protection, and despite all the fundamental differences, perhaps we can draw an analogy between building this kind of community defense and that which we provide by maintaining a high immunization rate against diphtheria. Because each individual influences the adjustment of others, just as individuals transmit disease to others, it may not be utopian to visualize the day in which one can figuratively immunize against mental disease. What we mean is, if more and more people understand mental phenomena, become well adjusted, and behave accordingly, there will be less opportunity for maladjustments to develop in others.

In the social sciences, we may expect rapid developments from research in unraveling the many facets of human behavior and their interrelated functioning. Emphasis must be placed on the need for more research in this area and financial support for the study of the complexity of human beings. But have we as practitioners in our own professional fields really utilized the research that has been done? Perhaps we have been caught in this world of magic and we are seeking an all-purpose answer to the process of education, without thoughtful diagnosis of the problems involved.

Just as physicians are expected to perform diagnostic tests before treating a disease and epidemiologists to spend the necessary time in diagnosing the problem of an epidemic before instituting community treatment, so the public health field has a right to expect from the health educator a diagnostic approach to the field of human behavior. That is why we raise the questions: Are we using the research that is already available to help us diagnose the problem? What are our goals? What are we moving toward?

In the World Health Organization Expert Committee report *Health Education of the Public*[3] it is stated:

> To accomplish his goal, the educator should have a first-hand knowledge and appreciation of the people with whom he plans to develop a health education programme. He should be familiar with the nature of the culture; the ways of life of the people; their goals in life; and their values, beliefs, traditions, customs and taboos with respect to health and illness. He should understand the objectives for which the people are willing to strive, and, conversely, the aspects of life that mean very little to them or that they are as yet unable to understand. Such understanding of the way of life of the people is important in setting the limits of any educational effort. What are the people willing and able to accept? What will they reject? What are the social and economic conditions

which must exist before certain innovations or educational changes can be undertaken?

Along the same line, social science has pointed out to us that in effective education, these are some of the things we need to diagnose:

1. We need to know the individual's behavior, his beliefs, his motivations, his goals, and ways of carrying these out. Hochbaum,[4] in his paper "Why People Come to Get X-Rayed," says:

   To us, early detection means better prognosis or shorter, simpler therapy. But many people are found to worry less about prognosis or difficulty of treatment and to worry much more about other things; some about losing their jobs and income, others about the shattering of their careers, still others about the financial burden on their families, and the like. Many of these people do not feel that early detection of tuberculosis would do much to alleviate these problems. For them, detection of tuberculosis—early or late—may, with good reason, appear threatening rather than beneficial and, therefore, they tend to avoid being X-rayed.

2. We need to know the individual's attitudes and past experiences that facilitate progress or create barriers to change. Kelley[5] says:

   We do not get our perceptions from the things around us, but the perceptions come from us. Since they do not come from the immediate environment and obviously cannot come from the future, they must come from the past. If they come from the past, they must be based on experience. The things around us have no meaning except as we ascribe meaning to them. They are nothing until we make them something and then they are what we make them. This can only be determined by what we are and where we have been.

3. We need knowledge of the group's goals, traditions, beliefs, practices, values, and cultures. Paul[6] cites the failure of a broad-scale publicity campaign in a Canadian town for the purpose of altering attitudes toward the mentally ill.

> One of the concepts they had sought hard to communicate was that no sharp line divides the sane from the insane, that personality types fall along a continuum running from the fully normal to the fully abnormal, and that released hospital patients are, therefore, not essentially different from other people and should be treated accordingly.
>
> But people in the community clung hard to their black-and-white concept of normality and abnormality. Never certain about their own sanity, they apparently erected a wall of defense that sharply divided the sane from the insane. In trying to undermine this popular attitude, the educators were arousing deep insecurities. The citizens showed outward apathy, attempted to withdraw, and ultimately expressed open hostility to the educators.

Paul says, "The lesson is clear. Before trying to change old health habits and ideas, it is wise to ascertain what they are and, more important, what psychological and social functions these beliefs and practices perform."

4. We need insight into the leadership-followership patterns established by the people. Sanford[7] describes leadership as a

relation: "Psychological factors in the follower as well as psychological factors in the leader help to determine this relation." Closely identified with the leadership-followership patterns are the accepted patterns of communication.[8] Lindgren[9] defines communication as "a process which is concerned with all situations involving meaning. Communication is thus concerned with an individual's attempt to express himself to others, to understand the events which occur around him and to understand himself." Lewin[10] puts emphasis on the gatekeeper and his influence in people's lives as a determining force in the broad area of communication and change.

5. We need to consider the objective advisability of change and the individual's or group's acceptance of change. In the Report of the Subcommittee on Evaluation of Mental Health Activities[11] the statement is made: "In considering the basic assumptions it is pertinent to ask by what right we ask change in others and how sound is our available knowledge." It was observed therein:

> As we react against advertising methods in their use of fear and pressure and promise of total cure, we differentiate ourselves as professional groups—teachers, social workers, sociologists, psychiatrists—dedicated to purposeful change of attitude by the fact of our primary concern for the individual. We have no axe to grind, no special interest of our own to further. Even so, we must stop to wonder at our own temerity and arrogance in asking change of others. We do not know what we think beyond today nor in what direction we are moving.

Introducing change, therefore, is something to be thoughtfully considered. The social anthropologists point out that the cultural patterns of people constitute a complex but firmly integrated whole. When change is introduced into one phase of living, such as health, it may completely destroy other phases of culture that provide real security to the people.

Again, we look to social science for clues to the ways the concept of change can be introduced with a minimum of difficulty and conflict. The manual *Cultural Patterns and Technical Change*[12] recommends that:

> Where specific technical practices are to be introduced into a culture or part of a society which has not hitherto used them, it is desirable to strip these technical practices of as many extraneous cultural accretions as possible. . . . Extraneous and culturally destructive effects can be avoided by stripping such scientific technique to the bone, to the absolute essentials which will make it possible for other people to learn to use it, and to handle it in a living, participating, creative way.

Such a diagnosis takes time if it is to be effective. We look to the day when social scientists will improve the instruments and investigative procedures to the point where precise determination can be made more readily. Meanwhile, how well have we used the methods already available? How effective have we been in using a diagnostic approach to human behavior?

Ahead of us lie comparatively unexplored areas: civil defense, with its emotional overtones of death and destruction. Will survival depend to a large extent on the ability of people to act quickly and effectively in times of emergency? Suburbia, with its problems of moving populations, which brings with it the impact of large groups on administrative setups geared to other days and different situations; medical education, with its demand for creative, imaginative experiences to enrich the quality of medical and community leadership; patient education, in hospitals, clinics, and doctors' offices, in which ideal learning situations are often blocked by apprehensions and misunderstandings in emotionally charged situations;

alcoholism, with its serious social and economic implications; varying population groups and the educational and social problems accompanying integration; new industrial areas; overcrowded schools; inadequate housing; limited rehabilitation facilities. These are the challenges.

How shall we meet them? We suggest that we meet them head-on, fully cognizant of the fact that we may stumble and fall; secure, however, in the knowledge that if we are willing to record our mistakes as well as our successes, we will make a valuable contribution. Again, we owe a debt to the research field for this objective approach to problems.

We have placed emphasis on diagnosis as the first essential in determining programs. Do we need to turn our attention to strengthening our profession? We suggest (1) that we analyze the kind of training given to health educators in "the light of our knowledge" of the kind of job to be done; (2) that we work toward the day when we will have more training in the social sciences so our health educators of the future will be comfortable and secure in working in this area; (3) that we think of training in a formal setting as only the beginning of a series of experiences; (4) that we plan carefully for that next step in career development by providing rich, creative experiences with mature guidance and supervision; (5) that we create opportunities for public health workers and social scientists to work together to solve practical problems; (6) that we test our programs step by step on an exploratory basis; and (7) that we record our efforts, carefully providing a firm foundation for the future.

Summary

The content of health education of the future is going to require changes in behavior. It is the responsibility of the educators to help adapt or find ways of applying the indicated behavior change in the way least upsetting to the established behavior patterns and within the potentialities of the people.

The methods will be much more precise, depending more on scientific determination of the situation, the need for change, the barriers to change, the testing of methods, and the objective measurement of behavior change. This means a closer working relationship with social scientists in practical field operations.

This has meaning for training. For health educators, more training in social science so they feel comfortable and secure working in the behavior area; for all public health workers, opportunities for understanding people, the role of the health educators, and the role of social scientists; for social scientists, opportunities to work with public health people in helping to solve practical problems.

Discussion Questions

1. Derryberry speaks of comparatively unexplored areas in public health? What are these?

2. How insightful do you think his viewpoint is in light of the tragic events of September 11, 2001, and our current health challenges, such as disaster preparedness and the threat of bioterrorism?

3. What implications does his viewpoint have for continuing education of the current health education workforce?

4. Is it still necessary today to change human behavior to prevent motor vehicle crashes?

Notes

1. M. Derryberry, "Today's Health Problems and Health Education," *Public Health Reports*, 69(12), 1224–1228, December 1954.

2. B. Mausner and J. Mausner, "A Study of the Anti-Scientific Attitude," *Scientific American*, *192*(2) 35–39, February 1955.

3. World Health Organization, Technical Report Series No. 89, *Expert Committee on Health Education of the Public, First Report* (Geneva: World Health Organization, October 1954).

4. G. M. Hochbaum, "Why People Come to Get X-Rayed," *Paper presented at the annual meeting of the National Tuberculosis Association*, Milwaukee, Wisconsin, May 25, 1955. (Mimeograph.)

5. E. C. Kelley, *Education for What Is Real* (New York: Harper, 1947).

6. B. D. Paul, "Contributions of Social Service," in *Signs of the Health Times* (New York: National Health Council, March 1955).

7. F. H. Sanford, "The Follower's Role in Leadership Phenomena," in *Readings in Social Psychology* (New York: Holt, 1952).

8. K. W. Back, "Influence Through Social Communication," in *Readings in Social Psychology* (New York: Holt, 1952).

9. H. Clay Lindgren, *The Art of Human Relations* (New York: Hermitage House, 1953).

10. K. Lewin, *Resolving Social Conflicts* (New York: Harper, 1948).

11. *Evaluation in Mental Health*, Report of the Subcommittee on Evaluation of Mental Health Activities (Washington, D.C.: U.S. Department of Health, Education and Welfare, 1955).

12. M. E. Mead, *Cultural Patterns and Technical Change* (Paris: United Nations Education, Scientific and Cultural Organization, 1953).

22

Education in the Health
Aspects of Family Planning

General Considerations

Family planning activities have expanded rapidly and extensively during the past decade in many countries of the world. The impetus for this growth has come from several sources. Health professionals have shown that fertility regulation reduces mortality and morbidity associated with pregnancy and childbirth and contributes indirectly to the general welfare of the family. Thus, family planning has become an important part of the general health service designed to promote the health of the family and society.

Demographers have shown the rapid expansion in population resulting from relatively recent decreases in mortality without corresponding reductions in natality. Their analyses and predictions of the future size of the population and its attendant problems have stimulated many countries to promote family planning as a primary means of reducing rapid population growth.

Economists studying the future demands for commodities and services have shown the impossibility of raising the economic level of a society where the population increase swallows up the economic advance. Family planning has been advocated as one of the

Originally published in *Pacific Health Education Reports*, 1971, 2, 16–50. Reprinted with permission.

ways of reducing population growth and contributing to increased economic development.

Agricultural analysts concerned with producing the necessary food and other agricultural products required by the people of a country have shown that the potential increase in agricultural production will not be adequate for the predicted growth of the population. They too have turned to family planning as one of the means of keeping agricultural production and consumption in balance.

Agencies concerned with accelerating economic and social betterment in developing areas have utilized the findings of the various analysts and have supported and sometimes stipulated extensive family planning services as a part of their development aid.

Promoters of human rights and the status of women in societies of the world have urged family planning information and services as a basic human right. U. Thant has indicated that ". . . information and availability of services in family planning is increasingly considered as a basic human right and as an indispensable ingredient of human dignity."

All these forces have resulted in the rapid development of family planning activities, particularly in countries where population growth is recognized as a problem.

Family Planning Depends on Many Services

The pressures of rapid population increase have stimulated a number of countries to initiate and expand family planning as a unipurpose priority program with little consideration of the level of other services upon which the successful operation of family planning activities may depend. Furthermore, adequate attention has not been given to the contribution family planning can make to achieving other objectives when all the elements necessary for its success are given their proper relative emphasis. For example, many of the methods of family planning, regardless of whether the objective is population control or improvement of health of mother and children, depend on health and medical services for success. The most effective contraceptives—IUD, pills, vasectomy, tubectomy, and the management of sterility—require medical service and/or supervision. Consistent contraceptive use until a pregnancy is planned, conception is achieved, and a successful delivery has occurred demands a continuing health service to follow up in its plan; a program concerned primarily with population growth will not only achieve its objective but will also contribute to improvement of health of the people. This principle has been clearly set forth in the resolutions adopted by the World Health Assemblies.[1,2]

The development of effective family planning is influenced by the educational level of the people. Competent workers are required to staff the program. It is difficult to recruit and train personnel to perform effectively the many necessary functions in family planning when their educational status is low. Long-range considerations for family planning, as for other aspects of health programs, will provide for improving education as a basis for existing and future personnel recruitment.

The above illustrations emphasize the importance of long-range comprehensive planning and the need to provide for a balanced extension of various development services when family planning without adequate supporting services leads to wastage of manpower and other resources.

Implied in the above is also the need for cooperative endeavors among many agencies using multi-disciplinary approaches from the beginning of any family planning efforts.

Family Planning in the Health Care System

Some kind of health system exists in every country, state, province, or community. This system is part of a larger complex represented in the community as a whole. Since family planning is a relatively new activity that is being developed, it may be well to examine briefly the various facets or subsystems of the community that it affects or into which it must be integrated.

Components of the System

1. *Preventive health services:* The local health services constitute one of the major units or subsystems into which family planning should be integrated. The maternal and child health staff may provide the direct services to families. Other staff in the health services can inform those who do not use family planning services of the value of family planning as a health measure. The sanitarians and other male workers constitute an important segment of the health service staff to stimulate the acceptance of family planning. They can be especially effective with the men of the community.

2. *Hospitals:* Another important subsystem is the hospital, where advice and services can be given to the postpartum women or to eligible women using other services, such as the outpatient, medical, surgical, and pediatric departments. But all staff—obstetricians, gynecologists, pediatricians, internists, urologists, nurses, and aides—should be alert to recommending family planning services as needed by families. Another pregnancy shortly after the birth of a child or when increase in family size would heighten other health hazards to members of the family is a particular period of need. The attitudes and advice of physicians to their patients have a strong influence on what families do.

3. *Private physicians:* In many countries private doctors constitute another important subsystem. Their favorable reaction and promotion of family planning among their patients is essential to full success in the program.

4. *Paramedical personnel:* Private midwives, traditional birth attendants, and auxiliaries who operate in the community outside the government health service constitute another

important subsystem. Their complete understanding and support of the health values of family planning are essential. If they see the service as interfering with their income, they may advise and work against family planning.

5. *Voluntary organizations:* The voluntary agencies, especially those whose major concern is family planning, constitute another important subsystem of the providers of services. They frequently are the initiators and promoters of activities that precede the services provided by the official parts of the system.

6. *Individuals of reproductive age:* Married women in the reproductive period, and especially the younger women, make up an obvious and important subgroup with which the family planning program is concerned. In some cultures the sexually active girls who are unmarried are a particularly important segment of the clientele subsystem. Not so widely recognized are the sexually active males, both unmarried and married. Both sexes are eligible to receive the service and should be included in program planning.

7. *Youth:* School-age children and youth are another group for whom relevant education in this area should be provided. Learning experiences may be integrated into various courses and subjects such as human biology, health education, family life education, and population education.

8. *Leaders and opinion makers:* Another very important group is the opinion makers, such as community leaders and officials, who legitimize the program and support or strengthen the health services of which family planning is a part.

9. *Correlative groups:* Other subgroups of the community are those groups concerned with ecology, social welfare, and environmental health. They see family planning as another tool to reduce the problems with which they are concerned.

The System in Operation

The components of the system are much more easily defined than the interrelationships of the subgroups and how they function within the larger system. It has been observed that many subunits operate independently and some even competitively.

There are smooth and supportive relationships between some units and often frictions between others. Much of this lack of coordination of the subsystems arises out of rapid expansion of the program, emphasis on certain subunits of the system, and failure to recognize the role of others. An essential function in which education plays an important part is to bring about active, coordinated, and supporting roles by the various units of the system.

Family Planning Depends on Decisions and Actions by People

Regardless of the primary objective of family planning, its final success depends on people, the decisions they make, and the actions they take. More specifically, the program is effective to the extent that people become convinced of the desirability and benefits of family planning and voluntarily decide to accept and continue some form of contraception according to their plan for the size of family they desire. This dependence on people, their decisions and actions, is just as true for programs emphasizing reduction in population growth as for those devoted solely to improvement of family health.

Despite the importance of people and their reactions, planning the educational task of assuring the voluntary participation of people has been given limited attention. Major emphasis in the planning of most programs has been given to the mechanics of securing facilities and personnel, and providing services. While these mechanisms are essential for introducing family planning activities in health programs, the educational aspects are equally important and need to be given meticulous attention from the beginning. Most of the educational plans have been very superficial, and also mechanistic. They have developed on the assumption that people can be pushed or coerced into participation through massive information campaigns or through financial or other comparable incentives. Family planning efforts seem to have "overlooked that the program was dealing with human beings, and human beings do not like to be treated as objects or as means of achieving a target of IUD insertions."[3]

Operating programs have seldom taken into account that the people' experiences with the services they are given and their reactions to the personnel and promotional campaigns have a strong influence on their acceptance and practice of family planning. Few, if any, educational plans have utilized systematically the research on human behavior, the principles of learning and health education enunciated in various technical World Health Organization publications and others that deal with enlisting the participation of people in health programs.[4,5,6,7]

In most countries where family planning programs have been operating for some time, reduced consumer acceptance and discontinuance of contraceptive use is occurring. The initial ready acceptance by a few individuals has not spread to the large number of those who need and could use the service. This reduction is becoming a serious concern to program administrators.

Family Planning in the Health Context

The objective of family planning in the health context is to regulate fertility in a manner that promotes positive health—i.e., physical, mental, and social well-being—and reduces the risks of mortality and morbidity of both mother and children, and lessens health-related pressures on family and community. The procedures to reduce such risks will vary for such factors as culture, socioeconomic status, parity, prenatal care available, nutritional status of the mother, and the like. In general, however, the risks will be reduced if the following objectives are achieved:

1. The first pregnancy occurs between 20 and 24 years of age.

2. Children are spaced at intervals of about three years for mothers who breast-feed and one to two years between completed lactation and the start of a new pregnancy.

3. Pregnancies do not occur after age 35 and in some cultures after an earlier age.

4. Unwanted pregnancies do not occur, thus eliminating their consequent sequels.

5. The number of pregnancies is sufficiently small to prevent maternal exhaustion.

6. Infertility is given professional medical treatment by competent personnel.

The organization, activities, and contraceptive methods to realize each of the above named objectives will vary from country to country and among areas within countries. These differences will determine the educational tasks to be done. For example, in order for women to have the first pregnancy occur between 20 and 24 years of age, the following are some of the measures that may be undertaken, depending upon the particular cultural settings: promote marriage at a later age; discourage intercourse without contraception; discourage pregnancies during teenage years; provide contraceptive services; and provide pregnancy testing and counseling. For spacing of births, the measures that might be used would include: seek out women recently delivered and promote family planning with them; promote family planning shortly after delivery; promote family planning at the postpartum visit; encourage extended period of lactation followed by contraception; prescribe use of condom by male; encourage abstention (separation of husband and wife for one year or more); encourage the practice of coitus interruptus. To prevent pregnancies late in the reproduction period, the procedures to be advised might be: encourage tubectomy of female; promote vasectomy of male; prescribe continuous use of pill or interrupted use with other contraception; insert IUD to be worn continuously or interrupted with other contraception; promote continued use of diaphragm; encourage male to use condom; promote the practice of coitus interruptus.

Uniqueness of Family Planning as a Health Service

Although family planning is primarily a health service, and the most effective contraceptive procedures require medical service or supervision, it still differs in many ways from the usual health services that are provided to prevent illness or to restore health to those who are sick. Some of these unique characteristics are detailed below.

Multiple Methods of Contraception

Perhaps the most unusual characteristic of family planning is the multiple alternative actions that people can be advised to take in order to realize its benefits. Several of these were mentioned above. This variation in action is in sharp contrast with the kinds of advice given to people to prevent or alleviate an unwanted health condition. Immunization for specific communicable diseases, a cervical smear for uterine cancer, insulin for diabetes—these are very specific actions that are advised in such programs. But in family planning the advised action may change with age and marital status. Either male or female can act and the family realizes the benefit.

What each is advised to do depends on the method of contraception that is adopted. Yet national programs have been known to emphasize one method almost exclusively. When something unexpected happens, such as numerous side effects from the IUD, there is a sudden shift to another contraceptive method. Physicians in different clinics have advocated one method to the exclusion of others. The above and other differences described below greatly complicate the educational task, for people want to know specifically what they must do before they decide to take action. Knowing what they must do is paramount if they are to continue action over a long period of time.

To complicate the educational task still more, some programs offer the individual a choice of contraceptive methods, known as the "cafeteria approach." This choice is offered without sufficient information about each method or specific assistance from professionals suggesting the one must suitable to that individual. This latter procedure is defended with the argument that the individual should have freedom of choice. From an educational point of view, the choice for which there should be the greatest freedom is the decision of the individual or family to prevent or postpone a pregnancy. The best contraceptive to achieve this objective is one that is chosen with technical professional guidance, the one that fits into the family's culture, available means, and manner of living.

Need for Family Planning Is Not Perceived as a Problem

The health education component of most health programs focuses on preventing or controlling a problem that is either already recognized by the people or can easily be interpreted as a potential health problem to them. With the exception of sterility management, family planning focuses on the prevention of conception, and this is not recognized as a health problem or need. Neither is it easy to interpret prevention of birth as a health problem to the people and especially to couples whose goal is to have many children in their family. Spacing and fewer children are recognized as needs by a few but not necessarily as health needs by the majority.

Family Planning Arouses a Number of Emotional Overtones

In almost all societies, sex, pregnancy, and reproduction are associated with certain taboos. Males may discuss certain aspects with males, and females with females. There are certain subjects in almost all cultures that custom prevents being discussed in mixed groups or even discussed at all. Individuals who have been socialized to these taboos may not feel free to discuss the subject with a stranger or a member of the opposite sex. This reticence to discuss family planning and contraception greatly increases the difficulty of the educational task. It also calls for careful selection and preparation in family planning of health workers. If they have grown up with these same social customs, they may find it difficult to handle their own feelings when giving educational advice about reproductive processes and contraception.

Moral and Religious Considerations Are Associated with the Subject

Some methods of family planning or services to certain segments of the population are proscribed by certain groups on religious or moral grounds. These opinions greatly complicate the educational task to be done. They may influence both the workers and the individuals in the community. For example, in a society where pregnancy outside of wedlock is considered immoral—yet many unmarried girls, especially teenagers, are becoming pregnant—education on ways to prevent such pregnancies is unusually complicated and even forbidden. Workers whose religion forbids interference with conception are often in conflict when their job requires that they provide or advocate contraceptive procedures. This conflict in the workers may have a negative effect on their educational contacts with people.

Family Planning May Interfere with Other Drives

The objective and methods of family planning may interfere with the full satisfaction of two universal basic drives—procreation and sexual intercourse. This further complicates health education about the subject. Families tend to want children immediately upon marriage. Where marriage is at an early age, the goal of family planning for health benefits is to delay pregnancy to the age of minimum risk. Also the spacing of children for health benefits may interfere with a family's desire or goal to have a large family. This is particularly true in societies where large families are expected or accorded social status. The methods of family planning either detract from the

spontaneity of the sex act or may be accompanied by highly undesirable and sometimes dangerous side effects.

These unique characteristics of family planning emphasize the
difficulty of education to promote the practice. To be sure, there
are problems associated with education about some regularly advocated health measures. For example, some are temporarily painful
(for example, immunization) or require the avoidance of a long-
established habit (for example, smoking). But the promotion of
none of these involves the difficult behavior change that is required
in family planning practice.

Purposes of Education in Family Planning

Health education in family planning is concerned with people and
the factors that influence them to practice family planning. More
specifically, the purposes of health education are the following:

1. To develop within the community a social environment and
   attitude wherein family planning is an accepted and advocated practice among leaders and opinion makers in the
   society—in short, to legitimize the practice.

   A few innovators will try a new practice and some may continue it for a period regardless of the social norms, but in any
   society the pressure to conform is very potent. Hence, one of
   the first educational tasks is to locate and inform the "gatekeepers" to action among the people. It is particularly important that all, or at least a majority, of the medical and allied
   professionals become aware and convinced about the health
   values of family planning so that they support rather than
   appear neutral or, as in some instances, advise against the
   practice among their patients.

2. To help people comprehend the health and other values
   of family planning and how it helps to satisfy their needs

and wants as a family. People should be thoroughly informed about the ways in which the practice will help them realize their life goals. This implies the educational task of learning what the goals and aspirations of the people are, diagnosing why they may not be practicing family planning at the moment, and then helping them to recognize how it contributes to achievement of their goals. Broadcasting information—assuming that the appeals will be meaningful to the people without some attempt to determine first the attitudes, beliefs and goals of the people—is not likely to help many of them become convinced that family planning is a service they need.

3. To inform people so they know and understand that their continued practice of family planning is necessary if they are to realize the benefits desired. This implies a thorough understanding of how to use the contraceptive method they have chosen. The information should be so complete and understandable that it will prevent or at least impede the development of subsequent doubts that might become rich soil for the spread of rumors by those ill-informed or opposed.

4. To assure that the overall plan includes provision of psychological support to those who accept use of a contraceptive, so that they will continue its use effectively. They should also know that they can turn to a substitute method if they wish to discontinue an unsatisfactory one. It is a new experience for individuals or couples who decide to use contraception for the first time. Sympathetic support and assurance from all the staff is an important educational influence for continued practice.

5. To assure that all family planning services and interactions with staff are satisfying to the individuals. This involves providing services at a time and place convenient to the people and in a manner that preserves their human dignity. It also embraces coordination of all resources upon which the people

depend for their information and services so that they have
a consistently favorable experience. In this connection, it
should be emphasized that people learn very definite and
often long-lasting attitudes from their experience with health
personnel who provide services to them. Their incidental
learning from these experiences may frequently be more effective and lasting than the overt teaching or advice that is
given through planned educational activities. Health education is concerned that the interaction between staff and the
people is a satisfactory one and that the people are pleased
with the service; that the staff is sensitive to the people's
apprehensions and to the ways various experiences they have
affect their decisions to accept and practice family planning.

Many efforts have foundered when the services were planned
and provided before there was support by the opinion makers
in the community. Others have not been as successful as
hoped because the training of the service personnel has not
included adequate preparation in family planning or sufficient
consideration of the way people will react and the necessity
of providing the services in a way that pleases them. Others
have faltered because people were coerced to accept a practice
without understanding how it benefited them (except maybe
through some incentive payment) or did not believe there
was a need to continue the contraceptive method chosen.

Each of these foregoing five purposes differs from the other,
according to the group with whom the education is carried out, the
information to be provided, the action to be taken, the timing
of the action, or the educational methods most likely to be effective. Planning for the accomplishment of these purposes should be
an integral part of the overall program planning. The degree to
which they can be achieved not only affects the objectives that are
stated in the plan but also contributes to the timing of many of the
service activities.

A Systematic Approach to Education in the Health Aspects of Family Planning

The previous sections have described the wide variety of methods of family planning, the unique characteristics of the program, and the detailed educational purposes of family planning. These are indicative of the many considerations that must enter into the development of an educational plan.

To facilitate the formulation of an effective plan, leaders and staff on health education services have developed a systematic step-by-step approach to the planning of education in health programs. The procedure is the same regardless of the health problem to be solved.[8,9] A description of the way these steps apply in family planning follows.

Participate with Administrators in Formulating the General and Detailed Objectives of the Health Program with Respect to Family Planning

The need for health education to participate in the development of the objectives of the program has already been mentioned. For example, health education staff, from their contacts with the people, can contribute information to the administrators on the contraceptives that are likely to be acceptable. They can also ascertain the time and place of services that are most convenient to the people. Likewise the educator's inquiries within the community can provide evidence on the readiness of the people to accept an innovation like family planning. If there is lack of interest or active resistance, it will influence the amount of educational effort and time required before substantial numbers of people decide to practice family planning. Such facts influence administrative decisions about the period in which a given program objective can be achieved.

It cannot be emphasized too strongly that the objectives need to be stated in clear and precise terms, including the possible contraceptives and the other services to be offered. Such statements as "family planning services for everyone," or "reduce the birth rate by a given amount," or "reduce the number of illegal abortions" need to be made more specific before the planning for effective education can take place.

Even the term *family planning* is lacking in precision. It is most often used as a euphemism for promoting contraception. Few programs appear to be focused directly on helping a family plan the number of children they want at the times they want, or should want, them. Practically none is concerned with determining whether couples want no children and, if so, helping them to realize that goal. Evidence for these statements is the fact that staff in their contacts with family members do not customarily ask how many children they want when their family is complete, and when they want to have their children, or even when they want the next child. These questions seem essential if an objective is to help couples plan their families. Some of the terms ordinarily used seem to indicate that the focus is contraceptive use rather than family planning. For example, the term *acceptors* is applied to those who begin to use contraception, *users* to those who continue the practice, and *dropouts* to those who stop. Even those who discontinue contraception in order to have a child according to their family plan are referred to as *dropouts*. In some countries, and particularly the United States, couples who want no children or no more children encounter many bureaucratic hurdles in trying to obtain a sterilization procedure.

These examples illustrate the need for objectives stated in specific terms and the role of health educators in helping to decide on the program objectives.

Development of Behavioral Objectives Based on Program Objectives

The actions various groups or individuals must take in order for the program objectives to be achieved must be specifically defined. For example, if the objective is to reduce the health risk by regulating the interconceptual space, and the contraceptives provided are pills and IUDs, the behavioral objectives would be to foster such conditions as the following:

1. All postpartum women and their husbands know the health benefits of spacing.

2. They understand the advantages and disadvantages of the methods being offered.

3. They know when and where the services may be obtained.

4. The majority of the couples decide to utilize the family planning services and accept one of the offered methods.

5. Those who accept a method continue to use the contraceptive until it is the optimum time for the next child.

The actions necessary to achieve the objectives are not limited to the couples or individuals being provided services but also include the specific functions of the service staff. In addition to the technical knowledge they need about reproduction, contraception, and skill in administering services—which would vary with staff responsibility—the behavioral objectives for the staff are as follows:

1. They understand and can communicate with men and women concerning any question they may have.

2. They recognize and deal effectively with unexpressed questions and anxieties of the individuals.

3. They provide services with privacy and with minimum embarrassment to the individuals.

4. At all times, they treat the women and/or men in a manner that preserves their dignity and feeling of self- esteem.

5. They provide services at times suitable to the individuals rather than at the convenience of one or more members of the staff.

6. They attempt to ascertain whether the individuals are pleased with the service and exert maximum effort to remove any misunderstanding or dissatisfaction.

As was pointed out in the section on the health care system, the actions of the various staff members must be coordinated and timed so that a minimum of lost effort occurs.

Conduct an Educational Analysis or Diagnosis

This step involves finding out where the people are with respect to actions defined in step 2 above and determining what factors are preventing them from taking the necessary action. Failure to act in order to benefit from family planning services is only a symptom. To be able to "prescribe" the proper educational treatment, one must identify the underlying causes. For example, if the people know about the benefits of spacing but are confused about contraceptive methods, there is need to clarify their confusions. If the educational diagnosis shows that they will not consider spacing because there is opposition by their elders or leaders in the community, then these gatekeepers must become convinced of the desirability of spaced births. Some of the questions usually investigated in the diagnosis are as follows:

1. What are the existing attitudes and traditions in the respective communities?

2. What are the people's goals, values, beliefs, aspirations, attitudes, wants, perceptions, and the like?

3. What do the people know about family planning and its methods?

4. Are they following any kinds of contraception now?

5. What are the reasons for their attitudes and actions regarding family planning?

6. Through what channels of communication do they learn about new ideas and new practices?

7. Do they learn about family planning through these same channels?

8. What has been their reaction toward other kinds of innovative ideas, particularly toward the use of preventive health services?

9. What are other agencies doing in family planning?

10. What staff and other resources are available or will be provided to render the necessary health services?

11. What educational facilities other than those provided by the health program can be enlisted to assist in the educational effort?

12. Are there any potential barriers that might interfere with the people learning and practicing family planning—such as language differences, illiteracy, cost, or previous unpleasant experiences with agencies introducing new programs or activities?

Some of the information required for the educational analysis can be easily determined. Some can only be obtained by competent specialists in health education, behavioral sciences, and communications.

Carrying out an educational analysis is analogous to the procedure followed by a physician in making a diagnosis before he prescribes treatment for a patient. Some information he needs is collected by his technical assistants; some he obtains himself; and on occasion he may seek information obtained by a specialist. It is also comparable to the tests a school teacher may administer to a new arithmetic class before she decides what is necessary to teach the students so that they learn the skills of multiplication. The educational diagnosis contributes an additional value to the program. It provides information useful to administrators in allocating resources. If large numbers of the people are informed and ready to accept family planning, then sufficient services need to be provided so that the people can begin to practice family planning. If the logistics of the services have not been scheduled to provide for those who are already convinced and are waiting for services, the people may decide that the practice is not necessary or desirable. If, however, almost all of them are uninformed or even perhaps resistant to any family planning, the educational services would be emphasized and the clinical services provided only when the people were ready to use them.

Establishment of the Specific Educational Objectives of the Health Program

The *specific* educational objectives differ from the behavioral objectives developed in step 2 in that they take into account what the people already know, what they are doing, and any barriers to their action that may have been uncovered in the diagnosis. For example, if there is widespread knowledge that family planning is a possibility and it is desirable, but the people do not like the family planning services provided, then working with the program administrator to improve the manner of giving the services is the primary educational objective. Or, if the women know about the IUD but refuse to wear one because of some rumor that is circulating, the educational objective becomes one of dealing directly with the spread of the rumor. The people can be provided with experiences to convince them that the rumor is false and also to establish within them confidence to try the device. Certainly, urging women to accept the IUD before dealing with the rumor is not likely to lead them to get one inserted, and it may reduce the effectiveness of subsequent educational efforts.

Setting the educational objective is not limited to specifying what different groups need to know and the actions they should take to carry out their family plan. Ascertaining what people know, believe, and are now doing permits much more realistic objectives for educational aspects of family planning than result when targets are prescribed at a central point of program administration without knowledge of the educational needs of the people and the amount of time it will take for them to become informed, to decide, and to act.

Development of the Detailed Educational Operations Plan, Including Plans for Evaluation

All the above decisions concerning information about the people, the objectives of the program, the specific educational objectives, and data on resources become the basic constituents in evolving the operational plan for education. In addition, the principles and procedures derived from educational and behavioral research are important factors in formulating the educational plan. Particularly relevant are the findings from research on such areas as learning, perception, diffusion, motivation, individual and mass communication, the behavior change process, and educational methods and materials—including visual and auditory aids.

The plan will incorporate decisions on several questions:

Preparation of Personnel

What learning experiences do the various health staff engaged in family planning need in order to perform their educational tasks? When and how can these experiences be provided? Staff are usually given training concerning the technology of reproduction and contraception and their technical tasks of providing service. They receive a minimum of preparation on the effect of their interactions with people. They are given very little explicit instruction on what kinds of information and assurances they should provide individuals. In other words, their preparation is limited in ways of working with people.

Of particular concern is the preparation given to medical personnel either in medical school or as continuing education. They need to learn the importance of encouraging the patients who seek their advice on various matters to plan their families. What educational experiences need to be provided physicians so that they give consistent information and guidance about the various contraceptives? Free discussion among themselves is highly desirable, but publicly debated controversies destroy confidence of the general public. The advice of the personal physician is often considered much more reliable by the people than information from an unknown or official government source.

Securing Community Sanction for the Program

How will the approval and support of other individuals and groups be encouraged, for example, clergy, village chiefs, political and financial leaders, heads of industry, voluntary agencies, professional societies, and other official organizations? It is important to create among respected and influential persons within the community a favorable environment toward the concept of family planning before attempts are made to educate the general population or before services are provided. In one area where there was religious resistance to contraception, the presentation of a carefully collected and analyzed series of data on the health hazards of having many children and frequent pregnancies resulted in religious support of a program. Only after the approval and support were given did the provision of services for education of the general public begin. The educational experiences planned to develop support of community leaders will depend on the diagnosis of their attitude and understanding. Possible methods include individual contact, group discussion, committee work sessions, conferences, or provision of pertinent data and information.

Education for Eligible Couples

What learning experiences, communications, and methods will be provided various segments of the population who can benefit from family planning, so that they decide to accept and practice contraception? Roberts and Griffiths,[10] after a review of a number of studies of knowledge, attitude, and practice, concluded that there are three groups in the reproductive age of the population: "ready accepters" of family planning (about 20–30 percent); the "unconcerned" (about 60–80 percent); and the "resisters" (10–20 percent).

The relatively small "ready accepter" group comprehends the value of family planning and knows the reasons for practicing it. They are already motivated to practice contraception. The information they want is where and when they can get services. Their interests in planning for the birth of their children provide the psychological drive to practice contraception consistently. In the initial stages of many programs the information and education efforts were patterned on the analogy of advertising and were concentrated on the dissemination of information through mass communications. The response of the people was similar to what happens in advertising—those who feel a need for the product advertised buy it, but many do not. The "ready accepters" began almost immediately to use the services and practice family planning. On the basis of their early response, the information program in some areas was judged to be successful. Often the mass communication activities were intensified. But when the interested individuals had accepted and were practicing family planning, the number of other eligible couples to begin using the service and to practice contraception declined.

Though some programs have been underway for a number of years the period of time has not been sufficient in any country to provide a large body of experience and data upon which to base successful educational efforts for the "unconcerned" group. The literature shows no country in which as many as 50 percent of the eligible couples (the most optimistic figures are nearer 25 percent) have developed a plan for their family and are practicing contraception to realize that plan. Some of this lack of success may have resulted because few educational programs have been developed in which there was a clear and specific statement of objectives developed from an initial educational diagnosis or appraisal.

Certainly, as Roberts and Griffiths[10] point out, there is need for more research, trial, and experimentation with innovative approaches. However, many suggestions can be derived from educational and behavioral science research, from the experience in various parts of the world, and from the limited research on educational problems in family planning. All these should be considered in planning the educational experiences for the "unconcerned."

One suggestion for developing the plan to educate the eligible couples derives from the research of rural sociologists on the adoption of innovation.[11,12] They have shown that individuals tend to go through specific stages in adopting a new practice. These stages have been labeled "awareness," "information," "evaluation," "trial," and "adoption." Bogue[13] has suggested a revision in the model to include six prerequisites before a new practice will be incorporated as part of normal activity. The adoption model he proposes asserts that a person will tend to adopt a new idea for practice when (1) he has been informed, (2) he has been motivated, (3) credibility has been established, (4) he has perceived the practice as being socially legitimate, (5) a positive attitude has developed toward the new practice, and (6) self-referral or self-involvement has taken place.

Neither the sociologists' model nor Bogue's modification has been tested to make sure it operates in family planning. However, analysis of the educational needs of the people using the stages in either model suggests specifics that would seem to be useful in an educational plan. The stages in the diffusion theory derived from the original research of sociologists on the adoption of innovations and their possible meanings for family planning are as follows:

1. *Awareness:* People must become aware that the new practice of innovation is possible. In innovations that have been studied, mass communication is one of the most forceful and frequent methods by which people become aware of the innovation. It would appear that in a number of countries the extensive mass communication efforts on family planning have been quite successful, according to KAP (knowledge, attitude, and practice) studies. These investigations, wherever they have been made, reveal that in almost all countries having family planning activities, a majority of the people are aware of family planning and many know

that pregnancy can be prevented. Studies have shown that in some countries the proportion of the people who have such information approaches 90 percent.

The educational diagnosis for a particular area would reveal whether this is true for that area. Studies show that fewer know about the specific methods that might be used and still fewer know where services may be obtained. Determination of the degree of awareness for a particular area would be learned from the educational appraisal or diagnosis. It would seem, then, that the need to acquaint people with the possibilities of family planning has been met with large segments of the population in countries where activities have been underway for some time.

2. *Interest:* After awareness, on their way to adoption, people become interested to seek detailed information about the practice. In this stage, people acquire the facts they want and feel are essential for them to decide whether the practice is for them. Depending on the concerns of the people, they may seek information about reproduction, meaning of contraception, and various methods and their advantages and disadvantages. They may want assurance that any negative information that they may have heard is false. They will also want to know how well the practices can fit into social and traditional patterns of behavior that may exist in their society. Some of the information desired or needed can be furnished through mass communication media and published materials, but most of it is specific to the individuals or groups for which the education is being planned. Consequently, face-to-face discussion, either on a person-to-person basis or in discussion groups, is indicated.

3. *Evaluation:* When people have acquired information they want, the next stage is to evaluate mentally the practice of innovation in terms of its usefulness to them—whether it fits with their goals, values, and aspirations, and whether its

benefits outweigh its disadvantages. This mental evaluation is a process all individuals go through when contemplating a decision. At this stage, the information that individuals want and need differs from what they received in the ones preceding. They are aware of the possibilities of family planning, and they have acquired the information they want. The kinds of useful educational experiences at this stage are personal support and encouragement from sources that the individuals trust. Neighbors, relatives, and friends, or other individuals who have adapted the practice and have found it satisfactory, are strong influences at this time.

The educational message at this stage also changes. The individual no longer needs information about the advantages of family planning or details about contraceptive methods. Instead he or she wants to know that the practice will be safe, that others have adopted and are using contraception satisfactorily, and that he or she will not be subjected to social disapproval by those who are important to him or her. Few, if any, programs have modified their educational efforts as the informational needs of the people changed.

Experience in some of the family planning programs has shown that satisfied users of family planning methods, particularly the pills and IUDs, can be favorable educational influences with others in their community. But operation of this favorable influence will not usually occur automatically. In most cultures, people do not discuss freely their sexual and contraceptive practices. If, however, the educational operation plan provides for recruiting some of the "ready accepters" or recent adopters of the practice and enlisting their participation in the educational activities, they can become positive educational agents in this and the succeeding stages in the process.

4. *Trial:* A positive evaluation leads to a preliminary trial of the practice—does it work for them? It is at this stage that

psychological support for continuation of the practice is needed. Concerns about side effects or questions about use are most likely to arise at this preliminary trial stage, and the provision of specific information that will satisfy their concerns and answer their questions is essential. One of the serious deficiencies in the programs around the world has been the large number of women who began the practice of family planning—the taking of pills or the insertion of an IUD— and then either discontinued or had the IUD removed. The same is true of men who began using the condom and for one reason or another discontinued its use. Much of this negative decision at the trial stage was due to the failure of the educational plan to provide the kind of experiences, counsel, support, and discussion that the people needed to remove their doubts and dissatisfactions.

More recently program administrators have recognized the necessity of educational experiences and support at this point in people's decision making about the practice.

It should be emphasized that proper educational experience at this stage in the decision-making process is crucial. Those individuals who, after trying family planning, find the experience to be unsatisfactory are likely to become not only nonusers, but they may also join the "resister" group and may become a negative influence in the community. Their influence is likely to be strongest among their friends and neighbors who may be wavering in their evaluation of the practice and their decision to give it a trial. Individuals who become dissatisfied during their trial stage are much more likely to communicate their negative reactions than are those who have a satisfactory trial and have adopted family planning.

5. *Adoption:* The last stage is adoption of contraceptive practice in order to achieve the couple's family plan. Adoption involves not only acceptance but also sustained practice.

The educational effort at this stage is centered on providing periodic advice and assurance in case doubts or concerns might arise. In programs where the primary goal is health of the family, education at this stage in the adoption process should also include advice to the family about when they should stop contraception in order to have their next planned child, and the actions to take in case pregnancy does not occur. It should also help the couples to follow proper prenatal care so that mother and baby may experience a healthy delivery and uneventful postpartum period.

The sociological research on the processes people experience in the adoption of various practices reveals that not every one goes through all these stages when they adopt a new practice. Certainly, this would be true of the couples who adopt and practice family planning. However, as has been shown above, consideration of the specific stages helps to define more clearly the educational needs of people. It delineates the change in the information needed at different stages and suggests elements of the people's educational needs that may be overlooked in a less analytical approach to developing the educational operational plan.

It also helps to give some perspective to the period of time that may be needed to interest the unconcerned group and help them go through the process of deciding to avail themselves of the benefits and services of family planning. Few people make decisions to act in a new way without time to weigh the consequences of the change. Because of this time factor, programs that provide continuing educational experiences over an extended period are likely to help more people be ready to accept and practice family planning than the short-term intensive informational exposure that has characterized many of the existing family planning programs.

A further suggestion from family planning research can be summarized in the concept that "contraception is a family affair": Studies have shown that where there is interspouse communication on family planning, there is greater acceptance of this practice.[10] Education of the male is especially important in those societies where the male is the dominant partner in family decision making. The educational plan should encourage interspouse communication on family planning methods. In some programs, discussions have been held by the health worker with husband and wife together. In other societies, where this is not possible, plans have been developed for a male educational agent to discuss the subject with males and a female worker with the females. Neither of these methods of educating the male is designed specifically to foster interspouse communication. Innovative program methods are needed that will encourage husband-wife discussion about family planning. Despite the advantages shown for involving the male in the decision-making process, many educational and service programs still concentrate almost exclusively on the female.

Other suggestions that arise from data on operating programs are these:

1. Those programs that have involved groups in the community in interaction among their neighbors and friends on the desirability of family planning have reported greater success than those where the stimulation, information, and guidance have come solely from the health worker. This is particularly true when the interaction has produced commitment to one another that they will accept and practice contraception.[10]

2. Programs in which the other concerns of the families are given attention in the educational contacts have had greater success in encouraging more of the "unconcerned" to practice family planning than have unipurpose contacts.

Education of Children and Youth

What provision will be made to acquaint youths, both in school and out, about the health aspects of family planning? What efforts will be made to inform them of the advantages to health of delaying or spacing pregnancies and of having small families? Most programs to date have concentrated on the woman and to a lesser extent on men of the reproductive age. This was to be expected since it is the adults in the reproductive age who must take the immediate primary action. However, education for those who will move into the reproductive period can be facilitated by some planned educational activities for young people at the time they show interest in the process of human reproduction and are looking forward to the establishment of a family of their own. Countries differ in their ideas of what should be included in the education of children and youth in this broad area of family living, human reproduction, sex education, and population education. Not only are there differences among countries, but within any given country widely varying opinions are held. Any comprehensive educational plan would consider these segments of the population and determine, within the culture and mores of the people, what information and experiences can be provided the young, and at what age.

Methods and Materials

Decisions about the educational methods and approaches to use with the population eligible for family planning should follow the guiding principles for the selection and use of methods and media that are given in the First Report of the Expert Committee on Health Education of the World Health Organization.[4]

There are, however, two important considerations with respect to methods that need to be emphasized because they have received so little attention in the majority of programs developed to date.

The first of these of particular importance is the involvement of community or neighborhood leaders and the groups from which they come as an essential part of the educational process. It has been shown that where community leaders are recruited and trained, they can be potent influences with their neighborhood group in providing understanding of the benefits of family planning and in stimulating groups to practice it. Where there is maximum involvement of community groups as an educational activity, the focus of the educator becomes working with the leaders of the respective groups. First he must locate the leaders—those who are recognized by the individuals of the group. They may or may not be the individuals who seek leadership roles or are readily visible to a worker who is not a member of the community group.[14] The leaders important for education are those to whom individuals in the community turn for advice and guidance when they are considering important decisions. After locating the leaders, the health educator undertakes to recruit them to work in the family planning educational effort. Some may be interested to participate; others may not be for various reasons.

The interested leaders are then given training to function as educational agents within their respective communities. The training is designed to provide them with the necessary information about family planning and the available services—and to help them develop a complete understanding of the program and its benefits.

During the training period, the advice of the leaders is sought about the ways in which they would like to conduct the educational activities within their respective groups. The health educator may assist the leaders in their first educational attempts until they feel secure in working on the family planning program. As soon as it is feasible, responsibility for the further education of the group is turned over to the leaders, with freedom to request help from the educator whenever they feel the need. Important to the success of this type of involvement of groups through their leaders is public recognition of the leaders' contribution to the program.[15]

A second consideration that needs emphasis is the fact that people learn from every experience they have, whether education was intended or not. The learning may be desirable or undesirable from the point of view of the program, depending on the satisfaction that accrues from the experience. Some examples are the following:

1. Exposure to meaningful messages in mass communication can alert people to the possibilities and benefits of family planning.

2. Health practitioners and researchers during the surveys or inquiries convey messages to the people and leave impressions on them.

3. Contact with health workers in the regular service leaves impressions about and attitudes toward both health workers and health services; it also provides opportunity for exchange of information about family planning.

4. Group and individual discussions within the family and with health workers, neighbors, friends, and other clients (especially with satisfied users) can help in clarifying procedures and removing doubts and fears.

Evaluation

What mechanisms will be set up to evaluate the educational effort? Decision on the procedures to evaluate the educational activities is an integral part of the development of the operational plan. Despite the fact that measurement of the impact of educational activities is difficult to quantify, consistent efforts should be made to obtain as reliable measures of progress as are possible. It should not be overlooked that "whenever a decision between alternatives [about program operations] is made, some evaluation is taking place, although it is often subjective and based on insufficient data and inadequate analysis."[4]

Evaluation may serve a number of purposes. Roberts[16] summarizes these as follows:

We evaluate to aid further planning and to improve programs, to increase our understanding of health education practice, to add to the body of knowledge upon which our work is based. We evaluate to help achieve opera-

tional efficiency and, related to this, to obtain data that
permit interpretation of program effectiveness so as to
obtain administrative support, community support, even
financial support. We evaluate for reasons associated
with motivation—to give staff and volunteers satisfaction and a sense of success. To give priority to these purposes . . . we evaluate primarily to study the effects of
practice so that we can turn our findings back into practice and improve it and, at the same time, strengthen the
scientific basis of practice in health education.

Workers concerned with improving evaluation processes in public health have identified three types of evaluation based on the
data used and the purpose the different types serve. Descriptions of
the three types, the methods they employ, and the way they apply
in family planning follow:

Evaluation of Effectiveness

This type of measurement is designed to yield answers to the question, "How well has the program achieved its objective in the time
period that activities have been underway?" Essentially evaluation
of effectiveness requires the following:

1. *Precise and clear objectives:* The objectives may refer to what
   the program is trying to accomplish, such as the reduction
   of mortality or morbidity of mothers and children. Or they
   may be the behavioral objectives of the program, such as
   an increase in the number of couples consistently practicing contraception. The procedure is the same regardless of
   which aspect of a program is being evaluated. If possible
   the objectives should be stated in quantitative terms. The
   same precise objectives developed for program planning and
   implementation serve as the first requirement for evaluation
   of effectiveness.

2. *Decision on the kind of data that will be accepted as evidence of accomplishment:* If the objective is to produce favorable attitudes toward the program by influential leaders, will public statements by the leaders be used as evidence or will a more precise measurement based on a planned poll be undertaken? If the objective is to help people practice family planning consistently, will the data be the number who practice contraception over a stated time period, or will the number who practice consistently plus the number who stop contraception to have a planned child be accepted?

3. *Baseline data gathered before the educational effort is initiated:* If such is impractical because of the urgency to get a service program underway, then some form of control group for which the same services are provided must be decided upon, in order to know how much change is due to the educational effort and how much would have taken place anyway.

4. *Collection of similar data at the time of evaluation:* In an ongoing program, periodic evaluations of effectiveness should be undertaken. Plans for these evaluations should be a part of the operational plan.

5. *Determination of success in achieving the objective:* A comparison of the data collected before the initiation of the program with the data obtained at the time the evaluation is made provides a measure of the effectiveness of the educational input.

Evaluation of Efficiency

In this type of evaluation, the major concern is the cost of achieving a given objective. For example, a program may have the objective of educating eligible couples to practice spacing of their children. At the time of evaluation, 60 percent of the couples are following the practice consistently. But the cost of achieving this result—including personnel salaries, services, materials, transportation, and any other expenditures—is found to be exorbitant. The efficiency of such a program would be low.

Another program might achieve a slightly lower percentage, with costs 50 percent less than that of the first program. Its efficiency would be higher even though its effectiveness—the proportion of individuals who practice contraception—was lower. Still a third program, using blitz methods of campaigning and mass recruitment of candidates for sterilization, may be relatively inexpensive for the result accomplished; yet it might leave such negative attitudes within the community that future efforts of the same kind would yield almost no results. Thus an activity that seemed efficient at one time may turn out to be extremely inefficient if measured later.

Evaluation of efficiency uses the data required for measuring effectiveness and in addition collects information on the cost of all efforts to produce the level of effectiveness. By comparing the costs with the achievements, one can determine the cost/effectiveness (usually termed "cost/benefit") ratio and decide whether the outcome is worth the cost. Efficiency evaluations have most often been used in the attempt to measure the relative costs of different educational procedures and the results they produce. All too often, single measurements of the value of the experimental procedure have been made rather than repeated measurements so that the effectiveness and efficiency of the procedure in producing lasting results could be judged.

Evaluation of Process

Process evaluation detects weaknesses in specific activities of a program and permits revisions before resources and time are dissipated without producing results. It requires a clear delineation of all the conditions necessary for effectiveness. For example, to achieve the objective of families spacing their children, some of the conditions necessary for effectiveness are that eligible couples must know about (1) the health advantages of an interconceptual space of two to three years, (2) a safe and effective method of delaying pregnancy,

(3) how to use the method, and (4) where to obtain the contra-ceptive service. These conditions can be considered sub-objectives of the main one. Each activity in a program has a purpose or sub-objective, and the extent to which it is realized affects the degree of success of the total program.

Returning to the example above, if, after a planned educational effort, a majority of the people do not understand the health advan-tages of family planning for spacing or do not know how to use a contraceptive or where to obtain the needed health services, then it is not likely that the couples will accept contraception for spacing.

Faced with such an unsuccessful result, further process evalua-tion will examine many aspects of the educational activity. For example, answers will be sought to such questions as the following:

1. Was the information clear and comprehensible to the people?
2. Was the channel of communication such that they were exposed to the information?
3. Was it considered a reliable source of information?
4. Were there social, economic, and cultural barriers that pre-vented acceptance of the idea?
5. Has there been adequate involvement of the people to rouse their interest?
6. Were there adequate and acceptable services available to the people?

If the purpose of each activity has been clearly specified, then continuous evaluation of its effectiveness can be made while the program is in progress. Reasons for any inefficiencies can be sought and appropriate modifications made to eliminate them. Such changes will contribute to the ultimate effectiveness of the program.

One procedure of process evaluation that has been fruitful in improving the educational activities is the recording of interviews between staff and individuals. These recordings have revealed errors of information that were given to the individuals by staff, questions that were not answered, and confusions that were not removed. They have also revealed unexpected problems of people that the staff had not been trained to handle. Such data can be used immediately for in-service training with staff.

Effective Education for Family Planning Requires an Organized Health Education Service

The previous sections have described in considerable detail the multiplicity of factors that enter into the planning and direction of efforts to help people learn, to make decisions, and to practice family planning. These same general factors and steps enter into planning the educational aspects of all other health programs. They prescribe the competencies in personnel that are required to develop and operate the educational activities for any health program, including family planning. The more important ones are as follows:

1. A primary concern about people, regardless of their education, economic level, or status in society. This implies a confidence that people will take constructive health action when they fully understand its implications, provided it does not conflict with other goals they have that are more important to them.

2. An understanding of the influence of attitudes, beliefs, interests, motives, values, perceptions, expectations, knowledge, social norms, and traditional mores, of associates, family, and relatives upon an individual's behavior and willingness to change.

3. Familiarity with the leadership patterns of communities and the influence they exert on people's behavior.

4. Skill to conduct educational programs that elicit support from the "gatekeepers" and "opinion leaders."

5. Skill in training indigenous educational leaders in the community, in transferring leadership to them; skill in becoming an educational consultant to the leader and the community of which he is a part.

6. Ability to assess the influences affecting behavior and to use the findings in providing educational experiences for the people.

7. Understanding of and skill in applying research on behavior change to help people learn to improve their health behavior.

8. Competence in analyzing the feasibility of program objectives in terms of the likely participation of the people.

9. Ability to develop in detail a statement of the desired behavior of staff and the people and to interpret these into educational objectives and activities.

10. Understanding of the communication process and ability to apply communications theory in developing an educational program.

11. Familiarity with the value and limitations of all types of educational and informational methods and media.

12. Ability to produce and pretest informational materials and to plan for their effective use.

13. Skill in evaluating the educational activities and re-directing those found to be ineffective.

14. Ability to assist in the development of staff education programs.

15. Competency in planning and providing experiences related to the educational functions of various categories of staff.

16. Skill in negotiations and coordination with organizations having interests and activities in educating the public about health, family planning, and related health problems.

Few, if any, workers could be expected to be expert in all of these skills and abilities. What is needed is a health education service with diverse abilities among the staff. It should be directed by a qualified specialist in health education with additional staff, including other specialists in health education, in behavioral sciences, and in communication media, as well as technicians.

Such a service, because of its specialized competencies, is able to provide better educational services for each health program, including family planning, than the different health programs can provide independently.

The health education service should be an integral part of the national ministry or department of health. Administratively it should be placed at that level in the organization structure where it can be directly associated with—and of service in administrative and program decisions concerned with—informing the people about the activities of the health ministry and with enlisting the desired action and support of the people in the various health and related programs. The health education service should also be so placed that all of its technical divisions have ready access to it for the assistance they need in the planning, implementation, and evaluation of the educational aspect of their respective programs. More detail on the organization and administration of a health education service appears in the report of the World Health Organization Expert Committee on Planning and Evaluation of Health Education.[5]

In addition to the health education service at the national, provincial, or state levels, it is desirable to have personnel competent in health education, related behavioral sciences, and communications taking a responsible part wherever health and family planning policy determinations are made, where significant program planning takes place, and where important education and training for health workers and others are provided.[5]

Because family planning is relatively new and rapidly expanding, many countries have bypassed the national health education service of health ministries and set up an independent health education unit to work exclusively on family planning. There are several reasons why such competing organizations tend to detract from the effectiveness of each other. Some of these are as follows:

1. In every country there is a shortage of well-qualified health education staff and, especially, experienced personnel who can plan and direct health education activities. Setting up competing services will tend to result in one or the other having inadequately qualified personnel. Neither will be sufficiently staffed.

2. If there are differentials in pay for personnel in the competing systems, dissatisfaction of personnel will arise, and instability of employment will occur. High turnover of personnel almost always leads to inefficiency.

3. Much more specialization in staff competence can be brought into the health education service when the resources that are available are pooled.

4. Separate health education services in health ministries or in independent governmental agencies for family planning compete for use of the same information media, often putting out competing and sometimes conflicting advice to the public.

5. A comprehensive health education service with ample resources to contribute to all health programs at various administrative levels of a governmental health service can, in time, be perceived as the source of competent health education. Family planning education can benefit from this perception.

6. Separate organizations compete for the attention of the same people. When individuals are surfeited with bids for their attention, they often disregard all attempts to provide them with meaningful information and guidance.

7. An effective, generalized health education service will be familiar with leaders, volunteers, and other resources in the area served by the health services. These will have been discovered through the educational effort on various health programs. Such information will be useful to the health administrator and staff concerned with family planning, and the cost of independently locating such resources will be eliminated.

Integration of the Generalized and Family Planning Health Education Staffs

A single, competent health education service within the organization of governmental health services functioning at national, provincial, or state levels can serve family planning as well as the other priority health programs. If the family planning administrator decides to use the generalized health education services, his perceived urgency of the program may result in impossible and unreasonable demands to produce immediate educational results. Even if a large amount of staff and resources are made available, it may be necessary to rearrange and perhaps reorganize the health education service to provide the essential educational (including communications) input required for family planning. Resistance to change by the existing staff and to the priority demanded for family planning may interfere with the quality and effectiveness of educational activities that could be provided.

If, on the other hand, an independent educational unit has already been established for family planning, and it is decided to amalgamate it with the generalized health education services, several problems may arise that will need to be considered. Since the family planning educational unit may be, and often is, as large as or larger in staff and resources than the generalized health education service of a health ministry, there is likely to arise competition for the leadership of the unit. Similarly, there may develop unhealthy competition between staff with similar jobs in the two units. The pressure for family planning education, because of the high priority that family planning has been given, may arouse resentment and passive resistance in the generalized health education staff.

In some situations, the generalized health education service has been pressed by responsible authorities to provide educational service for family planning, but no additional staff or budgetary resources were made available for the requested assistance. In others, the administrators have determined the specific educational effort that should be devoted to family planning without consulting the health education services. The educational outcome in both of these kinds of situations is not likely to be effective.

Listing these difficulties is not intended to detract from the desirability and increased potential effectiveness of a generalized health education service that contributes to family planning as well as to other priority health programs. Instead, they are mentioned because most of the difficulties can be obviated, or at least diminished, if they are recognized. Plans can then be made to solve them before they grow into serious personnel problems. Joint staff planning and decisions on ways to provide maximum informational and educational services to all programs will do much to reduce the problem. Provision of educational opportunities to those who are asked to perform tasks different from their previous job is another essential strategic step.

Coordinated Work by All Agencies
Is Essential to Effectiveness

In every country in which family planning has been initiated, there are voluntary agencies making a major contribution to the overall national objective. In some countries, the official agency contributes resources for activities of the voluntary agencies. In others, voluntary agencies supplement the work of the official agency. Also, in many countries, international multilateral agencies, groups from bilateral assistance organizations, and foundations are assisting family planning in a variety of ways. It is vitally important that the educational (including informational) efforts of all the groups and agencies be planned jointly and carried out in a coordinated manner.

Little benefit is derived from a program limited to information conducted by one agency when the timing of the information has not been geared to the scheduling of services by the official department. Also, the public can become confused when one agency may be promoting IUDs and another is stimulating the use of the pill. In one community, male workers from one organization were urging men to submit to vasectomy, and the female workers from another group were encouraging the women to use IUDs. Both were working with the eligible couples, but each was degrading the method being promoted by the other. Education of the people on the ways they can benefit from family planning is difficult enough without the confusion that will arise from such competing efforts.

Coordination and cooperation in the educational and informational activities require planning together. Each agency agrees to assume responsibility for those activities it can do best with the resources at its disposal. The focus is on the task to be done rather than on the coordinating mechanism, such as a council or committee. Too often a mechanism is developed before there is agreement on a problem and its solution, and the council or committee becomes unduly concerned with the minutiae of organizational structure and status. In such cases, attempts at joint program efforts are ineffective.

Cooperation seems to be much more difficult to achieve than competition. It is a responsibility of all those who work in education for any aspect of health activity to help foster coordinated efforts. Cooperation will increase the educational impact on the people and minimize the negative effects of competing efforts.

Need for Studies and Research in Education on the Health Aspects of Family Planning

The absence of a well-developed scientific base on which to build health education services for important health concerns—communicable disease, medical care, dental care, and others—has been well documented in publications of the World Health Organization.[17,18] The lack of educational and behavioral research on family planning is even greater. This limitation in research findings is all the more lamentable since improved health of the people and the success of family planning services depend upon their voluntary continued participation. Because of the unique characteristics of family planning, the relevance and applicability of research findings on education for other health problems require further study.

The lack of research in depth on family planning education is partly due to the relatively few research workers in health education, communications, and related behavioral sciences who have become sufficiently interested to conduct action-oriented investigations in this field. In addition, there is a lack of facilities for preparing research workers to conduct educational and related research in family planning.

Of the studies that have been made, the largest group deal with knowledge, attitude, and practice and are usually referred to as KAP studies. As has been pointed out, these show a fairly high level of knowledge and favorable attitudes but much lower reported practice. Validation of reported practice is very difficult, but it is generally conceded that consistent practice is even less than appears in the reports.

A second category in which a number of studies have been undertaken is in the area of communications. Most of these studies have concentrated on the mechanics of the communication process, the message, the channel, or the media. Few studies have given consideration to the interactions of the receiver and the sender or the perception of the message by the receiver. Psychological research indicates that the reactions of the recipient of a message are far more significant for behavior than the mechanics of the delivery or the contents of the message. Some of the problem areas in which research is badly needed have been listed by Roberts.[19] Additional areas that have become apparent recently include the following:

1. What is the influence of education about "planning the family" on the practice of those behaviors that reduce the risk of child-bearing? When should such education begin, and what should be the intended attitude and specific educational measures that can make "planning the family" a more meaningful and realistic concept?

2. How much information and understanding of the reproductive process, contraception, and male and female physiology are essential for consistent practice of family planning?

3. What is the maximum number of the eligible population who will accept and practice family planning? What intensive educational efforts are needed to bring about this result? The actions that should be taken to increase research on educational aspects of family planning are similar to those described for generalized health education research, as appears in the report of the WHO Scientific Group on Research in Health Education.[20]

Summary

Family planning programs have expanded rapidly during the past decade in many countries of the world. The achievement of their goals depends both on the voluntary participation of the people and the provision of adequate services. Stimulation of action by the people requires educational services that are as well planned and conducted as are the contraceptive services. Yet program administrators have concentrated mainly on recruiting personnel and providing clinical services and contraceptive supplies. To date the systematic planning of educational services to enlist the crucial participation of the people has been given limited consideration in program development; yet the decisions and actions of the people are crucial to the program's success. Activities that will help people decide to adopt family planning and related health practices and to follow these consistently require detailed and systematic planning, direction, and supervision as well as available, acceptable services. Some of the specific elements that enter into such educational programs have been described and competencies of staff delineated.

There is a dearth of specific educational and behavioral research on fostering the practice of family planning to guide programs. Stimulation of such research is badly needed.

Discussion Questions

1. What are the components of a family planning program according to Derryberry?

2. What are some key strategies and stages described in this chapter for developing a health education–related family planning program?

3. How important are partnerships among agencies in promoting effective family planning programs?

4. Why is cooperation among agencies often difficult, in your view, when it comes to health activities and family planning programs?

Notes

1. World Health Organization, *Official Records of the World Health Organization*—No. 163, Part I, p. 21 (World Health Assembly Resolution 21.43), Geneva, May 1968.

2. World Health Organization, *Official Records of the World Health Organization*—No. 197, Part 1, p. 13 (World Health Assembly Resolution 22.32), Geneva, July 1969.

3. Joan Rettie (Regional Secretary, Europe and Near East, International Planned Parenthood Federation), "The Role of Europe in the Third World: Population Policy and Its Role in AID Programmes" (mimeographed), paper read at the Council of Europe's Experimental Youth Center, April 1969.

4. World Health Organization, Expert Committee on Health Education of the Public, *WHO Technical Report Series No. 89*, Geneva, 1954.

5. World Health Organization, Expert Committee on Planning and Evaluation of Health Education, *WHO Technical Report Series No. 409*, Geneva, 1969.

6. World Health Organization, Scientific Group on Health Aspects of Family Planning, *World Health Organization Technical Report Series No. 442*, Geneva, 1970.

7. World Health Organization, Expert Committee on Dental Health Education, *Technical Report Series No. 449*, Geneva, 1970.

8. World Health Organization, "Suggested Outline for Use by Countries in Discussing Health Education of the Public" (mimeographed), Geneva, 1959.

9. World Health Organization, Regional Office for Southeast Asia, Intercounty Workshop on the Methodology of Planning, Implementation, and Evaluation of Health Education, New Delhi, November 1967.

10. Beryl J. Roberts and William Griffiths, "The Need for Educational Innovation and Research in Family Planning," in Pakistan International Family Planning Conference, *Population Control: Implications, Trends, and Prospects,* pp. 391–403, Dacca, 1969. Edited by the Conference Reporting Committee (Naffs Sadik, Chairman), Islamabad, Pakistan: Pakistan Family Planning Council.

11. H. F. Lionberger, *Adoption of New Ideas and Practices* (Ames: Iowa State University Press, 1960).

12. Everett M. Rogers, *Diffusion of Innovations* (New York: Free Press of Glencoe, 1962).

13. Donald J. Bogue, "A Reexamination of the Process by Which People Adopt Family Planning," in Pakistan International Family Planning Conference, *Population Control: Implications, Trends and Prospects*, pp. 369–77, Dacca, 1969. Edited by the Conference Reporting Committee (Naffs Sadik, Chairman), Islamabad, Pakistan: Pakistan Family Planning Council.

14. A. Govindachari and K. R. Sastry, "A Comparative Study of the Two Methods of Identifying Leaders," *Bulletin of the Institute of Rural Health and Family Planning*, Vol. 2, July 1967, Gandhigram, Madras, India.

15. K. Ranganathan, V. K. Srinivasan, and Betty L. Mathews, "An Action Research Study on the Role of Community Leaders in Promoting Family Planning in Rural India," *Action Research Monograph*, No. 1, 1965.

16. Beryl J. Roberts, "Concepts and Methods of Evaluation in Health Education," *International Journal of Health Education*, 5(2), 2–12, April–June 1962.

17. World Health Organization, PAHO/WHO Inter-Regional Conference on the Post-Graduate Preparation of Health Workers for Health Education, *WHO Technical Report Series No. 278*, Geneva, 1964.

18. World Health Organization, Scientific Group on Research in Health Education, *WHO Technical Report Series No. 432*, pp. 22–38, 1969.

19. Beryl J. Roberts, "Research in Educational Aspects of Health Programs: Its Relationship with Professional Education and Practice," *International Journal of Health Education*, Supplement, *13*, 10–13, January–March 1970.

20. World Health Organization, Scientific Group on Research in Health Education, *WHO Technical Report Series No. 432*, pp. 22–38, 1969.

Part V

Influencing the International Health Field

Overview

The three chapters in Part Five represent Mayhew Derryberry's philosophy of health education and its application to public health in a variety of international settings. He influenced the public health field not only through his own consultation work in Latin America, India, Africa, and Japan but also through the assignment of his senior health education staff in the Public Health Service to organizations such as the World Health Organization and what is now the Agency for International Development (USAID) in the Department of State.

From 1959 through 1961, Dr. Derryberry spent much of his time serving as a consultant for international organizations. In anticipation of the World Health Organization's Twelfth World Assembly, which would feature health education of the public, Derryberry stimulated wide participation by people of the United States in holding seminars, conducting technical discussions, preparing documents, and submitting recommendations. He was active at the assembly.

Each chapter selected for this part presents a particular message addressed to the needs of his audience. It is self-evident that the relevance of these messages has an even wider audience today. In Chapter Twenty-Three Derryberry illustrates how the nature of problems to be solved requires change in educational strategies. For example, if a particular situation required the provision of a safe water supply, not every affected citizen was required to understand and act on the problem. Instead, voters would respond by securing the legal authority or the sanitary facility necessary to address and resolve the issue for the entire community. Today, however, solutions to the problems of both individual and public health require the participation of all citizens.

Dr. Derryberry speaks of phases of health education programs, using the previous example as an instance of the first phase. The second phase is the larger and more difficult task of changing individual behavior to achieve improvement in personal and family health. This requires solving the broader problem of persuading each citizen to accept and use health services. We can liken these examples to the concerns we face today in environmental protection, individual health promotion, and the challenge presented by diseases such as acquired immune deficiency syndrome (AIDS). Derryberry's pragmatic examples identify barriers to behavioral change and the facilitators of change. We may ask, Is this being done today?

In Chapter Twenty-Four Derryberry captures the attention of his audience by starting out with successes in the area of sanitation—the field of his audience. He continues to use examples from malaria control and other sanitation concerns in order to help his audience more quickly comprehend his points on the sequence as well as the process of learning. Again, his judicious use of questions creates an attitude of partnership between the reader and the health educator. This personal involvement through relevant experience is characteristic of how Derryberry worked and taught.

In Chapter Twenty-Five he departs from descriptions of the specific program elements in health education to address the organization and management of programs encompassing large-scale use of individual educational methods. This paper sums up the vast experiences of countries all over the world in developing programs of health education. Derryberry sets forth a framework in which the principles of learning can be clearly understood and applied. He cautions against taking on too much too fast and stresses the importance of systematic procedures for communicating successful ideas.

These papers take the reader along on the journey that Dr. Derryberry traveled as he grew and matured in health education and in his commitment to the importance of people participating in decisions affecting their own health. Society's responsibility to adapt its problem-solving approaches to current needs is seen in a cross-cultural context.

23

The Role of Health Education
in a Public Health Program

Since the beginning of the public health movement, public
health education has been essential to progress. In the early
years, when the basic objectives of public health were the passage
of sanitation laws, the organization of a health service, or the provision of a safe public water supply, the principal task of health education was to secure the support of leaders in the community.
Although not every citizen was required to understand and act on
the problems, voters usually protected the entire community by
securing the legal authority or the sanitary facility.

Today public health is concerned with diseases that cannot be
controlled without the effective participation of all the people. Our
educational efforts must be broadened to include every individual
in order that all may understand and act upon the principles of
healthful living. There are two important phases of the health education program. There is the initial task of securing public support
for the concept that protection and improvement of the health of
the people is a social responsibility. This phase does not require
every individual member of the population to participate. The second, larger and more difficult task is to accomplish the changes in

Originally published in *Public Health Reports*, November 14, 1947, 62(46),
1629–1641. Reprinted with permission. Presented at the Second Pan-American
Conference on Health Education, Caracas, Venezuela, January 1947.

individual behavior that will result in improvement of personal and family health. When the first phase has been accomplished and there has been established a public health department or a health center where all the people may secure modern services for prevention of disease, we face the broader problem of persuading each individual citizen to accept and use these services.

A wide variety of services may be included in a modern public health program: immunization clinics, advice to pregnant women and to mothers, information on nutrition, chest X-rays for the early diagnosis of tuberculosis, broad programs for the diagnosis and treatment of venereal disease, and even the more recently developed programs for the diagnosis and treatment of cancer and mental health problems. These services can improve the health of only those who know how to act on the health problems involved. Everyone must become familiar with the advantages of immunization against smallpox and diphtheria and secure such immunizations for himself and his children. People must be brought to realize the importance of early diagnosis of tuberculosis, and they must respond in order to assure a favorable outcome for themselves as well as to protect others.

Because the methods are fairly simple, requiring little inconvenience to the people, health education in the United States has had fair success. A large proportion of the population has availed itself of vaccination against smallpox and diphtheria. Even for tuberculosis and the venereal diseases, discovery is relatively simple and requires little inconvenience.

In recent years, treatment for venereal diseases has been greatly simplified through the use of sulfa drugs for gonorrhea and of penicillin for both gonorrhea and syphilis.

But a different sort of educational problem faces us in securing the participation of all the people in programs that require more complicated procedures, greater amounts of time, and more fundamental changes in individual behavior. So far as we know now, no community action like the control of water, food, or milk will, of itself, have any effect on maternal deaths or deaths from cancer, for example. To be sure, the facilities for adequate health supervision and treatment must be in the community, but only those people who apply for examination and care will derive any benefit from the community resources. Successful work in a broad public health program, therefore, is much more difficult because, in addition to securing adequate facilities, it is necessary to inform all the individuals in the community and stimulate all of them to use the facilities.

I have emphasized the importance of this task in health education—changing individual behavior—because our future success will be commensurate only with the degree to which we are able to help people understand their health problems and actively use their new knowledge in solving such problems. In the past, individual understanding of public health problems was believed to have had a more specific role in the improvement of public health than it actually had. Community action and a rising standard of living have combined to produce dramatic results in saving lives and improving health, chiefly through creating a safer environment in which the individual has lived longer but with comparatively little change in his behavior. As soon as health programs began to provide services that require action on the part of the individual citizen, the professions met with both implicit and explicit indifference on the part of the public. It came as a great surprise to many public health workers that the people did not accept their precepts with the reformer's zeal. Only through a clear and sympathetic understanding of this individual attitude can health educators of the future hope to free the people from the personal opinions and behavior that are inimical to health. Therefore, we must patiently seek the manifold causes and as patiently seek the best means of breaking down the psychological barriers restraining people from acting to protect or improve their health.

Perhaps the most significant contributing factor to indifference is the general level of health in the population. By this I mean that whether the general health level is high or low, attention to health competes for interest and action with such paramount demands as earning a living; providing shelter, food and clothing; bringing up a family; and participating in the numerous institutions of the community, many of which are related to health remotely or not at all.

If the public is satisfied with its health status, changes in individual behavior are likewise resisted because such changes are often accomplished only with great inconveniences. We have all heard stories of grateful families in remote areas who have walked many miles over mountain trails to come to the health center for needed care. And it is true that once people become dissatisfied with their health status, they will make great sacrifices to better it. But these are the success stories of health education. The slim attendance at clinics, the "lost cases" in a venereal disease control program, as compared with estimated numbers of people in need of such services, are evidence that inconveniences—distance, discomfort, even painful experiences—are a substantial barrier to changed behavior. Closely related to these broad psychological barriers are the influences of established modes of behavior in individual families and of cultural patterns in the broadening social fields—the community, the region, the nation, and so on. Unless and until some member of the community demonstrates that a change in the mores is both beneficial and acceptable, habitual behavior will not be abandoned, or, if it is, only with great reluctance. Until acceptance is complete, the return to usual behavior will occur frequently, much to the dismay of public health workers who have not taken into account the tremendous magnetic power exerted by the human need to conform and to belong in one's own social group.

Because health practices are so intimately concerned with fundamental human drives, many of the cultural beliefs and practices in every society are related to health. It is this kind of "health education" in proverbs, folklore, prejudices, and pragmatic experiences that is passed on from one generation to the next. In recent years, health educators have learned that many deep-seated habits, often detrimental to individual and family health, have been formed from early experience and are retained with strong emotional bias. In a recent article[1] Lawrence Frank points out that much of the resistance to programs designed to secure better nutrition, better adherence to precepts of personal hygiene, and improvement in sexual relations may be found in the emotional experience of childhood when the infant is being conditioned, against his will, to eat, sleep, eliminate, and deal with other people in accordance with the adult concept of acceptable behavior.

Not only do early experiences with family and teachers produce emotional resistance to health education and services, but experiences with physicians, nurses, and other health personnel may result in highly emotional attitudes. Aside from the pain associated with immunizations, a visit to the dentist, and other treatments given by physicians and nurses, other experiences may turn a family away from the health center or the doctor's office as definitely as if a "No Admittance" sign had been put on the door. The type of experience I have in mind is the long wait in uncomfortable seats and forbidding quarters before seeing the doctor and followed by the apparent impatience of the doctors and nurses with human frailty and lack of understanding, as well as their failure to take into account the basic intelligence and willingness of human beings to deal with their own problems.

Happily, such experiences occur much less frequently today. Doctors have come to understand that the patient's problem can be solved only by mutual understanding and cooperation. Indeed, the whole concept of health education now and for the future must be the securing of mutual understanding and cooperation among all concerned, in order that the health problems of individuals and of the community may be solved effectively.

This recital of indifference to modern health practices and of the difficulties that health educators may encounter is not intended to discourage efforts to influence individual behavior toward more healthful living. Our lack of success in the United States has made us realize, however, that such attitudes must be the basis of consideration if our programs are to become more effective. Only through clear understanding of our difficulties can we plan realistically the use of the available tools and resources for health education.

What are some of the resources that can be utilized? The one that comes most readily to mind is the public information programs making use of mass media such as newspapers, pamphlets, lectures, radio, posters, exhibits, motion pictures, and other visual materials. At the risk of duplicating in part some of the later sessions of this conference, let us consider the part that information plays in effecting changes in individual behavior.

An effective mass information program is an important part of any successful health education activity. It involves analyzing the information problems, selecting messages suitable to various audiences, and planning strategic use of media and distribution channels. The information program is most effective in securing acquiescence and a degree of support. It may be likened to the softening-up process accomplished by artillery bombardment before the infantry advances. In emergencies, a carefully developed mass information program may be all that is necessary to stimulate appropriate action on a specific problem.

For example, when an epidemic threatens, the radio or the newspapers can direct a large proportion of the population to the sources for prevention and care. In Seattle, Washington, last spring, when virulent smallpox was introduced by returning troops, 85 percent of the population responded to appeals through press and radio, and presented themselves for vaccination. But in the less dramatic health problems—the day-by-day business of healthful living, the singular tragedies of preventable death—the mass, impersonal media need to be supplemented by other types of education effort.

Since Thorndike in his psychological investigations has shown that no learning takes place without interest, the previously cited general lack of interest in health accounts for the fact that large portions of the public do not respond to mass information. The citizen must be sufficiently interested to *read* the news article or pamphlet, to *listen* attentively to the radio or lecture, and to *view* actively the motion picture in order to learn what to do and then be motivated to do it.

Unfortunately, the individuals whose health behavior is most in need of improvement are all too frequently the ones who are least inclined to read, listen, or pay attention. To obtain perspective on this problem, we have only to examine our own knowledge, attitude, and behavior on some other valuable social objective, such as fire prevention, safe automobile driving, or theft. Despite extensive education programs on such objectives, many of us still violate the suggestions offered for our individual welfare.

The best illustration of the place of mass informational technique was the experience of the United States government in selling war bonds. The most extensive use possible was made of all known information media, including news articles, billboards, radio exhibits, pamphlets, motion pictures, and the like in an effort to induce people to buy bonds, not only for financing the war but also for curbing inflation. When final tabulation was made, it was found that over 80 percent of individual purchases were made on personal solicitation, which shows the need for intimate and personal contact in order to induce overt action in a large proportion of the population.

General discussion of the limitations of mass media is not to discredit their use in a well-rounded health education program, except to remind you that bombardment is not sufficient to take a city. Rather, it indicates the need for more careful evaluation of the proportion of total health education effort that one will devote to mass procedures and the amount that one will allocate to the other types of educational activity.

A second and equally important resource for health education is the schools. Representing as it does the institution that society has chosen to inform each generation of the accumulation of scientific fact and of the applications of this information to improved living, the school might well assume a major role in health education. Its teachers understand the learning process and are skilled in educational techniques. With the help of the scientific health worker to provide the content, the school should be the most potent instrument in effecting changes in the behavior of people. As a public institution it should provide a model health environment for those who attend or visit it and should encourage nothing but the most acceptable health practices within its boundaries.

Although the school has great potential for effective health education, not only of the children but of adults as well, we have discovered in the United States a need for improvement of our school programs. Too often, there is the tacit and unwarranted assumption, both by public health and educational workers, that if you teach the child proper health practices in school, he will go home and teach his parents. Parents usually regulate the activities in their households, including many practices that affect health. If these procedures are not in accord with the health principles the child has learned at school, he will find it very difficult to change them or his parent's attitude toward them, since they have become habitual practices with which the family is satisfied. It takes more than "I learned at school that we ought to eat more vegetables" to change the dietary habits of a family.

Another assumption often voiced by professional workers is that if the child in school is taught the principles of personal health, he will practice them in his daily living. But most of the behaviors that are taught (bathing, sleeping, eating, and elimination) are carried on at home under parental influence. The child is unable to practice the changed behavior he learned in school, and, as a consequence, the routines of his parents become his. It has also been assumed that if children learn what to do about adult health problems, they will practice them when they grow up. This overlooks our tendencies to forget quickly information that is not immediately applicable. Then, too, the rapid advances made by medical science bring about some modifications in the behavior the adult learned at school when a child and indicate a need for constant education in all age groups so that all can keep pace with the contributions made by medical science.

Thus, the influence of the school in changing the health behavior of the population is severely limited if it does not expand its program to include education for the adults as well as for the children. Unfortunately, too many of our schools in the United States observe an age limit and do not attempt to meet the educational needs of all the people in the community.

A second hindrance to developing fully the health education potential of the schools in the United States has been the failure to train our teachers in the functional facts underlying healthful living. A survey of their training in the biological sciences and in health education convinces us that our major problem in the United States is to find ways in which teachers may be better prepared to assume responsibility in health education.

One last weakness in the health education work of schools in the United States has been the misplaced emphasis on esthetic practices, or personal etiquette, to the exclusion of more significant health behavior and community health problems. Too often, teachers have stressed having the hair combed and a clean handkerchief but have neglected to explain such health practices as washing hands after going to the toilet or staying at home when one has a cold or other evidence of acute infection. In many areas, our schools have not provided a model sanitary environment; nor has their schedule of activities, including adequate time for lunch, coincided with their classroom precepts. It is gratifying to see that the needs of children for an opportunity to practice in their schools the best of health habits are being recognized. An increasing number of our schools are being equipped with adequate sanitary facilities, including soap, hot water, and towels. Many are offering hot lunches, efficiently prepared and served.

Last but not least of the potential influences for effective health education in the schools is the medical service. If conducted with the intention to give an appreciation of good medical practice and to advise parents on the health of the children, the medical service can do more to stimulate proper use of medical resources than any similar effort devoted to didactic instruction. If, however, it is conducted in a perfunctory, routine fashion, with little attention to the questions of parents or children, an unfavorable attitude will be built up toward utilizing professional advice, regardless of the competence of the physicians and nurses.

This critical review of our past practices has been made in order that we may sharpen our efforts to realize fully the potential value of the schools in health education.

The doctors and nurses, themselves, both in the health department and in private practice, are a third potent resource for health education. We have indicated their contribution in the school health service. They exercise a similar influence in all their other services to people. In fact, it may be said that every visit to the clinic or the doctor's office, every visit by the public health nurse, is health education, for the visit provides the most powerful type of learning, namely experience. If the experience is not satisfying, there will be a tendency to avoid seeking health and medical care the next time that the individual or a member of his family needs it. Medical and nursing personnel, therefore, need not only the skills and knowledge of their professions but understanding and ability in the art of dealing with people.

The educational influence of a competent medical and nursing staff reaches far beyond their patients through praise of their efforts by those they have served. Other members of the public health staff also have rich opportunities for educating the people. The engineers, sanitarians, and sanitary inspectors often have a difficult task in persuading particular groups of the population to comply with sanitary laws and regulations. Recently in the United States, persons engaged in restaurant inspection and law enforcement activities have stated that health education is a necessary tool in assisting them to achieve their objectives.

In the United States we are coming to realize, however, that future progress in health education, even within the schools or through the use of mass media, depends upon community-wide participation. Thus, the prime resource for future health education effort is in the various organized groups of the community. And this same utilization of community organization is essential in other social programs.

Many organizations, such as the Red Cross, tuberculosis associations, and welfare and professional organizations, have definite health objectives. Other civic, social, or industrial groups can often be interested in the health program and can render valuable educational service in the community. Within these organizations will be found many of the recognized community leaders—individuals who have won the respect of the people for their wisdom and for valuable advice in the past. Their influence is great. The community leaders do not always have the attitudes and opinions with respect to health that are approved by modern science. But if effort is spent in giving them a thorough understanding of what is needed and how problems can be solved, they can contribute immeasurably to better understanding among all the people. They can also become a powerful motivating force for community action and for changed behavior through their own acceptance of scientific methods and practices.

In most communities, the clergy will be found among the influential leaders; their cooperation is a valuable resource for health education. This source of support is all the more important in communities where church institutions include schools and hospitals.

In rural areas, leaders in agricultural work will often prove the most influential group in stimulating people to changes of behavior. As a rule, if a county agent or a home demonstration agent has helped the people of a rural community in solving some important economic problem or in meeting a crisis, he or she is an accepted leader without whose support the health education program will meet with apathy if not outright resistance. How can we mobilize these potential resources of a community, a region, or a nation for their maximum contribution to the health of the people? First, there must be a joint planning on common problems by all of the interested groups. The importance of planning together cannot be stressed too strongly. Attempts at cooperation too often fail because one person or one organization develops a plan and then endeavors to get the others to follow. Naturally, those who have tried to follow along become apathetic to the plan, for if it succeeds, the person who drew up the original blueprint is the only one to enjoy the satisfaction of achievement, while those who cooperated lose any real feeling of participation. They feel they are merely contributing to the planner's success.

All too often individuals or groups have their own problems and are unwilling to set aside their special interests temporarily to join with other groups in attaining an objective of more general interest. If there is joint planning on a common problem, all are working toward the same goal. Independent action produces competition of a sort that is fatal to the success of a health plan; namely, competition for the attention and action of the people, many of whom already lead overcrowded lives. Thus, the available resources for health are dispersed in many directions. On one side the people are urged to do something about tuberculosis; on another, to do something about getting a hospital, and on still another, to do something about nutrition. They are confused. In the meantime, there is the constant barrage of patent medicine and quack advertisements that call upon them to buy innumerable products, take this or that medicine, use this or that device for their health. In their wonderment, the people decide to wait until the various groups make up their minds on what is best to be done. Too often, they rely on a friend's advice, fall back on the practices that their parents or grandparents used, or yield to the pleas of the advertisers.

Cooperative planning is an essential of success in health education. It means joint consideration of and common interest in all the possibilities for the solution of a problem, and mutual agreement on the resources that each group will contribute and on the activities that each will perform. When there is such planning, continued cooperation is practically assured. Ivah Deering, in her book *Let's Try Thinking*, says, "People do not lightly set aside plans they have helped to make."

Participants in a cooperative venture must have an interest in each other's purposes, plans, resources, limitations, and responsibilities. Each has his own field of competence, which must be respected by all the others. Each also has his limitations, which not only he but all the others must recognize without implying criticism. Cooperation is impossible without this basic understanding and tolerance.

In the United States we have found, too, that in a successful health education program, there must be periodic and frequent checkups on progress and additional planning by the cooperating parties. It is not enough to agree on objectives, plan what each shall do, and then each go about the scheduled task. There is need for working together continuously, reallotting duties and changing methods of participation according to the changing status of the program.

There must also be technical leadership. Too often, unguided effort of enthusiastic people has ended in failure or in wasteful programs. To call upon the experts who know the good and bad points about any procedure and who can give the facts is not to underrate the people and the intelligent decisions they make, provided they have the facts upon which to act.

Finally, there must be a proper sharing of credit. Abuse of this requirement is perhaps the most frequent factor that interferes with cooperative effort. Some people appear to feel that credit to themselves and their organization is more important than the achievement of the objective. Certainly, we do not suggest that credit is unimportant. We must account for our own activities and for the expenditure of funds in terms of accomplishment. But it isn't necessary to claim credit for all the results of a cooperative program. Actually, a division of credit with other participants results in more appreciation of our own part in the program.

The special role of education in a health plan, we believe, is to secure this meaningful cooperation between many groups and individuals with diverse interests and capacities but with a common purpose—conservation of human resources. Another essential is an understanding and appreciation of the special qualifications that the many different types of professional workers can contribute to health education. Perhaps one method of bringing about better working relationships among professional groups is to have in the various agencies persons who have been trained in more than one special field. This idea has been put into practice in Puerto Rico, where the health department has employed people who had a background in education and trained them in health. The education department, the extension service of agriculture, and the labor department also did the same. So in these different organizations, there are one or more individuals who know education, who know public health, and yet are part of the organization. These people can interpret the contributions of their organizations to the other groups. In this way, the program can go forward through all the major channels that reach the people.

A few community-wide health education programs were initiated prior to World War II and have proved their value. The need for the maintenance of a high level of health during the war gave a great impetus to further development of programs in which the public was stimulated to participate in the solution of individual and community problems. A type of health worker seldom used before that time was recruited to conduct such programs in each community. These workers were college graduates, with basic training in the natural and biological sciences, education, and sociology. Most of them had taught in schools. In addition, they had taken one or more years of graduate training in a school of public health. Although not physicians or nurses, they have been well grounded in the fundamental public health sciences and also have acquired skills in community organization and methods of teaching. For want of a better name, these workers are called "public health educators."

In reality, they are extension workers for health—extending to people a better understanding of how to use the findings of science for healthful living.

When the public health educators began these programs in various localities, they first sought out all of the community organizations. In many cases, this meant visiting personally a large number of individuals, for the communities in the United States have a multiplicity of organized groups. The object of these visits was to find out if the leaders of the organizations were interested in community health improvement and, if so, to invite them to participate in a joint endeavor for determining and achieving objectives in health education.

The interested community leaders then met with the local health officer and the health educator. They told what *they* considered to be health problems in the community and obtained from the health officer the facts on the extent of the problems, what was being done to solve them, and what remained to be done. The various organizations then agreed on what problems should be tackled first and what each could do to help. One would agree to organize study groups in the community; another, to take care of the publicity; still others, to visit and secure the support of other organizations not then participating.

Soon it was recognized that methods had to be found whereby *all* the citizens could be reached directly. During the war, it was possible for the community leaders, aided by public health educators, to utilize the citizen organization created by the Office of Civilian Defense. Thus, in many communities a study group on health problems was organized in every city block, with a "block leader" in charge. The doctors, nurses, and engineers of the health department, as well as public health educators, met with these leaders to give them the technical advice and assistance they needed.

I should like to emphasize the importance of technical assistance. In order that sound information may be passed on to each citizen, community leaders and block leaders need to be carefully prepared for their task. We have found that with the interest and participation of the health department staff, the majority of the "block leaders" develop ability to conduct effective study groups, passing on correct information to a surprising degree.

All of the known tools for education are used: pamphlets, motion pictures, exhibits, and the like. These are secured by the public health educator. During the study of a specific community problem, mass media are employed; generally local newspapers and radio stations respond readily to the requests of community leaders for space and time.

These public health educators also undertook to assist the schools in coordinating their health education program with the activities of the community for better health. They worked closely with teachers, supervisors, and administrators.

The outcome of such community-wide health education has been satisfying. A recent demonstration resulted in 87 percent of the population turning out for chest X-ray examinations in a city where traditional methods, employed year after year, had brought only a few hundred people to tuberculosis clinics. During the demonstration, volunteers—organized by the community leaders— visited *every* family in the city, explaining the program and making appointments for the X-ray examinations.

The employment of qualified public health educators in local health departments is rapidly being accepted as desired practice by local health officers. Through such workers, the health officer finds it easier to reach his community, both for effective cooperation in carrying out his program and for understanding the individual and group needs of the community. Indeed, the role of the public health educator might be stated briefly as: to build a bridge of cooperation between the health services and the community at large, over which two-way traffic may pass. The traffic is composed of interests, needs, and resources of the community flowing toward the health agency, and the expert knowledge, services, and needs of the agency flowing toward the community. This interchange of information, aims, and activities results in more effective efforts to achieve the common purpose, namely, better individual and community health.

At the present time, there are some 200 public health educators working in local departments in the United States. The demand for additional workers far exceeds the supply, and, unless some method is found to accelerate training, it is likely that the demand for public health educators will continue in excess of the number of available, qualified workers.

Objective evaluation has not yet been made of the effectiveness of these public health educators and of the programs they are building. Such evaluation is the number one problem on our agenda for the future. We are confident, however, that real progress is being made in increasing community understanding and stimulating action, since concrete results have been observed in several areas.

Summary

1. All progress in public health requires education. When the problem is to provide a community facility or to improve some universally used product, such as the water supply, education of a majority of the people may result in the necessary legislation, authority, or funds.

2. Many diseases, however, can be controlled only through the intelligent action of all the people. The task of health education is to stimulate that action. Psychological, economic, and social barriers exist that make the task difficult.

3. A wide variety of resources, tools, and methods are available, however, to overcome the difficulties and to accomplish the task. These include mass information, the schools, and community leaders of all types. Each of these resources has its own limitations; a planned coordination of all resources is needed for effective health education.

4. The development in the United States that gives greatest promise at the present time is the trained public health educator in a local health department, whose specific task is to bring about this coordination of all community resources for the improvement of individual and community health.

Discussion Questions

1. How does Derryberry see the role of community, that is, each individual, in the implementation and support of public health programs?

2. What are some important resources for promoting effective health communications among communities?

3. What is the role of health education in a health plan according to Derryberry?

4. Why, in Derryberry's view, is the task of stimulating health actions that can prevent or control disease and injury so problematic?

5. How can some of the principles that Derryberry describes be applied to violence prevention, a public health problem rarely considered in Derryberry's time?

Note

1. L. K. Frank, "Health Education," *American Journal of Public Health*, 36(4), 357-366, 1946.

24

Health Education Aspects of Sanitation Programs in Rural Areas and Small Communities

Over the years, sanitarians[1] have made great strides in reducing disease through their efforts at controlling or eliminating those factors of the environment that favor transmission. They have built central facilities for water supply in which the water is made safe through filtration and chlorination; they have installed sanitary systems for sewage collection and disposal; they have drained or treated swamps and other mosquito-breeding places, and the like. These activities have brought about dramatic reductions in disease incidence, disability, and mortality, particularly in centers of population where such centralized services are practicable. The results have been accomplished largely by the sanitarian's own efforts. After securing official approval and the necessary resources in materials and labor, the sanitarian has been able to use his understanding of biological phenomena, his ability in engineering planning, and his executive skill in directing the activities of others to effect the desirable environmental changes without necessarily gaining the widespread understanding or participation of the people themselves.

But in villages and rural areas the same types of centralized and environmental improvements are not feasible. Although the basic

Originally published in *Bulletin of the World Health Organization*, 1954, *10*, 145–154. Reprinted with permission.

principles of sanitary science still apply, many of the actions that are necessary to break the chain of disease transmission must be taken by the people themselves. Such actions may include providing themselves with sanitary facilities, changing their personal behavior, and/or carrying out specific sanitary measures such as DDT residual spraying for mosquito control. In such situations, skillful application of the sciences of human behavior is as essential for success as the competent use of the sanitary sciences.

Application of the behavioral sciences—an essential part of effective education—follows the same broad pattern as is used in applying the sanitary sciences. The basic steps in the process are as follows:

1. The essential facts on which to base a program are obtained. The information needed includes not only facts about the particular situation but also the broad scientific generalizations that apply to other situations.

2. A program is planned. With the known facts about the situation and an understanding of what may be expected from various courses of action, decisions are made, and a plan most likely to be effective is developed.

3. The planned program is put into operation.

The remainder of this chapter will be devoted to some of the specific factors to be considered in each step of the process of program planning as it applies to education.

The Assembling of Essential Facts

There are many items of information about the people of any community that must be ascertained before an educational program can be effectively planned. Some of these, stated as questions, are the following:

1. What problems do the people recognize and have an interest in doing something about?

People are willing to act with reference to any situation only when they are dissatisfied with what they have and desire a change. For example, if the people of a community feel that malaria is their major problem and do not recognize the seriousness of enteric diseases, they will more readily participate in activities to cut down the incidence of malaria than in those focused on safe water or excreta disposal. Actually, any attempt to get them to work on reducing diseases of the intestinal tract when their major concern is malaria control is likely to be met with passive or even active resistance. If, on the other hand, the people are unconcerned about any of their environmental health problems as the sanitarian sees them, then the first task of the sanitarian becomes one of finding ways to create a desire for change by awakening the people to their sanitation problems. This must necessarily precede education about how the problems can be solved.

Finding out what problems trouble the people provides guidelines for beginning the sanitation program and determines in part what should be the educational effort.

2. What information do they already have about their problems? What do they perceive as the cause and the possible solutions?

Foster[2] writes: "The public health specialist is not operating in a vacuum, his subjects do not feel he is bringing light on a problem about which they know nothing. Rather, he is working in an area in which the subjects have definite and hard-to-shake beliefs." Some of these ideas may be correct, but even if they are not, the people are just as sure they are correct as the sanitarian is sure they are mistaken. There must be full knowledge of the people's information as a basis for planning an educational program. For example, people who understand the relation of unsafe water and unsanitary excreta disposal to the enteric diseases need only technical advice and assistance in finding the way to protect their water or to dispose satisfactorily of their human wastes. On the other hand, people who see the enteric diseases as being associated with the seasons, the growth of some plant, or as a falling out of harmony with the forces of nature require an entirely different educational content and approach before satisfactory solutions to the problem can be achieved. In this latter case, not only must they learn the scientific facts about the causes and prevention of intestinal diseases, but some methods must also be found to help them fit the scientific information into their present concept of the situation. For example L. L. Williams tells of a rice-growing area in China where the people believed that sleeping in the lowlands caused them to contract malaria. To avoid the disease, the workers in the rice paddies had adopted the custom of building their homes in the highlands above the area in which the mosquito was prevalent. The workers traveled down from their homes each morning to work the rice and returned each evening. As soon as a knowledge of the beliefs and behavior of these people had been ascertained, an approach to their education about the real cause of malaria and its control became readily apparent.

3. What are the usual channels of communication in which the people have confidence?

In every society there exist methods by which information is communicated among the people. These channels of communication may include: (a) the village story reader or teller; (b) the homes of recognized community leaders, the carriers of prestige, where people gather for up-to-date and authentic information on various topics; (c) conversations of womenfolk at the village bakery and village well and during social visits or while doing field work; (d) news and views exchanged during the weekly market and during religious festivals; (e) the village crier, who informs the whole community of important news by shouting it out at night; (f) key persons such as the teacher, the priest, or the headman, who read the paper or other literature to the people and pass on instructions from authorities; (g) conversation of men in coffee houses, at threshing floors, during social visits, and while doing field work.[3] In other societies, there are many clubs, associations, religious institutions, voluntary health agencies, and the like through which information is transmitted. As a basis for planning, the sanitarian needs full data on the channels through which information reaches the people. He also needs to know if there are any parts of the population that are not reached through any of the existing methods for disseminating information. Even in societies where there is a multitude of organizations, studies have revealed large segments of the population who would not be reached through the existing groups or organizations.

4. Who are the individuals to whom the people look for advice?

   In other words, who are the leaders of the people? It is necessary to find not only the titular leaders, such as the mayors and governors, but also those whom the people follow—the natural leaders. The latter group is often overlooked, yet all too often it comprises the key individuals to whom the people turn for advice and counsel. In addition to finding out who these leaders are, it is essential to know what specific information they have and whether they have any interest in doing something about the problem.

5. What are the social, economic, cultural, and religious characteristics of the people—their value systems, customs, beliefs, and ways of working—that may influence their actions?

   The importance of some of these factors has already been discussed. However, their strong influence on the types of behavior changes that are possible merit special mention. The sanitarian may need the help of an anthropologist or social scientist to guide him in securing the kinds of data in the area that should be known before programs are planned. The following incidents merely illustrate the kinds of information that need to be considered. In certain cultures the number 3 is a ritual number; in others, it is 7. In such situations, the actions that would be suggested might be organized into three or seven steps. In some cultures, bad smells are thought to be a cause of disease. Such a belief can easily be used in connection with a sanitary program for garbage disposal, but it may interfere with a privy-building program, particularly if the area is hot and dry, where the feces left outside a privy dry up in a short time and quickly become odorless. In cultures where the people value the life of all living things, the advice to kill germs by boiling water is likely to be met with resistance. A thorough knowledge of the beliefs, mores, value systems, and other social and cultural factors will aid in tying the environmental sanitation program into the people's usual patterns of thought and behavior and will avoid the pitfalls resulting from misunderstanding and distrust.

6. What resources exist in the community that can contribute to the educational program? How do they function in the community?

Are there any related programs into which the environmental sanitation program can be fitted? The schools, where they exist and serve a large portion of the child population, are often a valuable instrument for any community betterment. In considering the schools, however, it must be recognized that the teachers, principals, and supervisors may have other interests than sanitation and may want the schools to concentrate on other problems that they consider more important. Other groups that may be willing to help, since environmental sanitation will also contribute to their overall objective of community betterment, are those conducting programs of fundamental education, economic development, agricultural extension, rural and vocational education, village self-help, and religious education. If the sanitarian learns all about such groups—their goals and methods—and assists them in their program, they will join him in the improvement of the sanitary conditions in the community. If, on the other hand, he chooses to go it alone, he may encounter competition rather than cooperation.

Planning for Behavior Changes in the People

The preceding section outlines the kinds of data about the community, its people, and their thoughts, feelings, and ways of working that are needed for effective planning. However, it is not necessary or desirable for the sanitarian to gather all the information himself. Instead, considerable impetus will be given the educational program if, through their own efforts or study, the people discover for themselves answers to many of the questions. Therefore, in planning, the sanitarian must first focus on the way in which he can most effectively work with the people. He is concerned with helping them to make such changes as they decide are desirable, not with doing the things he has decided are good for them. As he goes about this planning, there are a number of factors to be considered, which again are stated as questions.

1. How can the people concerned be brought in on the planning of the individual or group action required?

   The first consideration is: "Who are the people concerned?" Certainly the leaders, both titular and natural, for they will give guidance on the subsequent things that the people may do. In fact, their influence is so great that they have sometimes been called the "gatekeepers" to action. But in addition to these gatekeepers, there are the people themselves. The sanitarian must plan so that all, or as many as possible, of those concerned will participate. It is especially important that those who will have any responsibility for carrying out the program have a part in deciding what shall be done and how. Planning for this participation of the people is especially important where the sanitary behavior that will protect them is a practice that must be followed consistently—such as boiling water, using a sanitary facility, and the like—instead of a single action such as an immunization or the construction of a central water supply.

Obtaining the participation of the people in planning what shall be done is emphasized because the scientists of human behavior have established that people will do those things that most closely satisfy their needs in life as they see them; in other words, people will choose to do the things they want to do. When people have a part in studying and planning the ways in which they will solve a problem, they are much more likely to carry out the planned action. Ivah Deering expresses this fact in her book *Let's Try Thinking* in these two statements: "To think [a problem] through within and with the assistance of the group is to build under the subsequent action a foundation which will stand greater storms and stresses, for it is made up of understanding, cooperation, and common effort. Those who have had a true part in making decisions will not see those decisions lightly set aside."[4]

There is no standard blueprint of how the participation of the people can be obtained. The sanitarian will need to use all the information that has been accumulated and be resourceful in his methods and patient in his approaches, for people do not quickly change the practices of a lifetime.

2. Within the limits of achieving the sanitary goals, what are the various solutions that may be offered the people?

In other words, are there a number of ways of achieving the environmental improvements from which the people may choose, and what nontechnical decisions can be left entirely to them? Although it is essential that the people participate in the planning of the actions they will take, there are many decisions that cannot be left to them. Such decisions are those that are prescribed by sanitary science. For example, whether malaria is transmitted by mosquitoes or bad air is not a question to be decided by the people. Sanitary science has proved that the control of malaria requires breaking the chain from the sick person to the vector to the well person. Likewise, preventing enteric diseases involves proper personal habits, sanitary disposal of human wastes, and safe water. However, there is a variety of ways in which these control methods may be realized.

The wise sanitarian will advise on the technical aspects of achieving control but leave to the people the kinds of decisions that, although technically unimportant, are important in the ultimate actions of the people. For example, whether privies are built with or without risers is unimportant to the technician. Nevertheless, situations have been reported where privies with risers were built for the people, and none of the people would use them since they preferred privies over which they could squat. In any situation there will be many possible technical solutions to the problem. If the sanitarian communicates effectively the various methods, their advantages and disadvantages, then he can rest assured that the decision of the people will be the one best for them and the one they are most likely to carry out. In the educational phase of a sanitation program, almost all questions about methods of spreading information and securing action can be decided more effectively by the people. The sanitarian must take responsibility for the technical accuracy of the information. He may also advise on method based on his previous experience, but final decisions can be left to the people.

3. What informational materials are likely to be needed; how and when will they be used?

In every program, some means of spreading the information becomes essential as the program progresses. The sanitarian should consider in his planning what types of informational material may be needed; for example, in a population with a high proportion of illiterates, audiovisual materials may be required. To be effective, such materials should be locally planned by the people concerned, related to their needs, and, if possible, produced by them. Many workers have reported misunderstandings that have been transmitted or resistances that have been stimulated through the use of materials developed in another country, or even in another section of the same country, for people with a different social, economic, and cultural background. In almost every situation, resources such as local artists, writers, and printers can be found to produce economical and simple illustrative informational material. Enlisting the participation of such people not only provides material economically but it also contributes to the educational program. Individuals must learn the information before they can develop material to transmit it. Knutson[5] has developed a series of conditions that must be met in order for informational materials to be effective. With some of his associates, he has shown how materials might be pretested in the process of being produced to see if they satisfy the conditions for effectiveness. Through such checking, possible misunderstanding can be eliminated and the likelihood of effectively transmitting the message greatly enhanced.

Probably more important than the production of informational materials is the timing of their use. All too often, sanitation programs are initiated at a time convenient to the sanitarians. Since the people are the ones whose participation is needed for success, the timing of the entire program should be determined by them. They will know when there is a real felt need for information and what types of facts need to be presented. The program should be timed for some period when there is the least competition for interest and action. In this connection, the practice of conducting informational programs at fiestas or during carnivals, on the basis that the people can be reached (physically), may well be questioned. One might ask: "Will the people learn about health problems when their primary concern of the moment is having fun—in fact, escaping from the depressing situations of ill health with which they are daily confronted?"

4. How will barriers to the success of the program be overcome?

Are there economic limitations that will interfere with the success of the program? Is there a shortage of materials such as pipe, cement, or DDT that would limit wide-scale action by the people? In the event of shortages, how will the sanitarian meet an insistent demand that may arise if the educational program is more successful than he had contemplated?

Another barrier that may be present, and for which the sanitarian should plan, is the attitude of the people toward technicians. Do they see individuals from outside their group as people from whom they can obtain help, or do they see them as authoritarians who interfere with their customary routines and impose burdens upon them? All too often the technician's behavior justifies this latter attitude, simply because he has not carefully planned a way of work in which people will see his desire to be helpful.

5. What will be the criteria of progress in solving the sanitary environmental problems?

Will the sanitarian measure his achievements by the number of sanitary installations made in a given period of time, or will he accept as his criterion of progress the fact that the people have set goals for themselves? As engineers who are accustomed to setting target dates and being able to measure their success in objective terms of units completed, it is only natural that they should choose the former method of measuring accomplishments. If, however, the sanitarian is also concerned with lasting improvement in the sanitary behavior of the people, he will measure progress in terms of the extent to which the people accept responsibility for setting their own goals and then moving towards their realization. In other words, he will have a sense of achievement not in the number of privies built, or in the number of wells or springs made sanitary, but in the increasing responsibility assumed by the people to put into practice the technical information they have learned and in their mounting desire to take other actions for the improvement of their living conditions.

Operation of the Program

When careful study and planning with the people for the educational program have been done, few problems should arise in the actual operation of the program. The major task is to check progress in terms of the criteria that have been set. Here the sanitarian can be most effective in assisting people to accept responsibility for their own improvement. He can help to set realistic goals, ones that can be accomplished in a sufficiently short period of time to bring a feeling of achievement. He can help the people to see progress even though the goal was not attained, and he can assist in revising the targets and target dates in a way that brings satisfaction rather than discouragement.

As the sanitarian follows his plans for helping the people, he must be ever alert to any misunderstandings or hostile attitudes that may be developing. Such situations require a reevaluation of his own plans, a diagnosis of the source of the misunderstanding, and a finding of ways for the people to participate in correcting the situation.

Summary

In the conduct of a program for sanitation education, one makes use of the scientific findings of the social sciences (the sciences of human behavior) in the same manner that sanitary science is used in planning specific environmental sanitation improvement. In both situations, all the pertinent evidence is collected and related to the general scientific principles that apply. From such study a plan is developed, tested, put into operation, and watched to see that the expected results are being achieved.

Such an approach to education produces a dynamic program that recognizes the importance of an individual's own attitudes, and those of the group with whom he identifies himself, in controlling his behavior. It is more than a program of giving information through posters, newspapers, radio, or motion pictures. It takes into account an individual's past experience and the imprint that may have been left on his thinking and attitudes, the information as well as misinformation that he now has, his ambitions in life, and the way in which these factors influence what he will learn and do. It also recognizes the effect of customs, traditions, religious beliefs, and the part the group plays in determining what is socially acceptable behavior for a given individual. Finally, it accepts the principle that each individual has the right and responsibility to decide for himself the actions he will take for the benefit of himself and his community, and it provides a means by which decisions for action can be made based on scientific data and technical advice.

Discussion Questions

1. What broad patterns used in environmental sanitation problems can be generalized to effective health education?

2. What is important about this approach that is currently applicable to planning contemporary health education interventions or programs?

3. What are some of the strengths and weaknesses of partnerships in the global health context according to Derryberry?

4. How would Derryberry's approaches to sanitation be useful in preventing today's environmental health problems?

Notes

1. Throughout this chapter the word *sanitarian* is used as a generic term embracing sanitary engineers and other public health workers engaged in the practical application of sanitary science.

2. George Foster, *A Cross-Cultural Anthropological Analysis of a Technical Aid Program* (Washington, D.C.: Smithsonian Institution, 1951), p. 60.

3. *Experience with Human Factors in Agricultural Areas of the World* (Washington, D.C.: United States Department of Agriculture, 1949).

4. Ivah Deering, *Let's Try Thinking* (Yellow Springs, Ohio: Antioch Press, 1942).

5. Andie L. Knutson, "Application of Pretesting in Health Education," in *Pretesting and Evaluating Health Education* (Washington, D.C.: United States Public Health Service, 1952).

25

Health Education

A Mass Movement

An essential ingredient for the achievement of any nation's goals is the health of its people. Therefore every country of the world spends a considerable amount of its resources to provide for health care of its sick and the prevention of disease. This is as it should be, for as has been frequently said in these meetings, physically strong and mentally alert citizens are essential if a country is to advance intellectually, socially, economically, and politically.

The universal acceptance of the importance of health is almost paralleled by the way in which health programs are developed in the various countries of the world. It has been the history of almost all health programs that the technical health experts spend considerable time and effort in developing health services and facilities that will improve the health of the people. In the beginning those who are sick, in pain, and in need of medical care may flock to the facilities to cure their ills. Yet even these services for the sick are seldom used to their maximum advantage by all the people. But when services of a preventive nature are offered, relatively few people seek these benefits in the beginning. This sequence of providing services without their full utilization by the beneficiaries has proven true in all the countries on which I have been able to get

---

Originally presented at the Fifth Health Educators' Conference in Bangalore, India, June 30, 1966.

information. It is true regardless of whether the services were maternal and child care, nutrition, immunization, malaria control, early care of chronic illness, family planning, or mental health.

Faced with this failure of the people to take advantage of the proffered services, directors of health programs in all countries have made attempts to improve the participation and cooperation of the people. It is at this point that great divergence in methods to stimulate full use of health services and facilities has occurred in the various countries. In some countries intensive publicity campaigns have been undertaken. During the period of the campaign, some increase in use of services occurs, but usually there is still a large segment of the population who have not responded, and the participation of people gradually has declined when the intensity of the campaign has diminished.

Some countries have concentrated their health education efforts in the schools, with the reasoning that if we teach the children about health and health practices, they can go home and teach their parents. This last assumption has not proven to be valid, and little improvement in adult health practices has taken place where school health education programs have not been supplemented extensively by other methods designed specifically to reach the adult population.

In some countries, voluntary agencies have undertaken to stimulate full participation of the people, and when their method of approach has been one of involving leaders of various groups of the population, the response has been better, though not fully satisfactory.

Some countries have recognized the complexity of stimulating full participation of the people and have developed a corps of health education specialists who have been trained in health education program planning, in the use of mass communication methods, in the methods of stimulating community participation in health programs, and in the basic scientific facts of health. This has been a slower procedure, but in India, the Philippines, Colombia, Venezuela, and the United States, considerable progress has been made in the jurisdictions where these workers have concentrated their efforts.

Still another approach has been the establishment of Houses of Health, such as are found in the U.S.S.R., where lectures on health subjects are regularly given by doctors from the health services. Thus we see that some form of health education becomes sooner or later an essential part of the health programs wherever they develop. None of the countries have attempted to develop a mass movement such as is being proposed for India. However, from the diversity of programs that have been carried out, we are able to abstract a few basic principles to guide the educational effort that India's mass movement will require.

Wherever the programs have been successful, there has been professionally competent and dedicated leadership both at the national level and at intermediate jurisdictional and operational levels of the society. This requirement for success is quite adequately met in India. As a member of the Central Council of Health's Committee on Health Education, appointed by you, I have had the opportunity to study the way in which the Central Bureau has systematically gone about developing strong staff and a parent organization for this leadership role. It has arranged advanced training in health education for a small corps of officers to man the various sections of the bureau. To further qualify these staff for their leadership role, most of them in the past year or so have tackled difficult problems in the field where there was lack of participation in health programs and have learned from practical experience the situations that will confront the grassroots workers and how they can be met. Thus they have both theoretical and practical experience to bring to their task of providing national leadership for the movement. In addition, a small corps of competent workers have been professionally prepared for state leadership, and in most of the states these leaders are in position and developing the state bureaus.

The Central Bureau has further trained a small number of district-level personnel for their leadership responsibility in the districts. In the course of this training they have developed both a syllabus and a methodology of on-the-job training that can be used in other centers in the further development of leadership for this mass movement. Thus there has been the initial preparation of leadership, but the success of the mass movement will require further training of a much larger corps of devoted workers to push the movement ahead.

A second principle we learn from a study of successful programs in other countries is the need to start intensively in a small way and in a limited area. In general it can be said that wherever the health education effort has been to reach all the people at once, the program has had limited success. But the successful programs we read about and have seen are those where resources and effort were first concentrated in a village, a county, or a city. As the program succeeded there, it spread to other parts of the country. As someone has said, "Nothing succeeds like success." The health programs in Rio Piedras, Puerto Rico, in California, in Colombia, and in Fayetteville, North Carolina, all demonstrate the value of small intensive beginnings.

The mass education of China spearheaded by Jimmy Yen began in one area of Tinghsien Province and gradually spread through most of the country before the Communists took over. This method of concentrating program efforts in a limited area is not unique to other countries. During these meetings here, we have heard of a number of successful projects, all of which started in a village, a block, or a district.

But the temptation always is to try to cover too large a segment of the population immediately. India is a big country with a very large population. All Indians need health education, thus making the temptation even stronger to spread the initial efforts too thinly, even though the results may be less effective. Certainly this too-extended approach will delay in getting the mass movement rolling.

A third principle arising from a study of programs in various countries is to start with problems of concern to the people. All too often we technical people decide what it is the people need to know and do, and begin there. Let me recount to you a story.

During World War II we were asked to conduct health education about venereal disease among the citizen groups near a military training camp. When our health educator met with the leaders of the small towns around the camp, they expressed concern about such problems as tuberculosis, sanitation, nutrition, dental health, and so on. Not once did they express any concern about venereal disease. The workers helped the people learn about the problems of concern to them and plan what action they could take to overcome some of their problems.

After about four months, a worker suggested that they again consider the problems of importance to the community. Again no mention was made of the venereal disease problem. As a good health educator, the worker suggested that many soldiers from the camp were contracting venereal disease in the community. The important leader of the town said, "Do we have to talk about that subject? It is very distasteful to me."

So the health educator continued to help the community work on problems of its concern. Some two months later the community leader began to recognize the seriousness of the venereal disease problem and initiated a successful campaign to close the houses of prostitution in various sectors of the community. Only by starting with items of concern to the people was it possible to arouse their interest in a more serious problem to the nation's security.

A fourth principle (mentioned by the minister yesterday) is to start in those communities where the people are willing to participate in learning how to improve the health of their community. Again the temptation may be to concentrate in the more backward villages on the grounds that they need it the most. But as the minister so aptly said yesterday, there are many communities that are willing to put some effort of their own into this movement, so let the others wait until they become interested or until resources are adequate to reach out to them. No mass movement can be started with apathetic people. But it is possible for today's apathetic people to be fired with enthusiasm once they see what has been done someplace else.

A fifth feature that was common to successful programs in other countries was their mobilization of all possible resources to assist in the program. I have yet to learn of a health program in which adequate resources in terms of funds, personnel, equipment, and materials were allocated to health education. From my point of view as a health educator, it always seems that the bulk of the resources go into the service program, and if any are left over, they may be used in health education. (I admit to being a biased person.) But I am not sure that this is an unmixed blessing. Often, in the absence of other resources, the imaginative health educator has been able to enlist help from sources that might not otherwise have been tapped.

If health education in India is to become a truly mass movement, then every possible organization that can contribute to the goal must become *a partner* in the undertaking. I am not sufficiently familiar with all the official, voluntary, and professional organizations and agencies to attempt to enumerate them. Obviously schools and colleges, community development agencies, informational organizations, and all voluntary groups would be a part of the movement. Not so obvious but equally important is the role of the commercial agencies, agriculture, defense establishment, industrial firms, labor groups, religious organizations, and even political groups. Unless the talents and unique contributions of all the various sectors of the population become a part of the movement, its impact will not be as great as we might hope.

There is one note of caution coming out of other countries' experiences that I would like to bring to your attention. In some countries where the health education program has attempted to enlist other resources, the tendency has been to assign responsibilities to the outside resources and expect them to do as they are told. Wherever this has been done, the participation of the groups outside the health department has been minimal or even nil. In the paragraph above, I chose the word *partner* in the movement deliberately in order to emphasize the importance of equal sharing in planning and execution of the movement as well as participating in the credit for success.

Corollary with the involvement of all the people, whether through their organization or individually, is the use of all channels of communication to the people. Publicity of all kinds is essential. It forms the sensitizing agent to make people aware of health programs and how to benefit from them. If this publicity is sustained, it will give excellent support to the individual and group contacts that have been shown to be necessary to secure participation of all the people in any movement or program. The radio, cinema, newspaper, exhibitions, pamphlets, and the like are the obvious publicity media to use, but there are many other imaginative communication channels that should not be overlooked. Some of these—such as katha, tamasha, and other dramatic methods, as well as matchboxes—have been mentioned at this meeting. Their effectiveness needs to be determined.

Sixth in the list of suggestions from the other countries is the need for a comprehensive and systematic plan. In the preceding section we mentioned the need for full involvement of a host of organizations and groups as well as the use of innumerable communications methods and channels. If the way in which the groups work and their roles and responsibilities are not agreed upon in advance, the health education movement can dissipate much of the potential energy through duplication and even conflict in program operation. In the countries where successful planning has been done, much time in the beginning is utilized in arriving at an agreed upon strategy, the deployment of resources, and careful scheduling. This early use of time in planning without any apparent program operations has paid rich dividends in the end. Once more let me emphasize that this planning is done *with* the participating organizations and groups, not *for* them.

A seventh characteristic of successful programs in other countries was the constant revision in plan and procedure as the program proceeded. Such revisions were made on systematic review of operations to locate the weak spots in the plan, the delinquencies in per- formance by some unit, and readjustments in strategy and plan to overcome the deficiencies. In technical parlance this is called "con- current evaluation"; but the name is much less important than the function and its purpose. Although several other lessons might be drawn from a more extensive study of programs in other countries, time would not permit an elaboration of them here. There is, how- ever, one other suggestion I would like to make.

It does not come directly from a study of other countries but from my observations during my stay here in India. The suggestion is that there should be a systematic procedure for the spread of suc- cessful ideas. There are many outstanding local programs of one kind or another in India. Professor Rao told us of two yesterday. The Honorable Minister mentioned the voluntary assessment equal to 100 percent taxation for wells in one district, and I have seen many outstanding health education programs in different small villages or blocks. Yet I find that these success stories somehow never get communicated to other workers engaged in similar projects. I have no doubt that there are many exciting, imaginative, and successful programs going on about which few, if any, of us know the details. It is my conviction that in the ultimate buildup of health education as a mass movement, much more rapid progress can be achieved if ways are found to make others aware of the details of successful pro- grams in various parts of this vast subcontinent.

In conclusion may I again draw attention to the excellent back- ground documents that have been made available to us for the con- ference. I had the good fortune to be given an advance copy on my arrival. I can assure you that there is no idea I have expressed that isn't contained in those documents. The papers not only have used experiences in India and abroad, but they have also interpreted into practical operational terms behavioral science findings pertinent to the achievement of the goal that has been set.

The task ahead may be likened to the removal of a mountain. If we use our efforts to remove a stone here and there, the results may be totally unapparent and we may become discouraged. If, however, we concentrate in one sector, soon a dent will appear, and we will be able to see the possibility of ultimately removing the mountain.

The concept of developing health education into a mass movement is a most bold and gigantic undertaking, but with the highly competent leadership of the Central Health Education Bureau and the state health education bureaus, and with the imagination that Indian workers can bring to any task they undertake, I predict a huge success that will far exceed the health education achievements of any country in the world.

Discussion Questions

1. What is the essential ingredient for the achievement of any nation's health goals according to Derryberry? Why is this ingredient so important in his view?

2. What 7 principles were described by Derryberry that he believed could be helpful for developing successful health programs in the United States? Do you agree?

3. What specific role did Derryberry envision for the role of publicity in raising awareness about health programs and services? What are the limitations of this approach for changing behavior?

Part VI

Research in Public Health Issues

Overview

The spirit of scientific inquiry dominated all of Mayhew Derryberry's work. The search for more effective ways and means to
help people make their own choices in health promotion is the universal theme of the chapters included in Part Six. Equally important
was the way that Dr. Derryberry encouraged health care providers to
apply social science research findings in their own practices.

The first chapter in this part (Chapter Twenty-Six) addresses
the concept of evaluation of the three major components of the
school health program—service, instruction, and sanitation. Derryberry suggests pragmatic methodology for evaluating the interrelationship of these factors in order to reallocate scarce resources to
solve immediate medical problems, such as the need to change from
the ritual of physical examinations to the actual provision of medical treatment.

The research methodology as well as the findings reported in
Chapter Twenty-Seven deserves close attention and replication
today. The focus on comprehension of the message by the intended
audience is one of the most important yet least addressed elements
in educational program planning. The length of time that it takes
to read a message, the vocabulary used, the wide gap between what
the professional thinks is important and what the public is interested in, and the ways attention-getting devices misfire are all
addressed in this benchmark study.

In Chapter Twenty-Eight Derryberry presents his vision of how health educators should prepare to help society solve new health problems as they evolve. Derryberry frequently met with National Institute of Health researchers in order to learn about and understand the medical and public health advances that would soon be available for widespread application. In this chapter he discusses such timely topics as the Pap smear and curbing cigarette smoking. In 1958, these measures were five to eight years away from being considered for public health program implementation. Derryberry selected particular audiences for his addresses in order to clarify issues or advance professional goals. The address reprinted in this chapter was delivered to the physical education community because of growing confusion and perceived role conflict between the public health education and the school and physical education communities.

Dr. Derryberry developed a perspective that considers various concepts of the tasks to be accomplished and outlines the need for professionals to realign their thinking in terms of the fast changing character of community problems. This chapter reports findings from the first efforts in health education research, conducted by members of Derryberry's staff, including Hochbaum's study that is often considered the initial presentation of the Health Belief Model, Nelson's pioneering work in patient education, and Sullivan's work on the timing of information. These studies all documented the various ways in which people behave when faced with health decisions.

The last three chapters describe the nature of health education research in terms of past accomplishments, present studies, and future concerns. They acknowledge the contributions made by social scientists from the fields of anthropology, sociology, and psychology. The application of research procedures from other fields is given special attention. Derryberry also poses questions regarding the directions that should be taken for future efforts.

Of particular significance is Chapter Thirty-One—the last major address given by Dr. Derryberry to the health education profession.

In it he reviews for practitioners the importance of understanding the nature of research findings and their potential for application. He points out the dangers of manipulating research to meet provider goals. He questions the viability of short-sighted research that attempts to defend preconceived notions of patient care while ignoring the patient's own input and contribution. He articulates his ethical concerns for the health education profession. He raises the consciousness for all of us, practitioners and researchers alike, to make *explicit* the principles and theories that guide our research and practice procedures. He cautions against simply getting on the bandwagon, by routinely and mechanically copying the procedures used in reported studies, when our situations may be different and require new approaches.

In this final chapter Derryberry's voice is almost prophetic as he speaks of the strengths and weaknesses to which we can all respond from our own experiences. The responsibility rests with all of us to meet Mayhew Derryberry's ethical standards and expectations.

26

Methods of Evaluating
School Health Programs

Four million of the 13 million young men of this nation have been rejected as unfit for military service because of some mental or physical deficiency. That is how the medical groups in the Selective Service System have evaluated the results of all our combined child health services for the last two or three decades. Such an overall evaluation, as disconcerting and startling as it is, can be viewed only as a measurement of the results obtained from the several protective health services, including prenatal care, infant and preschool health supervision, the school health program, and any other community health services. The data serve quite well to point out that our activities designed to maintain the health of our youth have not been as effective as we believed or hoped, or as they should have been. But these results do not provide any direct cues for obtaining any better results. They do not reveal where the fault lies—with our parents, our schools, or our community organizations. Nor do they answer questions such as: "Why have we not been more effective? How can we improve? What activities need strengthening? What are we doing that should be changed? Is some new activity needed?"

Originally published in the *Connecticut State Medical Journal*, January 1945, 9, 19–22. Copyright 1984 by Connecticut Medicine. Reprinted with permission.

Answers to detailed questions as to "why" or "how" to improve require a thorough analysis of everything that is done by schools and other agencies to assure healthy, stalwart children. Let us therefore examine some of the ways in which an evaluating analysis may be made. This analysis will deal essentially with the school's contribution, since that is the subject of primary interest to this group.

In any program as complex as the one devoted to school health work, it is necessary to evaluate each activity separately to ascertain where improvement is possible. Later, it is also necessary to evaluate the interrelations of the parts to determine whether an effective synthesis of the several activities has been made. We shall therefore consider methods of evaluating each of the three major phases of the school health program—health service, health instruction, and school sanitation—and then suggest methods of evaluating the interrelations of the three phases.

Health Service

Among the complicating factors in the health service program are (1) the large number of persons concerned with the health of children and (2) the variety of interests and professional skills involved. There are the parents, the teachers, the school physician, the nurse, the family physician, and, in many instances, a dentist or a specialist such as an otologist, ophthalmologist, or orthopedic surgeon—not to mention the child himself. With so many and such a variety of people participating in a program focused on a single objective, there are many opportunities for slips—omissions, mistakes, or doubtful practices—that permit the alibi game of buck-passing. How many times have we heard: "If only the parents would do what they should," or "If the teacher knew enough about the condition and would help in the follow-up," or "That school doctor is no good; he is always finding conditions that need no attention." Our methods of evaluation must try to find out why there is a need for any excuses.

They must find out what part of the complex sequence of procedures, necessary to identify children with specific medical needs and then obtain medical services for them, is not functioning. Such appraisal is especially important because, unless the child really receives the medical attention he needs, the entire effort put into the health service program—including observation by the teacher, examination by the physician, and the follow-up—is completely wasted.

Too often school health programs have overlooked this fundamental truth—one that is so obvious it seems too trite to mention. As an example, witness the many programs and even legislative enactments that require an annual examination of children in specified grades or frequently of every school child. However, so far as I know, there is no state that requires by law or any program that even approaches the goal of seeing that every child actually receives the medical service that a medical examination has shown he needs. There is probably no community in the country with sufficient school health personnel to approach perfection in this respect. But even with present personnel, wouldn't it be possible to change the emphasis in the program so that more of the effort available could be expended in medical attention and less time and effort spent on examinations? Perhaps we might at least aim at the goal of having every child receive the medical attention that an examination indicates he needs. If that goal were made the main focus, there would be less effort devoted to examinations whose findings are only recorded with nothing else done about them.

Evaluating all the different procedures that go into achieving such a goal and deciding the relative emphasis to be given each procedure are certainly potentially fruitful activities. "But," say some, "how do you do it?"

The American Child Health Association developed a general methodology for such a survey in its study "Physical Defects—The Pathway to Correction." It showed how an intensive investigation of what had been done for specific children could be analyzed to find the places where the program was weak and where, in the language of the study, cases were shunted from the "Pathway to Correction" or medical attention.

Nyswander developed this methodology to a high degree in her work on "Solving School Health Problems." Each step in the program was submitted to an objective evaluation, procedures that were unfruitful were discarded, and new and effective ones developed. No situation was too insignificant to be looked into. Even the effectiveness of the wording of various types of notes sent home to parents as well as who signs them was submitted to test and the results evaluated.

In each case the evaluation method was set up to answer a specific question, such as the following:

1. Do the records contain sufficient information to insure an understanding of the medical needs of the children?

2. Why are so many medical records of children who change schools misplaced? Where do they go?

3. Why are there so many disagreements between the school physicians and private physicians in their examination findings? What can be done about it?

One could continue indefinitely, but in each case the general procedure was the same.

1. A breakdown in the service was detected, or the origin or source of a problem was located.

2. The problem was broken down into parts so that each part could be submitted to experimental analysis.

3. Data were collected that would evaluate each separate detail of the activity under review. Sometimes the finding was the presence or absence of some information on a record. Often interviews had to be conducted. Occasionally experiments had to be set up and the results appraised.

4. Once a solution was reached, the administrative application was tried out in a small area before extending changes to the whole system.

5. Training, supervision, and group work with the personnel were always used in installing new practices.

Nyswander not only perfected the general methodology for experimentally building effective programs, but she also demonstrated the importance of considering even what seem to be only tiny problems. She proved that in this field too, "A chain is no stronger than its weakest link." Most workers in school health have considered evaluation as an estimate of the program as a whole. They have usually felt that it was an activity carried on by an independent group and only done on special occasions. In her detailed studies of various minute but related steps in the school health service program, Nyswander showed that continuing objective measurement of various alternatives of procedure markedly improved the effectiveness of the total program.

Overall evaluation is important and should be done from time to time, but workers need not wait for such special studies to ask themselves, "Am I carrying on my job in the most effective way possible?" However, one should not jump to hasty conclusions or change too quickly. Each contemplated change in procedure, no matter how minor, should be studied thoroughly to be sure that it will produce the desired results or be economical of effort before it is accepted. Setting up the type of experiment or developing the kind of data necessary to prove the superiority of any new procedure is a technical task, and those who undertake such studies should seek advice of those skilled in experimental method in order to make sure that the results obtained can be interpreted in terms of practice. This should not deter workers from reviewing their programs and locating procedures that might be improved through experimentation. After all, as one of our Public Health

Service officers once said, "Progress is made only by those with inquisitive minds."

Health Instruction

Turning to the health instruction program, several overall evaluations on specific subjects have been made by various public opinion polls. The most extensive measurement was the study of "What the Public Knows About Health," covering in all one hundred thousand people of various ages tested at the New York and the San Francisco World's Fairs. The finding of most concern to this group was that students over 17 years of age are poorly informed about practical facts—those that have a bearing on their own health, such as the combination of most nutritious foods, susceptibility of youth of that age to tuberculosis, and that venereal disease cannot be cured with a few treatments—while at the same time they are well versed on facts of physiology and anatomy, such as that hormones are manufactured in the ductless glands or that the blood fights germs by means of white corpuscles—information that has little application to daily living. Such an evaluation raises several questions. For example: Are our courses in biology, general science, and health education giving too much emphasis to physiological and anatomical information and not enough to instruction in the actual care of the body? Knowing where hormones are made or the purpose of white corpuscles may be important, but will it help one to be more healthy than he would otherwise be? Can we assume that a student armed chiefly with the basic definitions and relationships of a science will make the proper application of his knowledge if he has had no practice in the method of doing it? Is it not possible or even very likely that our health instruction has focused too much on imparting facts and not enough on how to solve health problems?

Perhaps what is needed in the health instructional phase of our program is a redefinition of goals. So long as the main purpose is to impart information, methods of evaluation are simple. But measuring behavior, attitudes, or facility in meeting new health problems is much more difficult. Unfortunately, very little work has been done along this line. A tremendous opportunity for valuable contributions to methodology of appraisal is open to anyone who can find ways of measuring the success achieved with instructional programs.

School Sanitation

On the evaluation of school sanitation, no recent extensive study covering the country or any large part of it is available. From such data as are available, it would seem that Connecticut has made as much progress as, or more than, any other state. With the "School Building Code" that provides a general statement of principles covering design, construction, and operation of school buildings, and its use throughout the state, real progress has been made. Practically all schools are served by public water systems, and the number of schools with outdoor privies is extremely small. This is very much better than the situation in one state in which, at last count, there were 1,500 schools without any sanitary toilet facilities at all. There is, however, still room for improvement, and there is also the opportunity for the sanitation appraisal to be made as a part of the instructional program or even to be expanded to the development of a study of home sanitation by the students.

Coordination

How can one evaluate the coordination of these three different phases of the program? What are some of the items that need to be studied?

First of all is the staff. No program is better than its staff. One needs to evaluate the adequacy of the staff to do the job that is to be done. This appraisal means more than the number of degrees that they hold, the number of organizations that they belong to, or the length of experience they have had. It means a real check of the activities that they perform. Nyswander showed that a time-analysis checklist, through observation of the work of school nurses, uncovered innumerable places where only a small change brought about marked improvement in effectiveness. Carefully analyzed stenographic notes of instruction, history taking, supervisory remarks, or individual advice to parents will uncover many inadequacies of interrelationship. Often the instruction is too meager, in too technical terms, or does not reach all concerned. To what extent are the personnel keeping up with modern developments both in education and in public health practice? If some workers learn of newer procedures and want to make changes, and others cling to the old practices, confusion is likely to arise. Perhaps the only technique for evaluation of the staff's progressiveness is to watch their programs and measure the degree to which agreement or confusion prevails.

Detailed following of cases—including the information given to parent, child, teacher, nurse, or doctor and the use made of that information—will evaluate the degree to which the activities of each dovetail with the other. Franzen developed the technique of asking various members of the school health staff identical questions of common interest about the same child. The degree to which they all had the same information measured the cooperation of the staff.

Another technique for evaluating the coordination of the program is the extent to which there is group planning among the personnel. It is not enough to have a staff meeting periodically, unless each member contributes to the listing of problems and to the working out of solutions. Group problem-solving is difficult to accomplish but real progress will be made only when each of the several professional workers can learn to respect the members of other professions and recognize the contribution that each can make in the solution of the health problems of children.

Evaluation

Thus far we have described some of the phases of the school health program and suggested various techniques that might be used. I cannot close without a few words of caution. The health habits and attitudes of children, as well as their physical well-being, are quite difficult to measure. There is a distinct need for the development of more precise tools of evaluation. Until they are developed, we must be careful to view our interpretations in terms of the crudity of the methods of measurement.

Children's health conditions and behavior are the result of many factors other than the school health program. Interpretations of the results of any evaluation procedure must therefore be made against a broad background of social and economic environmental status. But despite the pitfalls of interpretation, we must not neglect evaluation. Only through continuous appraisal and revision of our activities can we keep our programs effective.

Discussion Questions

1. What are the key components of a school health program, and why is evaluating school health so important? What additional key components have been added during the last decade to expand and make more comprehensive the coordinated school health program?

2. What are some evaluation methods Derryberry believed were needed to evaluate school health programs? Can you enumerate others that might be important today?

3. Why is it so difficult to evaluate the effectiveness of health instruction in schools?

4. What does the lack of valid measurement result in?

27

Exhibits

Health educators have recently become increasingly concerned about the effectiveness of their efforts. No longer satisfied with their own subjective judgments of their work, they have begun to ask: Is this poster attractive to other people? Is this pamphlet interesting? Will this exhibit teach what we think it does? Does the public really examine our material, and do our messages get across?

It is difficult to get reliable answers to such critical questions about methods of health education. A given poster, exhibit, motion picture, or pamphlet might be considered excellent by one leader and be labeled poor by another, equally competent. Disagreements in judgment are, in fact, as common as agreements. Recognizing, therefore, that subjective evaluation, even by experts, fails to furnish an index of effectiveness, Homer Calver, of the American Museum of Health, suggested a comprehensive study of the exhibits assembled by the Museum in the Medicine and Public Health Building at the New York World's Fair. Firmly convinced of the need for more objective evaluation, the Museum and the Public Health Service undertook the study, from which a few of the practical conclusions may be given.

Originally published in the *American Journal of Public Health*, March 1941, *31*(3), 257–263. Reprinted with permission.

In this evaluative study, the analysis has been focused on the public's reaction to the exhibits rather than on the characteristics of the exhibits themselves. Thus, in order to measure the effectiveness of the exhibits, data were collected to answer such questions as the following:

1. Does this exhibit attract attention?
2. Does it sustain interest?
3. Can it be easily understood?
4. Does the audience get the message?

In order to answer the first two questions, the behavior of a random sampling of 3,000 visitors to the building was observed. In each instance, a member of the staff followed an individual through the building and recorded each exhibit at which the visitor stopped, together with the length of time (by stopwatch) he remained there. The summarized record indicates the relative popularity of the display and how well it retains the interest of those whose attention it attracted.

Answering the question "Can it be easily understood?" required the collection of several types of data:

1. How long did it take to read the legend? This factor, together with the average length of time individuals actually looked at the exhibit, gives presumptive evidence of the extent to which it was possible for the total message to be obtained.

2. Were the words used too technical for the public to understand? The relative difficulty of each word in the legends was checked against the frequency with which it was in common use, as shown by the Thorndike Word List of the 20,000 most commonly used words.

3. Was the exhibitor's objective readily apparent to the spectator? A number of individuals were asked what they thought

the exhibit was expected to teach, and their opinions were checked against the objective stated by the committee responsible for the exhibit.

Test questions based on the content of the several exhibits were used to measure whether the public learned the message. At a booth called the "Quiz Corner," individuals were tested, and the tests were marked according to whether a given exhibit had or had not been seen. By comparing scores obtained before viewing an exhibit and those obtained after viewing it, one index of the effectiveness of the exhibit is secured.

Such, then, are a few of the types of data obtained, and the present discussion will be limited to the items listed above. The complete scope of the data will be discussed in the final report, but the examples given here are believed to be sufficient to indicate the method of attack on the problem.

What practical conclusions can be drawn as a result of this study? Even though tabulations are still incomplete, several well-defined principles of exhibit construction are apparent from the preliminary analysis. Each such principle or indication of proper technic will be listed and discussed below.

Panels of Statistical Data, Graphs, and Tables Fail Signally in Attracting or Retaining Attention

The Pneumonia Exhibit in the Hall of Man was displayed on two walls set at right angles to each other. The right-hand wall presented statistical material, whereas the left-hand wall was made up of panels describing the disease and its course. Adjoining the statistical panel was one having to do with proper nursing. Out of 950,000 persons who viewed any part of the Pneumonia Exhibit, roughly 9 out of 10 (88 percent) spent some time examining the panel that described the disease, whereas only about 2 out of 10 (18 percent) spent any measurable amount of time examining the statistical panel.

Even the nursing panel, which might have been considered disadvantageously placed since it was nearest the corner, attracted and held the attention of 3 out of each 10 persons who visited the exhibit. The conclusion here is quite obvious—namely, that any message that might have been conveyed by the statistical panel was totally missed by four-fifths of its possible audience.

The Maze of Superstitions also included a statistical panel, and similar observations were taken in that exhibit. Among all those who visited the exhibit, the proportion attracted to the statistical panel was much less than half of the number that visited any other part of the exhibit. One-fourth of all who saw the exhibit looked at every part of it except the statistical panel. In this connection it should be noted that the criterion of "looking at" or "viewing" was the ability of an observer to detect the individual being observed in the act of looking at the exhibit for a period of time measurable on a stopwatch.

The Demography Exhibit, portraying various phases of population growth and distribution in the United States, although it occupied a prominent position in the Hall of Man, attracted fewer spectators than any other exhibit of comparable size in that part of the building.

The time required to read the legends in statistical panels was longer than for any other part of the exhibit. Nevertheless, persons who visited or looked at the statistical panels spent less time in such viewing than in looking at any other panel. It is apparent, therefore, that the statistical panels not only failed to attract the attention of a large proportion of the visitors, but they also failed to hold interest in those whom they did attract.

Statistical Panels Frequently Fail to Convey a Message

In order to test how much spectators learned, a series of questions based on the statistical exhibits were presented to visitors. The answers were segregated according to whether or not the individual taking the test had seen the exhibit in question. When the following true-false and multiple-choice tests based on the Pneumonia and Demography Exhibits were used, no significant difference could be detected between the answers of those who had seen the exhibits and of those who had not. In some cases the proportion answering the questions correctly was slightly higher among those who had seen the exhibits, but the result could not be called statistically significant. The questions used were as follows:

1. More people die from pneumonia than from cancer. (True or false?)

2. The pneumonia death rate is higher in middle age than in infancy. (True or false?)

3. Among the causes of death, pneumonia ranks: first, third, fifth, tenth?

4. The number of deaths caused by pneumonia each year in the United States is approximately: 20,000; 130,000; 250,000; 460,000?

5. One-eighth of the world's population now live in America. (True or false?)

6. The greatest number of foreign-born persons in the United States in 1930 came from: Germany, Italy, Russia, Ireland?

The conclusion stated just above relates to panels in which a number of facts are presented. In contrast to that conclusion, it appears, therefore, that if a single statistical fact is the major emphasis of an exhibit, it is much more likely to be learned. When the following questions were used to test the educational effectiveness of such isolated statistical facts, the proportion answering correctly was significantly greater among those who had seen the exhibits than among those who had not.

1. The percentage of the adult population stricken by syphilis is estimated to be: 1 percent, 3 percent, 5 percent, 10 percent.

2. The largest number of cases of syphilis reported as traced to one infected person is: 2, 24, 56, 106?

This small sampling would suggest the importance of limiting statistical material to one or two outstanding facts that are given prominence. This point is being emphasized because many health exhibits consist almost wholly of statistical material, and especially since it seems possible that those whose major interest is in statistics may have overestimated the public's concern for that type of information.

The Message to Be Conveyed Must Be the Focus of Attention

The exhibit called "The First Year of Life," through its arrangement, focused attention on a number of models illustrating the physiology of pregnancy. The sponsors of the exhibit, however, stated as their objective the education of the spectators in the hygiene of pregnancy. Material on the latter subject was arranged in front of and below the models and thus was not the normal focus of attention. In testing the effectiveness of the exhibit, the questions used were limited to the subject of hygiene. The result was that for each question, the number of correct responses was approximately the same, regardless of whether the exhibit had or had not been seen. Furthermore, this was the only exhibit tested on which we failed to obtain, for at least some of the questions, statistically reliable differences between those who saw and those who did not see the exhibit. Upon learning of these findings, the association sponsoring the exhibit decided to study the problem during the 1940 Fair. The conclusion stated above is substantiated by the fact that for questions based on the material in the models, significant differences were obtained in the responses of those who saw the exhibit as opposed to those who did not.

The Use of Even Common Professional Words May Be Misleading to the Public

Our study of the vocabulary used in legends indicates that even the most common professional words may be incomprehensible or unknown to the group intended to be reached. By selecting 50 words of varying difficulty from the legends of exhibits and asking classes of college students and a group of WPA clerical workers to define the terms, an unexpectedly high proportion of the terms were found to be completely misunderstood. For example, one-half of those responding had no idea of the meaning of "nephritis," and an additional one-fourth had incorrect ideas about the term. It was thought by some to mean nervous disorder; by others, rheumatism; and by still others, blood disease. Similar results were found when the test words were "strabismus," "placenta," and "therapeutic." Public health workers, to whom these are everyday terms, may well beware of their use in exhibits designed for the general public.

Even Expertly Designed Exhibits May Impart Misinformation

In one exhibit there were a number of pictures of contrasts in the appearance of healthy and abnormal conditions in children. With one exception, the pictures showed white children. In the illustration having to do with rickets, however, the two contrasting pictures were both of African American children. When the statement "Rickets is primarily a disease of African American children" was scored by those who saw the exhibit, it was regarded as true almost twice as frequently as by those who had not seen the exhibit. The variation of more than one factor in a series of contrasts in this instance left a completely wrong impression.

Similarly, in the exhibit on anemia, inadequate labeling was responsible for misinformation. In this instance, the misinformation was due to individual misinterpretations of unlabeled color

transparencies. One particular color transparency pictured the foods
that are rich in iron. However, since the individual foods were not
labeled in the picture, persons tended to draw their own conclusions as to what specific foods were meant. Of the number of persons asked to name the foods in the exhibits, universal agreement
was obtained for only three items. One particular picture, for example, was variously considered to represent apricots, new potatoes,
plums, tomatoes, and peaches. Another was thought to represent
prunes, mushrooms, kidneys, or chicken livers. Incidentally, a similar situation has been observed in the diabetes exhibit at the San
Francisco Fair. In this instance, the foods pictured as proper for a
diabetic were not labeled, so that a number of spectators, being
asked what meat was pictured, gave various answers, such as ham,
pork, lamb chops, and steak.

Tests as an Educational Technic

In the course of our study, we more or less accidentally discovered
what seems to be a valuable health education technic. It was carried
out with 35,000 visitors at the 1939 New York Fair and has been
repeated with double that number at the San Francisco Fair in 1940.
Seven tests on health information were used to determine what the
public knows about health. Visitors gladly took the tests but also
demanded to know the correct answers. Accordingly, brief answers
to all questions were prepared, and each such answer gave not only
the correct response but some explanation of the reason for it. Originally sent out to those who had requested them, the answers were
later given to the visitors immediately after they took the tests. We
have found that practically all who took the tests read the answers.

Additional interest in the technic is indicated by the volume of
requests for additional copies for unions, schools, Civilian Conservation Camps, and individuals who desired to give the tests to their
friends. Although we have no direct evaluation of the effectiveness
of the device in teaching health to the public, it does meet our first

two criteria of attracting attention and sustaining interest, at least until the material is read.

A practical adaptation of the technic has been worked out for use in community groups by a few health educators. Questions based on the material that is to be taught are given to members of group meetings at the beginning of the meeting. During the meeting, the major portion of the time is given over to discussion of the answers. This method has been found to arouse active interest in the material to be taught.

While it has been impossible in a brief paper to describe the many interesting and outstanding exhibits, an attempt has been made to caution against the hazards of presentation as well as to indicate the need for experimental study of our educational efforts. In this attempt, emphasis has naturally been given to some of the minor limitations in exhibits so that the need for care in selecting and organizing material may be stressed.

Discussion Questions

1 Visual communications are important in communicating research findings. Why do posters reporting health-related results frequently fail to convey messages accurately?

2. What are some factors that Derryberry believed should be considered in order to improve this type of communication format?

3. Are health fairs and exhibits "interventions"? If so, should they be evaluated for their effectiveness in changing knowledge, attitudes, or behavior?

28

Some Problems Faced in Educating for Health

Those of us engaged in the task of educating for health are becoming increasingly analytical and critical of our own efforts. Although we are able to see many changes in health behavior that result in improvement in the people's health, we cannot be satisfied because there are still a large number of individuals who neglect to put into practice those scientific findings that if properly used would improve their health. Our dissatisfaction is a healthy attitude and can be turned to constructive action. But to do so as a profession, we must intensify our efforts in analyzing how we can be more effective.

As a first step it is well to examine carefully as many of the facets of the task as we can. We shall restrict our analysis to a look at only three aspects of the overall problem: (1) differing perceptions of the task to be done, (2) the character of the health problems and their meanings for health education content, and (3) how people react in a few health situations and what these suggest for health education.

Originally published in *Professional Contributions*, No. 6 (American Academy of Physical Education), November 1958, pp. 78–87. Reprinted with permission. Address given at the 29th Annual Meeting of the Academy on March 29, 1958, Kansas City, Missouri.

Differing Perceptions of the Task

All of us know that we need to have a clear definition of the goal we want to reach if we are to be successful in taking the steps to obtain it. Perhaps all of us are in complete agreement as to the goal of educating for health, but as I listen to the conversations and observe the actions of the many professional people who are participating in the task of educating for health, I get the distinct feeling that not all of us agree on what is meant by the goal or how it may be accomplished. For example, some educators seem to consider that health education means imparting a definable body of knowledge about physiology, disease prevention, nutrition, personal and community hygiene, and so on. If they can show that their students have acquired this knowledge, their goal of educating for health seems to have been satisfied. Others appear to be more exacting. They demand that the information find expression in action shown by the health practices of their students. This kind of education is much concerned about the formation of health habits.

Many public health workers seem to consider health education to be the selling of health programs. As a consequence they often limit activities to advertising methods such as the mass media—radio and television, news releases, pamphlets, movies, talks, and the like. If they include action as part of the goal, it is usually public response to some specific direction the health workers are giving, such as "Get an annual medical examination," "Fluoridate the drinking water," or "Immunize your child against some disease." Another group appear to believe it is the job of health education to provide those experiences for children and adults that will help them to make sound decisions about their health behavior, so that they may more nearly achieve goals that satisfy them and are beneficial for society. There are altogether too few of the health educators who are willing to take this more difficult approach to the educational goal. These differences in understanding the task to be done are enough in themselves to detract from the effectiveness of the overall effort, but the existence of these differences is even more serious because it gives rise to ideas that are partially but not entirely true. The persistence of such ideas is a real barrier to effective health education. Let me mention a few, without elaboration—many more can be added to the list:

1. Health education is like every other subject and should be taught and fitted into the curriculum in the same manner as any other factual or skill subject.

2. All that people need when they are not following good health practices is health information. (Even though there may not be full acceptance of this verbal statement, the behavior of many of those educating the public would indicate such a belief.)

3. Health education is a task of persuading people to do things that experts have decided are best for them.

4. Health education efforts should be concentrated in the schools at the time when children are learning. There is not much to be done with older people, whose habit patterns are more firmly fixed.

These partial truths influence both content and method in health education. In order to be more effective in our efforts, we have a real job to do within the health and education professions to interpret more precisely what is involved in the overall goal of "educating for health," an objective to which everyone subscribes.

Changing Character of Health Problems

A second facet of the health education problem is the changing character of the health problems about which education is undertaken. These changes are of several kinds. First of all, there is the shift in the kinds of conditions that are the major causes of disability and death. A previous presentation to this Academy developed in considerable detail the advances that have been made in conquering the communicable diseases. It emphasized that the health problems of greatest significance today are the chronic diseases and accidents—in the home, at work, and on the highway. There was also an analysis of some of the educational problems that face us as we undertake to cut down on the misery caused by these conditions. There is no need to repeat the points made four years ago in that analysis.[1]

There is, however, an added factor in relation to these conditions that has real meaning for us as educators. The communicable diseases had a single direct cause—a bacterium, virus, or some other pathogenic agent. Because of this fact, it was possible to develop a specific preventive or control measure. When there was clear and conclusive evidence that a particular disease was due to a single cause and that a specific action (vaccination, elimination of mosquitoes, or a drug such as penicillin) would prevent it, the educational task was easily defined and in many situations was not too difficult.

But at the present state of our scientific knowledge, it appears that the chronic diseases, and certainly accidents, are caused by a multiplicity of factors. No single remedy is likely to be found to prevent or cure these problems that have so many different causes. If people are to understand multiple causation and be able to respond to advice that often must be complicated by an explanation of the combination of causes, then people are going to need a much deeper understanding of the biological, physiological, and chemical processes within the body. Does this mean more detailed scientific content in our health instruction? If so, the problem of health education grows more difficult, and the content we include may require revamping.

Another category of health problems coming to the fore today grows out of industrial and technological advances. In many communities, hazards are being created within our physical environment through the dispersal of industrial wastes both in the air and in the streams. Have we considered the educational aspects of air and stream pollution and water conservation, and the contribution that we as health educators might make to the abatement of these problems through informed and intelligent community action?

Also in this category growing out of new developments is the problem of radiation. A few years ago the term *radiological health* would have confused us all. Already the problem is of sufficient importance to justify the establishment of a full-fledged division in the Public Health Service. The discoveries about ionizing radiation have placed extremely valuable tools in the hands of the physician. In addition to the X-ray and other radiation-producing machines, the radioactive isotopes of the various elements are tremendous aids in diagnosis, treatment, and medical research. Promotion of such beneficial use of radiation, one of the important aspects of radiological health, adds a new dimension to educational needs.

To prevent impairment from exposure to unnecessary amounts of radiation is the other aspect of radiological health about which much information has been circulated recently. It appears that this is also an aspect with which we as educators should be more vitally concerned. Should we not try to become more conversant with this problem so that we can aid in defining the contribution of education to the development of a sensible but cautious attitude toward this valuable and powerful phenomenon?

Closely allied to the problems arising from new physical and chemical technological advances are the educational problems created by medical research findings that indicate a need for change in long-established health procedures. It is more difficult to think about change in an accustomed practice than in regard to new ideas. Consider, for example, the new knowledge about the effects of repeated exposure to radiation that has caused re-examination of the practice of routine X-rays as a case-finding device in the control of tuberculosis. After review by a committee of experts, it was recommended that:

1. Mass radiography of the chest, operated under competent auspices, is a fundamental technique in the detection of tuberculosis.

2. Mass X-ray case-finding should be applied selectively in groups at high risk of tuberculosis infection and disease.

3. All tuberculosis X-ray survey programs should have the prior approval of the applicable state or local health department.

4. Consideration should be given to the tuberculin test as an initial screening device in low-prevalence groups.

5. Every community should evaluate on a continuing basis its tuberculosis problem, needs, and resources so that local X-ray surveys may have efficient use and maximum effect.

6. Adequate safeguards should be utilized to protect all persons from unnecessary radiation.[2]

As was to be expected, this recommended change in the widespread use of X-ray in case-finding activities caused considerable unrest.

Our task as educators becomes one of helping to interpret the change, but isn't there a more significant implication in this situation? May we not expect other important research findings that may change certain behaviors that health educators have spent a lot of time encouraging? The director of the National Institutes of Health writes, "There are many persons who think that by 1975 we shall have:

1. Conquered most of the infectious diseases;

2. Learned to cure cancer by virotherapy;

3. Discovered a chemical basis for mental disease and manufactured an antidote to it;

4. Developed dietary or other means of protecting blood vessels and the heart itself from disease and premature failure."[3]

Although he personally does not share this optimism, the scientists whose opinions he is relating made such predictions only after review of research progress over the past ten to twenty years. As educators, what are we doing to help people accept change? What can education do to make it possible for people to distinguish scientific findings from the claims of quacks? How are we preparing people to change from accepted practices without losing faith in other advocated health practices where research has not indicated a need to change? But there is another kind of problem of educational significance that arises from the application of some of the accumulating research findings. It is one that calls for enlisting the participation of the healthy people of the community for the benefit of individuals who are or have been less fortunate. To illustrate: through improved methods of therapy, better hospital procedures, and in some cases the aid of tranquilizing drugs, patients of mental hospitals are being returned to the community in increasing numbers. There were about seven thousand fewer patients in mental hospitals at the close of business in 1956 than in 1955.

The meaning of this phenomenon in terms of the educational task may best be demonstrated through an analogy to a communicable disease. An individual is in an infectious community (one in which he is unable to adjust) and succumbs. He goes to the hospital (mental) for treatment and recovers or improves sufficiently to be sent back home. This places him in the same (infectious) environment. Instead of being treated as one who has been physically ill and permitted special considerations while he is recuperating, actually he is often expected to show more than normal stability by his employer, his social companions, and his work group. In his weakened state, in this more highly infectious environment, he has a relapse and is returned for further treatment. Is there a task for health education to help change this state of affairs, creating supportive attitudes among the people and dispelling the tendency to avoid former mental health patients—a behavior exhibited by so many of the public? Even though we would all respond affirmatively to the question, do we have enough know-how at the moment to bring about the change? What do we need to prepare ourselves to do the job?

Likewise, do we have a role in creating a more positive attitude toward psychotherapy and counseling than now exists? Only recently, a health educator who was concerned about the way he was relating to some of his associates voluntarily sought the aid of a psychiatrist. At no time did he lose any time from work, nor did his employer detect any lack of efficiency. When he applied for employment in an official health agency, he volunteered the information that he had been under the care of a psychiatrist, who incidentally had given him a clean bill of health. He almost failed to get the job. The fact that a health organization exhibited this reluctance to recognize preventive health behavior is an indication of the extent of the educational job ahead. Perhaps less dramatic, but of a similar nature, is the attitude of many people toward those who are handicapped in other ways. A group whose major task is working with people having all sorts of crippling conditions stated that one of the major problems they encounter is the lack of a constructive attitude among the normal population toward those less fortunate. Do we know what attitude and behavior will enable the handicapped to function in the most normal way? What might we do to contribute to the development of that attitude and behavior?

This description of the change in the character of some of the health problems of today is by no means exhaustive. It does, however, indicate a type of analysis that may contribute to a better definition of what kinds of education about health are needed.

Behavior of People in Health Situations

A third approach to analyzing the problem is a review of what we know or do not know about how people behave when faced with situations requiring health decisions. An increasing number of studies of the health behavior of people under a variety of circumstances are being undertaken. Such studies should be most helpful to health educators in locating the places where improved educational experiences are indicated.

One such study has just been published by Hochbaum under the title *Public Participation in Medical Screening Programs: A Sociopsychological Study.*[4] Drawing his sample from three communities where tuberculosis case-finding programs of different kinds have been conducted, he undertakes to determine the sociopsychological factors distinguishing those who voluntarily seek an X-ray from those who had never submitted themselves to an X-ray. He summarizes the critical findings as follows:

> The decision on the part of people, whether, when, and where to obtain chest X-rays is due largely to the interaction of three sets of factors: the "psychological state of readiness" for the decision to obtain X-rays, certain situational influences, and environmental conditions that provide the opportunity of X-raying. Three interacting specific beliefs or attitudes form the principal components accounting for the psychological state of readiness: a previous belief in his susceptibility to the disease, a belief in the possibility of having the disease at any given moment in the absence of noticeable symptoms, and a belief that early detection of the disease will avoid or ameliorate those of its aspects that are most anxiety-producing in his case.

Although these beliefs appear related to knowledge, this relationship is not a simple one. The possession of information concerning their content in itself is not sufficient to result in appropriate behavior, that is, seeking to be X-rayed. Certain additional psychological conditions need to prevail.

Do we know how to develop the "psychological state of readiness" so that people will react when the occasion demands? Have we considered how to develop sensitivity to the proper stimuli that suggest taking preventive steps without producing a tendency toward hypochondria or other anxiety states?

In another study (unpublished) of an exploratory nature, Dan Sullivan—working with the staff of the Wichita–Sedgwick County (Kansas) Department of Public Health—uncovered a number of behaviors among the people that have meaning for health education. Their study was concerned with the educational problems that arise in the control of rheumatic fever. Doctors, parents, public health nurses, and a school principal were interviewed concerning their respective understanding of the condition and needs of specific children who had had acute attacks of rheumatic fever. Some of the findings from the family interviews signify important health education problems. Some of the parents reported they were afraid to ask their doctors about matters that worried them because they felt the physicians were too busy to answer their questions.

A similar finding (unpublished) is reported by Elsa Nelson from her explorations in a medical ward of a hospital. She interviewed patients and the doctors who attended them. The patients stated that they would like to know about their disease and condition from the doctor. When questioned as to whether they had asked the doctor, they said, "No, he is always so busy. I don't want to impose on his time." When the doctors were asked whether they ever talked with the patients regarding their disease or prognosis, they replied, "No! They don't seem to want to know. They never ask any questions." These case reports certainly do not meet the requirement of a scientific sample, but since these reports were made, I have encountered a number of my friends who have not felt comfortable asking their doctor questions about things that were bothering them.

I feel certain that most doctors would respond to the people's questions. In fact, it has been observed that one physician has placed a sign on his desk encouraging people to ask him about any problem that was concerning them.

Do not these findings suggest an educational need to help people discuss their complaints in a more positive way with their doctors? Do we include some help on such problems in our health education?

In Wichita they also found, as one would expect, that the "teachable moment" was immediately after the condition was diagnosed. Those who had never heard of rheumatic fever sought information at this time. They sought it from neighbors (the "over the back fence" phenomenon we all deplore), from others who had experienced rheumatic fever in the family, and from publications. Some of the publications they mentioned were *Today's Health*, *McCall's*, encyclopedia, dictionary, nurses' magazines, and a doctor's medical textbook.

Elsa Nelson found that patients with similar diagnoses exchanged information as well as misinformation that they gleaned from the doctors' consultations near the bedside.

To be sure, educators cannot be at the side of every person when they or their close relatives or friends are sick, but are we doing any preparation of people to react intelligently and healthfully in such situations? How can we help people find the information they want from a reliable source?

Finally, let us look at a gross analysis of the public's reactions to some recent research findings. Four years ago the paper presented to this academy carried this statement from an outstanding epidemiologist: "If the polio vaccine proves successful, then public health as I have known it is a thing of the past." In the intervening period the vaccine has proved its effectiveness in greatly reducing paralytic polio, if individuals are vaccinated as recommended. Yet over one-fourth of the young people under 20 have not had a single injection, and less than one-half of this age group have had all three shots. It is estimated that about a third of the population over 20 have had shots. At the same time there are approximately 29 million cc. of the vaccine available. The American Medical Association, the National Foundation for Infantile Paralysis, and the Public Health Service are engaged in the promotion of this very simple and safe preventive measure. Yet the public's response is certainly far from enthusiastic.

Another, similar situation needs consideration. Within the year scientists have developed the Asian influenza vaccine, and the pharmaceutical companies have manufactured it in tremendous quantities. Approximately 45 million cc. of vaccine were used within a few weeks last fall in 1 cc. and 1/10 cc. injections. Although the threat of Asian influenza has subsided, the deaths from respiratory illness during the first two months of this year were approximately double the usual number occurring at this time of year. But very few people were vaccinated during that period—even though vaccine was abundantly available.

Here is still another finding. A comprehensive statistical study of cancer in Connecticut for the 17-year period 1935–1951 showed that 66 percent of the women with early diagnosis of breast cancer survived five years, whereas the percentage is only 33 for those who examined their breasts, followed the practice for a few months and then discontinued it.[5]

Soon the cytological test for early discovery of cervical cancer will become widely available. Here again the survival rate for early detected (localized) cancer of the cervix far exceeds that of the more extensive cancer.[6] To what extent will women consistently submit to this test when it becomes available? There are two other recent findings of a somewhat different character. The first of these is the tranquilizing drugs. These first appeared on the commercial markets in 1954. Since that time they have been taken by at least 20 million Americans. Accurate estimates of their use are not available, but in 1956, $150 million was spent on tranquilizers, and 34 million prescriptions had been issued. These estimates do not include the amount of pseudotranquilizing drugs that are being widely consumed without being prescribed.[7]

The extensive use of these drugs by many of the public is being made despite the informational advice that has gone out. In all the authentic information put out, the point has been stressed that the full effects of these drugs are not known and that there may be temporary or permanent damage. The problem of smoking and cancer is another case in point. A study group on smoking and health was organized in June 1956 to review the problem of the effects of tobacco smoking on health. It found that at least 16 independent studies carried on in five countries during the past 18 years show a statistical association between smoking and the occurrence of lung cancer. Following this report the Surgeon General issued a statement on July 12, 1957, in which he said, "In the light of these studies, it is clear that there is an increasing and consistent body of evidence that excessive cigarette smoking is one of the causative factors in lung cancer."[8,9,10]

One might have expected that such a straightforward presentation of fact backed by the findings of the highly competent study group would have influenced the use of cigarettes. However, data on consumption certainly do not indicate any reduction in smoking. In the calendar year 1956, people of the continental United States smoked 393 billion cigarettes for which they spent $4,840,000,000. In 1957, the number consumed was 409 billion and the amount spent was $5,115,000,000.[11] Even though the Surgeon General's statement was not released until July 1957, if it had had real impact, the number of cigarettes consumed last year should have been less.

The reactions of the people to these research findings raise serious questions for us as educators. Why are people so apathetic toward actions that have proven health value? Certainly it could scarcely be said that the information about their value has not been disseminated. On the other hand, why are such huge amounts of money spent for tobacco? Why are people so willing to take chances with the tranquilizing drugs before all the evidence is in?

Can it be that health is not very important in the value systems of our people? If so, what is our responsibility in trying to change value systems? What are the determinants of various kinds of health behavior? So far as smoking is concerned, should we focus on helping youngsters not to start the habit? Or do we need much more definitive data on smoking and the need it serves?

Summary

There is a real need to diagnose the problem of health education in order to determine the content that will have meaning to a particular audience and to select methods that will provide the most appropriate learning experiences if we are to become increasingly effective. Three ways of looking at the problem have been considered:

1. Varying concepts of the task to be done and the ways of doing it reduce the outcome from efforts now devoted to health education.

2. There are many changes in the character of the health problem we face that have implications for both health education content and method.

3. The decisions for action that people make with respect to situations involving positive or negative health outcomes provide cues to the needs in health education.

   Throughout this analysis there has run one central thread, implied although not made explicit. This thought is the urgent need for more definitive research on which to plan competently and carry out effectively programs of health education. If this academy will give leadership in such research, then the formidable problem of health education may be tackled with much greater confidence that the efforts of all of us will achieve the results toward which we are striving.

Discussion Questions

1. What are some of the behavioral beliefs that govern human behavior?

2. What is implied by the term "teachable moment"?

3. How can health educators help people to obtain health information when they need it and to take action in light of the facts?

4. According to Derryberry, what are three ways of looking at a health problem that warrant a health educator's consideration?

5. What in Derryberry's view will well-designed research of health education topics help to achieve?

Notes

1. Mayhew Derryberry, "Today's Health Problems and Health Education," *Public Health Reports*, 69(12), 1224–8, December 1954.

2. "X-Ray Case-Finding Programs in Tuberculosis Control," Public Health Service Statement, *Public Health Reports*, 73, 1, January 1958.

3. James A. Shannon, Director, National Institutes of Health, "Medical Research—1975," *Challenge*, Vol. 5(8), 18–22, May 1957.

4. Godfrey M. Hochbaum, *Public Participation in Medical Screening Programs: A Sociopsychological Study*, Public Health Service Publication No. 572, 1958.

5. Connecticut State Department of Health, *Cancer in Connecticut: 1935–1951*, 1955.

6. "Population Screening for Uterine Cancer by Vaginal Cytology," *Journal of the American Medical Association*, September 15, 1956.

7. National Institute of Health, *Tranquilizing Drugs: Progress Report*, Publication No. 65, December 1956.

8. Statement by Surgeon General Leroy E. Burney, U.S. Public Health Service, "Excessive Cigarette Smoking and Health," July 12, 1957.

9. Phillip Cooper and James B. Knight, Jr., "Effect of Cigarette Smoking on Gastric Secretions of Patients with Duodenal Ulcers," *New England Journal of Medicine*, 255(1), 17–21, July 5, 1956.

10. American Cancer Society and American Heart Association, *Report of Study Group on Smoking and Health*, March 6, 1957.

11. U.S. Department of Agriculture, Agricultural Marketing Service, *Annual Report on Tobacco Statistics*, September 1957.

29

Research

Retrospective and Prospective

The primary goal of health education is to increase people's knowledge of the scientific facts about health and to stimulate them to apply the knowledge in improved health practices. Research in health education, then, is concerned with the process by which people change their health behavior. It includes study of all the various factors in the process and the dynamics of the relationships between these factors. For example, health education research encompasses studies of the social and cultural characteristics of the people, the character of the health practice being advocated, and the educational methods and materials used in bringing about the change or improvement in health behavior. It is also interested in research on the effectiveness of efforts to bring about change. More and more research workers are turning their attention to the dynamics of the interrelations of the many factors entering into the change process. An elaboration of these types of research as taken from reports in the literature will indicate how far we have come in research and some of the problems that lie ahead.

Originally published in the *International Journal of Health Education*, October 1960, 3(4), 164–169. Reprinted with permission.

Knowledge

Some of the first attempts at studying the characteristics of the people consisted in measuring their knowledge, or lack of it, as well as such misinformation that they might have with respect to various health subjects. After such baseline measurements, a plan of health education of some kind was carried out, and subsequent testing revealed the change in knowledge that had taken place. Such studies have been more frequently conducted in the schools, for they are patterned after the way studies in other school subjects have been conducted. Such studies, where applied to an adult population, have proved disappointing in that improvement in the health knowledge of the people frequently did not result in more hygienic practices.

Social Factors

The anthropologists have contributed perhaps the largest number of studies to show that factors other than knowledge of health facts enter into the success of the health education process. For example, the work of Foster and associates in Latin America, Read in Africa, Freedman in Indonesia, DuBois and Dhillon and many others in India, not to mention a host of others, has emphasized the important part that the cultural customs of the people play in determining their response to health education activities. Religious practices and beliefs, concepts about disease causation and cure, value systems, social and power structure, and so on have been shown to exert real influence on the degree of acceptance of new health information and the way it is put into effect.

Almost all of the studies of the anthropologists have been conducted in cultures other than their own. Seldom is it possible to find a report of a study by an anthropologist who has investigated the value systems, traditions, and so on of his own country and reported their influence on the health practices of that coun-try. For example, the early settlers in the United States were pio-neers who gave little attention to potential dangers as they pushed westward. Their general attitude was: "Do not look for trouble; if you do, you will find it." Could it be that this cultural attitude is partly responsible for the relatively low percentage of people in the United States population who seek health exami-nation annually? Certainly, much information has been put out urging this action.

A number of studies have been reported on social and economic status, occupation, educational level, and so on of groups of people prior to education. The reports usually show comparative results in improved knowledge and practices in the various groupings of the population. Seldom have these studies probed to ascertain whether these factors had an influence in the dynamics of the educational process and, if so, the way in which they operated.

Individual Factors

Somewhat more recently there have been appearing reports on studies of the individual—his motivations, perceptions, attitudes, beliefs, and practices—and the ways in which these influence his response to health education. Leadership for these studies has come primarily from the social psychologists and mental health workers.

Not too much has been reported on how research findings about the people have been used in planning health education aspects of public health programs. Bogolepova and her workers have reported a number of studies of this kind. They first find the reasons that spe-cific groups (such as those with arthritis, cardiovascular disorders, rheumatic fever) are not following hygienic practices. On the basis of these data, they experimentally develop ways of educating the specific cases and then evaluate the success of their efforts.

The above description of types of studies of the people is suggestive of the many areas of investigation that need to be undertaken in order to improve the scientific basis for the practice of health education.

Motivation for What?

Earlier, I mentioned that research in health education was concerned with the character of the action that was being advocated. For example, is it an individual or a community action on which the health education effort is focusing? A dental program can focus on periodic dental examinations and treatment of individuals, or it might be focused on adjusting the fluoride content of the community water system.

Is the advocated practice a single action that the individual needs to take, such as vaccination, or is it a continuing hygienic regimen that must be adopted, such as reducing the amount of favorite foods one eats in order to lose weight or reducing children's sugar intake to cut down on dental caries?

Will the benefits of the action advocated accrue to the individual who takes it or to his child? It is usually much easier to get parents to have their children immunized than to submit themselves for immunization.

Is the action one that needs to be taken now or later, when some condition or symptom appears? Is the advocated action or actions for the purpose of preventing some potential future illness (preventive health behavior), or are the actions suggested as ways to relieve an already unhealthy condition (stress behavior)?

These questions must be taken into account in any research in order that study results will be comparable. I have seen reports on education programs for immunization where such distinctions were not made. The success of education with patients having different disease conditions that require changes of behavior under stress does not provide guidance for programs urging preventive health action upon a healthy population group. Perhaps the greatest number of reports of studies has appeared in the area of methods and materials. These studies are of several kinds:

1. The communication and persuasion process.
2. The various media of communication.
3. The different educational methods.

The Art of Persuasion

Most of the studies on the communication process have been done by social scientists. They have been concentrating on the theoretical concepts that underlie the transfer of information from one person to another, as well as the factors that influence changes in opinion. Their studies have been conducted using all sorts of subject matter content, including health. Some of the detailed items they have investigated are:

1. The communicator or the person originating the communication. What effect do his trustworthiness, his apparent intentions, and his group affiliations have on the degree to which the audience will listen to and accept his message?
2. The content of the communication. What appeals are used? What is the effect on the way in which the arguments are presented? Incidentally, much of their work centers on the use of fear or threat as a way of motivating acceptance of a communication. (In the light of their findings we may want to investigate much more thoroughly our own use of this appeal.) What is the effect of conflicting communications? Certainly here is a question on which we need more enlightenment in the field of health. All too often advertisements present varied suggestions contrary to those we, as health workers, are trying to communicate.

3. The effect of the groups to which the audience belongs. How acceptable to individuals are communications that run counter to attitudes held by groups of which the individual is a member?

4. The length of time people retain a communication—a message of information on which they act immediately and one on which they are to act when the occasion demands.

All these investigations by the theorists in communication need to be studied for their implications in health education. In addition, most of their findings need to be tested using health facts as the content of the communication before we can apply on a wide scale some of the concepts that they are developing.

Say It with . . . a Film? . . . a Poster?

Studies of the effectiveness of various materials and media tend to follow three general research designs:

1. The first type of study employs laboratory experiments in which the same information is presented to comparable groups using different media. The relative amount learned by those exposed to the different media is used as a measure of the comparative effectiveness of the media tested. Admittedly, the results obtained in the laboratory situation may not be directly applicable when used in field programs. However, I recall one experiment of this kind in which the relative effectiveness of sound films, silent films, and sound film strips was compared. It was found that the more economical the medium, the more effective it was; that is, the sound film strip was more effective than the movies, and the silent movie was more effective than the sound film. If this finding should prove to be true in practical field programs (and there is a theoretical rationale for the finding), then we could save

much money and still have effective audiovisual aids by using more widely the less expensive media.

2. The second type of study of materials focuses on exposing a given message in one or more ways and at different times to the same audience—or to comparable audiences—and then questioning a sample of the intended population as to whether they saw or heard the specific message, what they can remember of the message, and what they are doing about it. Not too many studies of this kind have been made in the health area.

3. The third type of study is based on the opinion of people about various media. Their opinion is obtained during an interview or in response to a questionnaire. People are asked such questions as: From what media did you learn a given item of information? On what media do you depend for information, and which media do you prefer? Such studies are relatively easy to carry out, but most of them have serious limitations. People seldom can remember where they first heard a particular information item. Even the media they say that they prefer may not be the media from which they learn facts. Hence, conclusions based on such data may be misleading. As we advance in our studies and research in health education, I hope we can become much more precise in our investigations of the media at our disposal.

All Methods Have Their Place

Studies of the methods of health education have usually employed the experimental–control group design. That is, comparable groups are given the information, using different educational methods, and the relative response of the people to the material is checked.

As a result of such studies, it is practically safe to say that in those cultures where the experiments were carried out, group discussion leading to decision is a superior method to giving lectures. Here is a problem where cross-cultural studies are needed to ascertain if this is a universal difference, or limited to specific cultural groups. I have talked with two health educators who were working in cultures other than those where these experiments were conducted, and they had been able to confirm the finding, though their methods were not entirely comparable with those used in the original experiments. It has also been shown that personal communication under certain conditions is better than the impersonal methods of mass communication.

We need to subject all our methods to rigid evaluation so that we can know more adequately their strengths and weaknesses. There is, however, *one pitfall to be avoided* in all studies of our methods and media. Often my public health colleagues ask such questions as "Are exhibits better than movies?"; "Are mothers classes better than individual conferences?"; or "What is the best way to do health education?" To my way of thinking, such inquiries are analogous to a layman asking a physician these questions: "Is aspirin a better medicine than paregoric?" or "What is the best treatment for illness?" All the methods and materials have their place. Their relative effectiveness, singly or in combination, will depend on the characteristics of the people with whom they are used, the kind of action that is being advocated, and the person who will use the materials. *We need to learn what educational methods work with what kinds of people to produce what kinds of actions.* It is in the dynamics of these interrelationships that much intensive work is needed.

We Must Not Mistake Effort for Accomplishment

The last area of studies and research on which more and more reports are appearing is evaluation. Increasingly, health workers are seeking objective evidence of their accomplishments in health education. Here again the reports include three types of studies:

1. Pretesting of materials and programs before they are put into broad-scale use.

2. Reports of the numbers of pamphlets distributed, the numbers of film showings, the number of inches of newspaper publicity, the number of people attending lectures, and so on.

3. Objective evidence of the increased information and/or number who took, or are continuing to take, the recommended action.

The pretesting of materials and programs is the kind of study that all practicing health educators can and should be doing. Knutson, Ward, Jacobs, Ford, and others have reported the steps they took in determining the extent to which material being developed could be read, understood, and comprehended and whether the action fitted into the people's ways of doing things. Few resources were necessary to make these determinations. The resulting improvement in the tested pamphlets, exhibits, and so on justified the time and effort.

For many years the volume of activities and materials distributed was reported as evidence of a program's effectiveness. Today not so many reports of this kind are submitted as evidence of success. As Clements has said, "We must not mistake effort for accomplishment."

Most of the evaluation studies that report changes in health behavior have been limited to the single-action type of behavior. This is the one kind of behavior that is easy to observe and count, such as getting an immunization, taking a shot of penicillin for yaws, or getting an X-ray for a tuberculosis case finding. Accumulating the evidence that people have changed their diet, are following a strict hygienic regime for arthritis, or are taking medicines at a prescribed time, is much more difficult. Nevertheless, we need to continue our efforts to find the methods of uncovering evidence of this kind.

The preceding discussion has centered on studies and research in the education of adults about health. There is a fairly large body of literature devoted to studies and research on health education in the schools, but the limits of this paper do not permit an adequate review of work in this specialized field.

Summary

The preceding description of studies and research has used as its frame of reference the elements in the educational process that a practitioner in health education uses as he plans his program. It indicates that most of the areas of concern have received some investigation. What has been done seems to point the way to much more useful and precise findings when the various elements are studied in depth.

The task ahead is to interest research workers in human behavior to test out some of their theories in the area of health behavior. Meanwhile, practitioners in health education can increase the precision of their own program efforts if they use to the fullest extent the limited research findings that are available.

Discussion Questions

1. What are some of the potential factors that could influence the health education process as described in this chapter?

2. What are some research areas Derryberry discusses that could improve health education processes?

3. Are these research areas relevant today? Why? Why not?

4. Derryberry calls for "pretesting" health communications before applying them in an intervention or campaign. How often is this done today?

30

Research Procedures
Applicable to Health Education

R esearch is in vogue. In fact, it is being carried on in such proportions that one could almost apply that old song title "Everybody Is Doing It Now." Furthermore, our current attitude seems to
be that if you have conducted a study and published its results, your
status is raised.

Let us look at the extent of research in the health and education fields in terms of financial outlay. Last year the nation's expenditures for medical and health-related research reached $1 billion,
55 percent of which were Federal funds.[1] For direct education
research, the principal private foundations and government agencies spent approximately $10 million, and if research related to edu-
cation is included, the total would be closer to $15 million.
Certainly these figures are convincing evidence that society will
support research in both the health and education fields.

But to what extent is research in health education being supported by these funds? There are no compilations to answer this
question, but it is my impression that activity in this field is far too
limited. Russell's[2] review of the *Research Quarterly* for the 10-year
period 1951–1960 reported only 59 studies.

Originally published in the *Journal of School Health*, May 1963, 33(5), 215–220.
Copyright © 1963 by American School Health Association, Kent, Ohio 44240.
Reprinted with permission.

The limited number, however, does not reflect an unawareness of the importance of getting more investigations underway. Committees of the AAHPER and the APHA have compiled lists of health education problems requiring study. The recently appointed Commission on Research of the AAHPER has attempted to establish priorities among the many subjects listed. In their paper presented last year at the American Public Health Association, Guthrie, Schultz, and Davis[3] again emphasized that more research is called for in health education. The Health Education Service for Schools and Colleges of the American Medical Association[4] has published a list of methods that can be used to check changes in knowledge, attitudes, and behavior of students relating to health.

First, let us look at studies of health knowledge, attitudes, and behavior. Have we focused too much effort on the measurement of health information? Have we too readily followed the pattern set by other subjects in the educational curriculum—for example, history, mathematics, and geography—without making necessary adaptations for the differences between health education and the other content subjects in the curriculum? For example, in the content subjects one of the basic goals is to impart information so that students will develop the ability to relate facts for greater understanding and skill in problem solving and decision making. But is it the major goal of health education to impart a specified body of information and to develop skill in problem solving or decision making? Before you answer in the affirmative, let us examine the question more closely.

Historical facts are stable, they relate the past. Their use may vary with new happenings, but the basic facts are constant. Relationships in mathematics are fixed; for example, 2 + 2 = 4. This is the same at school, home, business, or wherever you turn.

In geography, the places, their characteristics, products, and climate are generally constant, only the names and boundaries change. But how about information on health? What was true yesterday may not be true tomorrow. A few years ago everyone over 15 years of age was advised to get an X-ray annually to detect tuberculosis. Now it is recommended that we be tuberculin-tested.

Or there may be debate about what is true. Whether to use killed or live virus vaccine is an issue at the moment. Controversy marks the relationship of smoking to cancer and other health conditions. Furthermore, what is stated as fact in the school may not be practiced at home.

What kind of research on the status of health knowledge of children will have universal applicability under these circumstances?

One educator, who has reviewed many reports of studies about health knowledge and attitudes in both child and adult populations, said:

> [I have] come to the conclusion that all one has to do to win fame is to develop a questionnaire, administer it, and report the results in various categories and cross-categories with a statement as to which are statistically significant by the chi square method and which are not. This material is then published in a professional journal and, quite regardless of the size of the sample or the universality of the situation, purports to become a signpost from which many other workers take their direction. As a rule, the authors make frank statements of the limitations of the study in the discussion, but only after the "conclusions," usually couched in general terms, leave the impression that the findings can be applied universally.

Before I am misunderstood, let me quickly assure you I am not saying that research on information and knowledge is unimportant. I am saying that it should be consistent with the role that information or knowledge plays in the goals we are trying to achieve. Certainly determination of the status of children's knowledge is a requisite for program planning. It also provides a baseline for program evaluation. But, alone, is it research? Even though the entire group of children in one locality is tested, can the results be generalized to other communities or the nation? Is this more like the contour survey made by engineers before they start a road, or the data a doctor collects for a diagnosis, than actual research? Yet 15 percent of the 59 studies reported by Russell were classified in this category, as were almost a quarter of the studies reported by the Research Council.

I do not contend that national studies based on adequate sampling procedures with comprehensive tests are not research and cannot be generalized. They can much more readily qualify as such, however, when they are the starting point for experimental programs to improve quality of health education efforts.

In addition, investigations into the development of measuring instruments that reflect those elements of information important to the aims of health education and their relationship to factors in the education environment can surely be classified as health education research. I shall have more to say about this kind of research activity later.

In the area of health attitudes, have we been clear on what we are looking for? What do we mean by attitudes in measurable terms? Are we referring to the verbal expression about some statements, informational material, or health practice? Or are we concerned about the criteria that operate when children choose what they will do? As one example, does health or popularity influence girls to participate in the Cherry Blossom Festival? Almost every spring I marvel at the complete disregard of health advice evidenced by pretty girls who aspire to be crowned Queen of the Festival!

Have our studies concentrated more on the status of attitudes than on change? When and how are fundamental health attitudes established? Have we done longitudinal or age-grade studies of attitude formation? As a corollary to these questions, have we even begun to determine the factors and influences that control attitudes so that we can get some guides on how to maintain favorable ones and change those detrimental to health?

My critical questions do not point the way to precise methods or procedures of investigation, but I hope they will stimulate probing to greater depth in our research efforts on attitudes. Turning now to the question of health behavior and behavior change, surely this aspect of health education deserves major emphasis in our investigating efforts.

Yet in our research, what behavior have we studied? Has it been: behavior at school through behavior inventories, observations, verbal responses, and so on; behavior in the home through questionnaires, checklists, diaries, and the like; behavior in social situations with peers or gang members; or the health practices of adults who have formerly been our students?

Let me ask these two questions: (1) Has the volume of research on health behavior been directly or inversely related to the importance of the social setting in which the behavior occurs? (2) Have we concerned ourselves with the "easy to measure" aspect of the problem to the neglect of the more important elements? Studies of behavior and its determinants at any age or grade level or over any period of time are vitally important. Experiments in improving health practices are most desirable in any situation where children are. But how much research have we focused on the dynamics of health habit formation either in the school or at home?

To summarize in one broad question: Have we adequately conceptualized research in health education?

I have not made a thorough search of the research literature in school health. But I have not found in any of the reports I have read a set of integrated hypotheses reflecting the many factors operating in school health education and how they influence the final outcome. You may ask what I mean by an integrated theory or series of hypotheses. Let me give you two examples. Rosenstock, Hochbaum, and Kegeles have proposed and tested to some extent a theory on determinants of preventive health behavior.[5] Kurt Lewin, in his presentation of a quasi-stationary theory of behavior change, suggests the framework of a model on which to build an integrated theory of health behavior.[6]

By and large, the approach has been a study here and there without relation to any broad matrix or conceptual framework of problems. Russell's study of authors substantiates this. He found that 44 authors (77 percent) contributed only one report during the 10-year investigation period and only 10 individuals contributed two research documents. It would seem that if investigators were working on a matrix of problems, a larger number would have completed more than one research project and reported it.

It is not necessary to produce an integrated theory or conceptual framework upon which all workers agree. Actually there is value in having more than one overall theory so long as the framework developed has its foundation in basic behavioral research. For once a series of integrated hypotheses has been stated, each can be tested through a systematic probing in various situations. Results obtained will permit validation of each hypothesis, modification of the model, or its complete rejection. This theoretical approach will sharpen our understanding of health education and the factors associated with it.

To develop such theoretical formulations is no easy task. It requires far more time and thought than writing out a questionnaire, test questions, or interview schedule, administering these to a group of people, tabulating the replies, and writing a report.

It demands, among other things, a thorough study of the literature both directly and indirectly related to health education and an understanding of how research findings are evaluated and related to one another. In short, such development is far more dependent on creative thinking than on how-to-do-it recipes for research procedures and methods.

Earlier I mentioned the development of measuring instruments as useful research activities. A large portion of our data instruments are questionnaires, tests, interview schedules, and observation checklists. Seldom have I seen published assurance that the influence of the instrument upon the information obtained has been kept to a minimum. In other words, would the results have been different had the questions been phrased differently?

The scaling of test items, the development of reliability for consistency and replication, regardless of time and method of administration, and reporting results of such investigations are essential steps in the construction of a psychometric instrument. Two techniques in this area seem to me to have particular value: the open-ended questionnaire or interview and the projective-type test.

Questionnaires and interview items to which the respondent must select a choice of responses can be tabulated with little difficulty. The respondent must try to figure out which words most nearly fit his opinion (sometimes when none does). Open-ended questions provide greater freedom for the respondent to state his opinion, thus permitting expression of a fuller range of his attitudes and behavior. Classification of such free responses is difficult, but with built-in consistency questions it can be made both objective and reliable.

The projective method of interviewing has been shown to elicit far more accurate data in certain situations. Hochbaum found that people in reply to direct questioning might state that a person could have tuberculosis without symptoms. But when shown a picture of an X-ray van and asked why some people were going in and others not, respondents might give as a reason, "He feels all right." This latter response has been shown to reflect far more adequately the respondents' true attitude.

So much for the product part of health education, that is, the effect upon information, attitudes, and practices. Let us turn for a moment to the process, that is, the curriculum, program, and activities.

In this area, present research seems to be chiefly surveys of normative patterns rather than experiments in procedure or controlled operation of programs. One can question the value and significance of such studies other than to provide measurements for gauging progress. Without experimentation, how can we know in which direction on the distribution curve of practices one should move? If the percentage of programs following one practice is 15, can we tell from the survey whether it should be 85, 100, or something else without some validation based on outcome? Controlled or rigorous experimentation is necessary to provide direction. The procedure is difficult; at times it may require compromise, but a more adequate determination than personal opinion of the relationship between program activity and outcome is badly needed.

How these relationships are established is important. One method that seems to be more widely used in school health research than in other areas of investigation is the jury or expert panel method. Here the investigator prepares a series of statements and submits them to a jury panel for a rating on a scale of 1 to 5 or "agree" and "disagree." The task of the researcher is to make up the statements, select a panel, send them the material, tabulate the responses, and report the results.

This may be a good way to get data for a paper or a doctor's dissertation, but it is far better evidence of how one group rated a series of statements at a particular time than of conclusions that have real validity for future planning and action.

As a conclusion to this critique of research in health education, I should like to share with you a study of the reasons for disapproval of some of the research proposals submitted to the National Institutes of Health (NIH).[7] These proposals were in the medical and related biological fields and were not specific research projects in health education. However, some of the reasons for disapproval given by the experts who reviewed the projects seem to highlight in a different way some of the earlier points made in this paper. A review of these reasons may help us improve the quality of our efforts.

Of the 6,000 applications for research grants received by the NIH during the 12 months ending June 30, 1959, approximately 2,000 were disapproved. A sample of 605 of these applications was studied with respect to the adverse comments made by the boards of scientists who reviewed them. Thirty-three different study sections were involved in the 605 disapproved applications. Hence, the adverse comments reflect a wide range of judgments. The reasons for rejection are grouped into four classes:

1. Those concerning the problem—the question that the proposed research would seek to answer.
2. The approach by which the answer would be sought.
3. The competence of the investigators.
4. Other reasons.

I shall report only the reasons most frequently given:

1. The problem is of insufficient importance or is unlikely to produce any new or useful information.
2. The problem is more complex than the investigator appears to realize.
3. The problem has only local significance, is one of production or control, or otherwise fails to fall sufficiently clearly within the general field of health-related research.
4. The research as proposed is overly involved, with too many elements under simultaneous investigation.
5. The proposed tests, methods, or scientific procedures are unsuited to the stated objective.
6. The description of the approach is too nebulous, diffuse, and lacking in clarity to permit adequate evaluation.
7. The overall design of the study has not been carefully thought out.
8. The statistical aspects of the approach have not been given sufficient consideration.
9. The approach lacks scientific imagination.

10. Controls are either inadequately conceived or inadequately described.

11. The investigator appears to be unfamiliar with recent pertinent literature or methods, or both.

Despite the critical nature of these remarks, I am aware that much sound health education research has been done and is underway. It is my philosophy that improvement comes not so much from a review of all the virtues in a situation but from a frank and unvarnished look at the places where constructive changes can be made. I am convinced that much progress through health education research will be made in the next decade, and that this group will contribute materially to that progress.

Discussion Questions

1. Compare and contrast the funding available to support health education research 40 years ago with that available today.

2. What are four classes of reasons for research proposals being rejected?

3. What can future health educators do to strengthen their chances for funding of critical research questions?

Notes

1. "Federal Expenditures for Medical and Health-Related Research, 1960–63," *Resources for Medical Research* (Washington, D.C.: U.S. Department of Health, Education, and Welfare Report No. 1, August 1962), p. 1, chart.

2. Robert D. Russell, "An Analysis of the Health and Health Education Research in the *Research Quarterly, 1951–60*," *Research Quarterly*, March 1962, p. 37.

3. Eugene Guthrie, Carl S. Schultz, and Roy L. Davis, "Research Needs and Bottlenecks in School Health," *American Journal of Public Health*, October 1961, pp. 1525–1531.

4. "Many Methods Useful for Evaluation in Health Education," *International Journal of Health Education*, April–June 1962, p. 93.

5. Irwin M. Rosenstock, Godfrey M. Hochbaum, and Stephen S. Kegeles, "Determinants of Health Behavior," White House Conference on Children and Youth, 1960.

6. K. Lewin, "Frontiers in Group Dynamics," *Human Relations*, 1947, pp. 143–153.

7. Ernest M. Allen, "Why Are Research Grant Applications Disapproved?" *Science*, November 25, 1960, pp. 1532–1534.

31

Research and Practice
in Health Education

The title for this paper is extremely general and broad. To deal with it in any comprehensive way would require the rest of the afternoon. But don't worry, I am conscious of your time restraints. I have, therefore, chosen three unrelated facets of the subject that to me seem to be relevant at this time. The first facet has to do with decision making on health practices. In her presidential address to the Tenth Annual Meeting of the Society for Public Health Education, Beryl Roberts developed from the behavioral science literature of the 1950s a theoretical base for decision making regarding health actions. She gave very little emphasis to the question of who makes the decisions since the major focus of her paper was community action, and the basic tenets of community organization are that the community makes the decisions. But today, when the major problems are chronic diseases and the actions much more individualistic in nature, the question has assumed major importance. Is it the provider of service or the consumer who makes the decisions?

Because of our professional training and philosophy, I am sure almost all of you would say without hesitation, "It is the patient or consumer who decides." This point of view was forcefully expressed by Bob Johnson in his presentation at this same lun-

---

Originally presented to the Public Health Education Section of the American Public Health Association in Washington, D.C., November 2, 1977.

cheon last year. He pointed out that there are "those individuals [who] would use education . . . to have learners accept already decided conclusions" and indicated how such use of education did not conform to the philosophy of health educators. Sigrid Deeds made this point emphatically at a session on who makes the decisions in health education.

As I read samples of research in preparation for this paper, I was struck with the preponderance of reports that accepted the position that the provider makes the decisions. First, there were the hundreds of studies on patient compliance. Certainly I didn't read them all, but most of those that I did read focused on some aspect of the patient or his family carrying out the practices decided for him by the physician. One pamphlet I picked up carried a whole section on "How to Motivate the Patient to Comply." Then there were several papers on behavior modification in which the experimenter (sometimes a health educator but mostly not) manipulated the situation, reward system, and other reinforcements to change the client's behavior so that he would comply with the authority or provider-determined practice.

These studies on compliance bring to mind Kelman's three processes of change: compliance, identification, and internalization. They raise the question: Should compliance be the educator's goal, or should we concern ourselves more with helping an individual or patient decide whether to internalize a different behavior into his goals, values, and habit system? If our answer is the latter, then our educational strategy (content and methods) becomes quite different from direct teaching or manipulation to enforce a regimen.

Other evidence pointing to the fact that providers are making the decisions is the number of articles reporting the development of teaching units and programmed instruction on such topics as diabetes, weight reduction, nutrition, hypertension, and so on, in which the emphasis is on how the educator can teach what the patient must know and do, not on how he can help the patient decide what he wants and is willing to do.

However, I did find some studies in which the educational emphasis and methodology focused on the patient or consumer making the decision. Steckel and Swain at the University of Michigan have used contingency contracting—a permissive form of behavior modification—to help individuals make those lifestyle changes required to reduce hypertension. They report 100 percent success with patients performing the acts that they themselves agreed to do. The secret of their success lies in their rigid adherence to laws of learning. They break down the ultimate change in lifestyle into specific sequential behaviors. They do not burden the patient with a myriad of changes that he must make all at once. Each behavior is so specific that it can be written into a simple contract. The desired behavior is one that the patient considers appropriate and realistic for him to achieve in the specified time, which is usually short. On completion of the contract, the agreed upon behavior change is reinforced with a tangible reward that the patient has previously selected and included in the contract. In short, the educator and patient agree on a specific behavior that he will practice for a short period for a reward that he selects in advance and is stated in the contract. As one behavior becomes established, a maintenance contract is made and a new behavior in the complex of changes is considered by the patient and educator.

Another approach to patient decision making is underway at Beth Israel Hospital in Boston. Here alternative treatments for a condition are entered into a computer together with full information about the probabilities of success of each treatment, its side effects, duration, cost, and so on. The patient studies each treatment, with the opportunity to ask the computer questions that it is programmed to answer. After the patient studies the different regimens, he selects the one most suitable for him, or he may even decide not to follow any one of the alternate treatment patterns. The success of these experiments is dependent on making explicit to the patient the results to be expected in whatever decision he makes. It is not "informed consent." It is informed positive decision, and psychologically the difference is much more than a semantic one.

The fact that far more favorable outcomes occur when people are allowed to make the decision validates our own educational philosophy. It also gives emphasis to the importance of the movement to develop the "activated" patient.

Let me now call attention to a couple of studies in family planning. Much of the effort in family planning has been focused on urging clients to practice contraception, spacing, and so on. A group at the University of Washington first concentrated their efforts on developing a tool on the "hierarchy of birth planning values" and have been using this tool with couples to help them decide about having another child and the method of contraception—in case their decision requires it. Belcher, Lee, and I also, conducted a study in which we helped couples decide if and when they wanted another child. When they had made their decision, we focused the education about family planning on helping them achieve their goal, which could include becoming pregnant at a time they had chosen.

A second facet of my subject deals with some of today's research methodology and the conclusions the methods generate that can be detrimental to sound educational practice. In much of the so-called health education research today, a specific educational intervention or strategy—such as a home visit, group discussion, or use of a pamphlet—is applied to a population, and the degree to which it induces the desired change in behavior is measured. The strategy is sometimes called a "package program" or "inputs." Either term implies a mechanistic approach to education. When the procedures prove to be ineffective, the investigators may report that education (not the specific procedures they used) is not effective. Such a conclusion is like reporting that drugs are not effective in treating disease when only one drug has been used in a particular way and without any diagnosis of the situation.

Carol D'Onofrio and Hamouda Hanafi encountered a report of this kind in the book *Compliance with Therapeutic Regimens* by

Sackett and Haynes. The conclusion as stated by Haynes was that educational strategies were less effective than behavioral strategies in producing compliance.

This conclusion could be easily interpreted by the unsuspecting as "education is no good." However, when the same studies were rated for adequacy of the educational interaction, it was found that improved compliance and therapeutic outcomes occurred in 100 percent of the studies where the essential educational procedures were followed with any degree of adequacy.

As practicing health educators, we must be ever on the alert, but not on the defensive, to make sure that studies in health education recognize the dynamic and interaction aspects of the learning process. We must point out to researchers that intervention without diagnosis is almost always doomed to erroneous conclusions. Larry Green emphasized this point at the Patient Education Symposium in San Francisco last month.

Let me mention two other closely allied research procedures that are of vital concern to us as health educators. The first is the use of improvement in health condition as a criterion of the effectiveness of any educational program or process. Green has described the fallacies that can arise when the advocated behavior may or may not result in improved health of the individual.

The other research procedure that may lead to erroneous results is having control and experimental groups equated only on physical diagnosis. If one is conducting a controlled educational experiment with individuals having a single disease entity, the experimental and control groups should be equated not only on their physical condition but also on knowledge, attitudes, value systems, motivation, and present behavior. These are the variables that will have a potent influence on the educational outcome.

One final comment on method. Behavioral scientists are interested in the variables that account for differences in outcome and how much each variable contributes to the difference. They use statistical methods to determine the general or average effect of each variable that they have included in their study. Having made these determinations, their research goals are satisfied. Although such conclusions are of importance to us practicing educators in our program planning, our unique research focus should go beyond such determinations. We need to search for the additional factors that influence the behavior of each individual. An illustration of this reaching beyond the models of behavior change is the work of Caron and his associates at a veterans hospital, working with clinic patients suffering from peptic ulcer. They found that in addition to the factors in the Belief Model, lack of understanding of basic physiology and the relations of the antacid treatment to their physiological symptoms caused patients to neglect their treatment. There were also misconceptions that had to be routed out before the patients could internalize and adopt the curative and preventive practices.

Is it possible that in our research we tend to stop when we have determined the averages and do not go on to investigate in detail those cases that deviate from the central tendency? Such detailed individual case study is expensive and difficult to carry out, but I suspect that it would add much to our understanding of health behavior and extend our theoretical concepts considerably. At least it is a hypothesis worth testing.

The third aspect of my subject is related to the use of behavioral research in practice. Many researches are reported in which the Belief Model, Lewin's Force-Field Model, the Diffusion Model, and more recently the Locus of Control Theory are used to explain the success or failure of educational efforts. But as all of you know, they serve quite a different function when we are planning and conducting practical programs. Each of the elements in the models helps us in our diagnosis to pinpoint educational needs and to suggest possible educational interventions. But when we report on such specific programs as case studies, do we make sufficiently explicit the learning and behavioral theories that guided our procedures? In my opinion, if such were done, our professional literature would be much more precise, and there wouldn't be as much tendency to copy mechanically the procedures in situations that are totally different.

There is one other way in which the basic behavioral research can be used to underpin our practices. I believe that it provides an effective method of gaining acceptance and appreciation of our educational expertise, particularly with other professional and research workers. Often, in attempts to interpret health education principles and methods, we try to simplify and explain them without reference to the basic research or science that we are applying. Since most health professionals and scientists think they know about education, learning, and teaching (many of them have been doing it for years), they feel entirely competent to challenge whatever we may say. If, however, we cite research models and formulations as the basis for our methods, they are likely to listen to the sound educational procedures that we may suggest.

Let me illustrate from the experience of several of us health educators this past spring, when we served as members of site visit teams to review institutions applying for NIH grants for Diabetes Research and Training Centers. We found that reference to specific research findings with a bibliography created a respect for the educational principles and behavioral models on the change that we were advocating. In fact, several of the scientists asked for references to the literature we cited. It is not possible to generalize from one experience, but I wonder if we use our science findings enough in explaining the procedures that we follow.

Summary

I have dealt briefly with only three aspects of my subject. They are as follows:

1. Decision making in health practices and who makes the decision.

2. Concerns of health educators about some current research approaches to health education problems.

3. Use of basic behavioral science research findings as guides to diagnosing educational needs, designing interventions, and interpreting health education principles to other health professionals.

Discussion Questions

1. Compare and contrast the methods described by Derryberry of helping individuals to decide to adhere to a prescribed regimen.

2. What do you think the best approaches might be to improve behavior change in light of current evidence and health education practice?

3. What is the importance of using social frameworks or models in the context of research studies in health education as outlined by Derryberry?

4. How can behavioral science contribute to the identification of health outcomes that are meaningful to measure?

5. What are some of the ethical issues today's health educators face in research and practice?

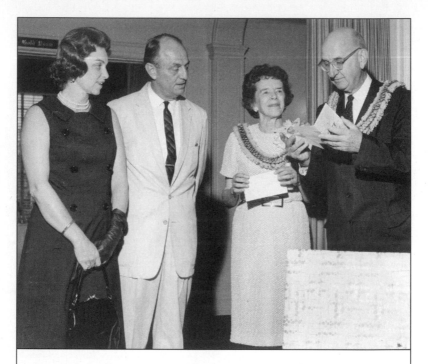

Photo, circa 1963, of Luther L. Terry, MD, Surgeon General of the U.S. Public Health Service, *second from left*, and Mrs. Terry, *left*, extending thanks and best wishes to Dr. Mayhew Derryberry, *fourth from left*, and his wife, Helen, *third from left*, on the occasion of Dr. Derryberry's departure from the Public Health Service to work on assignment in India. Courtesy of Mr. Clarence E. Pearson and the National Center for Health Education.

Appendix A

Published and Unpublished Papers of Mayhew Derryberry, Ph.D.

Published Papers (in chronological order)

Franzen, R., & Derryberry, M. (1931, December). The routine computation of partial and multiple correlation. *Journal of Educational Psychology, 22*(9), 641–651.

Palmer, G. T., Derryberry, M., & Van Ingen, P. (1931). *Health protection for the preschool child.* New York: Century.

Franzen, R., & Derryberry, M. (1932, October). Note on reliability coefficients. *Journal of Educational Psychology, 22*(7), 559–560.

Franzen, R., & Derryberry, M. (1932, November). Reliability of group distinctions. *Journal of Educational Psychology, 22*(8), 586–593.

Franzen, R., & Derryberry, M. (1933, October). Weight and skeletal build. *American Journal of Orthopsychiatry,* pp. 445–454.

Palmer, G. T., & Derryberry, M. (1934, March). Health service for white and Negro families. *Child Health Bulletin,* pp. 65–67.

Palmer, G. T., & Derryberry, M. (1934, May). Health service for white and Negro families. *Child Health Bulletin,* pp. 99–104.

Palmer, G. T., & Derryberry, M. (1934, May). An index of nutritional status. *Public Health Nursing, 26,* 233–234.

Palmer, G. T., & Derryberry, M. (1934, August 30). Medical and public health attitude toward smallpox vaccination and diphtheria immunization. *New England Journal of Medicine, 211*(9), 413–415.

Derryberry, M. (1934, November). Why do physical defects in children remain uncorrected? *Child Health Bulletin,* pp. 204–207.

Derryberry, M. (1935, March). Immunization and nativity. *Child Health Bulletin,* pp. 50–57.

Derryberry, M. (1935, May). Nutritional status indices. *Child Health Bulletin*, pp. 96–98.

Derryberry, M. (1935). Physical defects —The pathway to correction. In *Principles and practices in school health education* (pp. 151–158). New York: American Child Health Association.

Derryberry, M., & Van Buskirk, E. (1936, May 1). The significance of infant mortality rates. *Public Health Reports, 51*, 545–551.

Derryberry, M., & Daniel, J. (1936, June 12). The development of a technique for measuring the knowledge and practice of midwives. *Public Health Reports, 51*(24), 757–771.

Derryberry, M., & Palmer, G. T. (1937, May). Appraising the educational content of a health service program. *American Journal of Public Health, 27*(5), 476–480.

Derryberry, M. (1937, October). Teaching nurses to keep records. *Public Health Nursing, 29*, 557–559.

Derryberry, M. (1938, February 18). Reliability of medical judgments on malnutrition. *Public Health Reports, 53*, 263–268.

Derryberry, M. (1938, April). Taking the public with you. *The Health Officer, 2*(12), 615–621.

Derryberry, M. (1938, June). The nurse as a family teacher. *Public Health Nursing, 30*, 357–365.

Derryberry, M. (1939, January 20). "Do case records guide the nursing service? *Public Health Reports, 54*, 66–76.

Derryberry, M. (1939, January). How may the nurse become a better teacher? *The Health Officer, 3*(9), 253–268.

Derryberry, M. (1939, May). Resume of school health studies. *Journal of School Health, 9*(5), 125–129.

Derryberry, M. (1939, May–June). Administrative procedures that interfere with effective public health nursing. *The Health Officer, 4*(3), 18–23.

Derryberry, M. (1939, July–August). How to influence health behavior of adults. *The Health Officer, 4*(4), 114–117.

Dean, J. O., & Derryberry, M. (1939, September). A procedure for putting health department reports to work. *Public Health Reports, 54*(38), 1709–1718.

Derryberry, M., & Nyswander, D. (1939, October). The physician's and the nurse's part in health education. *American Journal of Public Health, 29*(10), 1109–1113.

Derryberry, M. (1939, November 17). Nursing accomplishments as revealed by case records. *Public Health Reports, 54*(46), 2035–2043.

Derryberry, M. (1939). The nurse as a teacher of tuberculosis to the family. In *Transactions of the 35th Annual Meeting of the National Tuberculosis Association*.

Derryberry, M., & Weissman, A. (1940, March 22). Using tests as a medium for health education. *Public Health Reports, 55*(12), 485–489.

Derryberry, M. (1940, June). Educational qualifications of staff members in health departments. *American Journal of Public Health, 30*(6), 645–651.

Derryberry, M., & Caswell, G. (1940, December 13). Qualifications of professional public health personnel—Plan and scope of the survey. *Public Health Reports, 55*(50), 2312–2319.

Derryberry, M., & Arnstein, M. G. (1940, December 20). Nursing visit transcripts as training material. *Public Health Reports, 55*(51), 2351–2355.

Derryberry, M., & Caswell, G. (1940, December). Qualifications of professional public health personnel—Health officers and other medical personnel. *Public Health Reports, 55*(52), 2377–2396.

Derryberry, M., & Caswell, G. (1941, February 7). Qualifications of professional public health personnel—Nurses. *Public Health Reports, 56*(6), 211–229.

Derryberry, M., & Caswell, G. (1941, February 21). Qualifications of professional public health personnel—Sanitation personnel. *Public Health Reports, 56*(8), 311–327.

Derryberry, M. (1941, March). Exhibits. *American Journal of Public Health, 31*(3), 257–263.

Levy, J., Derryberry, M., & Mensch, I. (1942, July). A new technic of health education for use in baby stations. *American Journal of Public Health, 32*(7), 727-731.

Derryberry, M., & Brockett, G. S. (1943, June). Preserving confidence in health instruction. *Public Health Nursing, 35*, 244–250.

Derryberry, M., Calver, H. N., & Mensh, I. N. (1943, June). Use of ratings in the evaluation of exhibits. *American Journal of Public Health, 33*(6), 709–714.

Derryberry, M., & Dean, J. O. (1944). Extension experience in public health. In *The contribution of extension methods and techniques toward the rehabilitation of war-torn countries*. Report of the Conference on September 19–22, 1944, U.S. Department of Agriculture.

Derryberry, M. (1945, January). Methods of evaluating school health programs. *Connecticut State Medical Journal, 9*, 19–22.

Derryberry, M. (1945, November 23). Health education in the public health program. *Public Health Reports, 60*(47), 1394–1402.

Derryberry, M. (1947, June). What is health education? *American Journal of Public Health, 37*(6), 643–644.

Derryberry, M. (1947, November 14). The role of health education in a public health program. *Public Health Reports, 62*(46), 1629–1641.

Derryberry, M. (1949, May). Analysis and evaluation of a tuberculosis control program—Health education. In *Transactions of the National Tuberculosis Association*, pp. 237–240.

Derryberry, M. (1949, October 14). Health is everybody's business. *Public Health Reports, 64*(41), 1293–1298. (Also published in *California's Health* [1949, November 30]; *Public Health News* [New Jersey Department of Health monthly bulletin] [1950, April]; *Atualidades* [Medico-Sanitaria] [1950, April]; *North Dakota Health News* [1950, June]; *Connecticut Health Bulletin* [1951, January].)

Derryberry, M. (1950, March). Health education and public relations. *American Journal of Public Health, 40*(3), 251–252.

Hoyt, C. J., Knutson, A. L., & Derryberry, M. (1950, November). What the people know: An evaluation of the information and attitudes regarding tuberculosis before and after the mass X-ray survey in Mishawaka. *Monthly Bulletin of the Indiana State Board of Health*, pp. 250, 262–263.

Hoyt, C. J., Knutson, A. L., & Derryberry, M. (1950, December). What the people know: An evaluation of the information and attitudes regarding tuberculosis before and after the mass X-ray survey in Mishawaka. *Monthly Bulletin of the Indiana State Board of Health*, pp. 281–282.

Derryberry, M. (1951, July). Health education in public health. *Health Views* (West Virginia Department of Health), *2*(3), 1–6.

Derryberry, M., & Knutson, A. L., et al. (1952). Pretesting and evaluating health education. Public Health Monograph, No. 8. Washington, DC.

Derryberry, M., & McKeever, N. (1952, November). Education for better health. *Journal of the American Association for Health, Physical Education, and Recreation, 23*(11), 21–22.

Derryberry, M. (1952). Dental health education as a part of the total public health education program. *Bulletin of the Virginia State Dental Association, 29*, 67–71.

Derryberry, M. (1953). Notes on exhibits as a health education medium. In *Pretesting and evaluating health education*, pp. 23–25. U.S. Public Health Service Publication No. 212. Washington, DC: U.S. Public Health Service.

Derryberry, M. (1954, May). Health education. *Bulletin of the National Tuberculosis Association*, pp. 95–96.

Derryberry, M. (1954, October). Rapporteur for the Expert Committee on Health Education of the Public. In *First Report*. Technical Report Series, No. 89. Geneva: World Health Organization.

Derryberry, M., & Skinner, M. L. (1954, November). Health education for outpatients. *Public Health Reports, 69*(11), 1107–1114.

Derryberry, M. (1954, November). New problems in public health: A challenge to health education. *Professional Contributions*, No. 3 (American Academy of Physical Education).

Derryberry, M. (1954, December). Today's health problems and health education. *Public Health Reports, 69*(12), 1224–1228.

Derryberry, M. (1954). Health education aspects of sanitation programmes in rural areas and small communities. *Bulletin of the World Health Organization, 10*, 145–154.

Derryberry, M., & McKeever, N. (1956, January). What does the changing picture in public health mean to health education in programs and practices? *American Journal of Public Health, 46*(1), 54–60.

Derryberry, M. (1957, November). Health education in transition. *American Journal of Public Health, 47*(11), 1357–1366.

Rosenstock, I. M., Derryberry, M., & Carriger, B. K. (1958, February). Why people fail to seek poliomyelitis vaccination. *Public Health Reports, 74*(2), 98–103.

Brugnetti, I., & Derryberry, M. (1958, October). History of a health education fellowship program. *Public Health Reports, 73*(10), 916–918.

Derryberry, M. (1958, October). Some problems in educating for health. *International Journal of Health Education, 1*(4), 178–183.

Derryberry, M. (1958, November). Some problems faced in educating for health. *Professional Contributions*, No. 6 (American Academy of Physical Education), pp. 78–87.

Skinner, M. L., & Derryberry, M. (1959, May). Some aspects of health education for medical students. *Journal of Medical Education, 34*(5), 529–535.

Derryberry, M. (1960, October). Research: Retrospective and perspective. *International Journal of Health Education, 3*(4), 164–169.

Derryberry, M. (1960). Health education—Its objectives and methods. *Health Education Monographs*, No. 8 (Society of Public Health Educators), pp. 3–9.

Derryberry, M. (1961, May–June). Better communications: An essential in today's public health. *Michigan's Health*, pp. 43–46.

Derryberry, M. (1961, May–June). The public health nurse in health education. *Texas Public Health Association Journal, 13*(3), 121–123.

Derryberry, M. (1963, May). Research procedures applicable to health education. *Journal of School Health, 33*(5), 215–220.

Derryberry, M. (1964, October–November–December). The role of field study and demonstration centres in health education. *Madras Health Education, 4*(4), 5–15.

Derryberry, M. (1966, January). A tough job even for Hercules. In *New approach to family planning: Proceedings of the Industrial Conference on Family Planning, Calcutta*. Calcutta: Indian Chamber of Commerce.

Derryberry, M. (1967, February). Voluntary health organizations in the U.S.A. *Swasth Hind*, pp. 35–39.

Derryberry, M. (1970). Health aides. *Public Health Reports, 85*(9), 753. (Introduction to a series of articles by others.)

Moore, A. R., & Derryberry, M. (1971, January–March). Education and training on health aspects of family planning. *International Journal of Health Education, 14*(1), 2–22.

Bloch, D., & Derryberry, M. (1971, July). Effect of political controversy on sex education research—A case study. *The Family Coordinator*, pp. 259–264.

Derryberry, M. (1971). Education in the health aspects of family planning. *Pacific Health Education Reports, 2*, 16–50.

Derryberry, M. (1972). Contributions of George T. Palmer. *American Journal of Public Health, 62*, 130–131.

Derryberry, M., Belcher, D., & Austin, M. L. (1972). *The planned family: Goal of family planning*. (A family planning brochure.)

Derryberry, M. (1974). Theory and practice in health education: A synthesis. In Dorothy Nyswander International Symposium: Papers on the Theoretical Issues in Health Education, University of California, Berkeley, September 27-28, 1974. Berkeley, California: University of California School of Public Health, pp. i–xi.

Derryberry, M. (1977, September). Assistance in planning a family. *Newsletter* (California Interagency Council on Family Planning), *2*(4), 1.

Derryberry, M. (n.d.). India in the vanguard. (Journal unknown), pp. 25–26.

Unpublished Papers

Unfortunately, complete bibliographic information is unknown or unavailable for some of Mayhew Derryberry's unpublished papers. Moreover, not all of his unpublished papers whose titles appear in this listing have survived, and those that have survived are not available in one location. His doctoral dissertation is accessible through New York University. Some of his surviving papers are held in archives at the American Association for Health, Physical Education, Recreation, and Dance, Reston, Virginia, or at the Society for Public Health Education, Washington, D.C. Other papers may be found in archives at the National Library of Medicine, Washington, D.C., at the Pennsylvania State University Special Collections Library, and at the University of California School of Public Health, Berkeley, California.

Social and economic factors associated with health protection for the preschool child. (1933). Thesis submitted as partial fulfillment of requirements for the Ph.D. degree at the School of Education, New York University, 451 pages (abstract, 3 pages).

An evaluation of the effect of public health education on the knowledge and practice of the Negro midwife. (1935, May 13).

Health for today's children. (1939, August 28). Presented at the In-Service Training Institute, Flint, MI.

The evaluation of health education content and material. (1939, August 29 and October 16). Presented at the In-Service Training Institute, Flint, MI, and the 68th annual meeting of the American Public Health Association, Pittsburgh, PA.

Health education by public health nurses. (1939, December 7). Presented at a meeting of the Florida Public Health Association, Jacksonville.

Is your health education effective? (1939, December 9). Presented at a meeting of the Florida Public Health Association, Jacksonville.

Health education—A function of public health departments. (1940, February 9). Presented at the Conference of State and Local Health Officials, Trenton, NJ.

Health information, please. (1940, October 31). Presented in Morgantown, WV.

Evaluation of exhibit material. (1941, May 15). Presented to the Science Museums Section of the American Association of Museums, Columbus, OH.

Organizing a health education program for an extra-cantonment area. (1941, October 12–14). Presented at the Institute for Public Health Education, Atlantic City, NJ.

Solving local problems as a contribution to defense. (1941, October 22). Presented at a meeting of the American Dietetic Association, St. Louis, MO.

America examines its public education system—Education and health. (1941, November 17). Presented at Woodrow Wilson High School, Washington, DC.

The role of education in national fitness. (1942, April 15). Presented at a meeting of the American Association for Health, Physical Education, and Recreation, New Orleans.

Health education in wartime. (1942, October 12–14). Presented to a group of
teachers, Los Angeles.

What the public knows about health (coauthored by Arthur Weissman &
George Caswell). (1942, December). Prepared for the American Museum
of Health, New York, 145 pages.

What is an adequate health education program? (1943, May 15). Presented at
the New England Health Education Institute, Boston.

The role of assistants in health education. (1943, June 18).

Methods and materials in health education. (1943, June 24).

Coordination of health education in the areas of official and unofficial organizations. (1945, October 10). Presented at the Mississippi Valley Conference
on Tuberculosis, Chicago.

Cooperation in health education. (1946, November 18–23). Presented in Edge-
water, MS.

The place of public health education in a public health program. (1947, October
6). Presented at a meeting of the American Public Health Association,
Atlantic City, NJ.

John Q. Public attitudes affecting tuberculosis control. (1948, June).

So you're taking a public opinion survey. (1950). (Manual for volunteer
interviewers.)

The Mishawaka Health Education Project. (1951).

The contribution of health education in meeting the health needs of the nation.
(1952, June 17). Presented for the Society of Public Health Educators
before the President's Commission on the Health Needs of the Nation,
Washington, DC.

Health education—A school-community job. (1953, October 17). Presented at
a meeting of school administrators, Norman, OK.

Improving programs of health education through research and evaluation.
(1953).

Soliloquy. (1955). Given in Baguio, Philippines.

State and federal partnership in health education. (1957, April 17). Presented at
the Biennial Conference of the State and Territorial Directors of Public
Health Education.

Preparation for Asian flu. (1957, October 8). Presented at the Del Prado Hotel.

Training for public health workers. (1957). Presented to the National Tuberculosis Association, Chicago.

Program planning in health education. (1959, October 24–25). Presented at a
meeting in Ocean City, MD.

Our heritage in school health. (1960, April). Presented at a meeting of the
    American Association for Health, Physical Education, and Recreation,
    Miami, FL.
Talk given to executives of the Paper Cup and Container Institute. (1960,
    May 12).
Studies and research in health education. (1960, October 31). Presented at a
    meeting of the American National Council for Health Education of the
    Public, San Francisco.
Some communication problems of the health practitioner. (1960, November
    15–16). Presented at the National Health Forum's Pre-Forum Workshop
    on Communication between the Practitioner and the Public, New York.
The public health educator's views on techniques in public health education.
    (1961, February 27). Presented at the Conference on Public Dental
    Health Education Activities of the American Dental Association,
    Chicago.
Health educator—Partner in health. (1961, March 7). Presented at the annual
    meeting of the Texas Public Health Association, Fort Worth.
Current research on changing health practices. (1961, May 10–12). Presented at
    a meeting of the Michigan Public Health Association.
Recent and current research in health education. (1961, June 6). Presented at the
    meeting of the New York State Public Health Association, Rochester, NY.
A look ahead at health education. (1961, June 8). Presented at the meeting of
    the New York State Public Health Association, Rochester, NY.
Some problems in health education. (1961). Presented in Japan.
Health education in the next decade. (1962, May 4). Presented at the Confer-
    ence of Health Education Secretaries, New York.
Interrelationship of voluntary and official health agencies in health education.
    (1962, September 26). Presented to the Missouri Health Council, Jeffer-
    son City, MO.
Partnership in public health education. (1963, March 25). Presented at the
    Conference of State and Territorial Directors of Public Health Education,
    Williamsburg, VA.
New challenges in health education. (1963, May 8). Presented at a meeting of
    the Health Education Section of the Southern Branch of the American
    Public Health Association, Biloxi, MS.
The patient and his family: A focus for health education. (1963, May 28).
    Presented at a meeting of the Western Branch of the American Public
    Health Association, Phoenix, AZ.

Evaluation in health education. (1963, June 9). Presented to the American Cancer Society Health Education Committee chairmen and staff, Chicago.

Welcoming remarks. (1966, January 19). Presented at the inaugural meeting of the Indian Association for the Advancement of Medical Education, Delhi, India.

The need for population control—An American view of a world problem. (1966, January 29). Presented at the Family Planning Conference of the Indian Chamber of Commerce, Calcutta.

Health education—A mass movement. (1966, June 30). Presented at the Fifth Health Educators' Conference, Bangalore, India.

Making health an individual and community affair. (1967, May 2). Presented to Delta Omega at the University of California at Berkeley.

Educational principles in mental health. (1968, May). Presented at a conference in Asilomar, CA.

Behavioral aspects of family planning. (1969, June 25). Presented to the Psychologists' Section of the 36th Annual Conference of the Western Branch of the American Public Health Association.

Ethnic and cultural perspectives. (1969). Comments on the culture of family planning during a panel discussion.

The emerging priority of health education. (1971, November 22). Presented at the 35th annual meeting of the Pacific College Health Association, Pacific Grove, CA.

Family planning concept in health care delivery. (1976, May 6). Presented at a symposium in Madison, WI.

Research and practice in health education. (1977, November 2). Presented before the Public Health Education Section of the American Public Health Association, Washington, DC.

Analysis and evaluation of a tuberculosis control program. (n.d.).

Effectiveness of cancer educational programs with pharmacists. (n.d.).

Health ways of health workers. (n.d.).

A potential source of health education personnel. (n.d.).

Public health education related to the knowledge and practice of the Negro midwife. (n.d.).

Appendix B

The Mayhew Derryberry Award and Its Recipients

The original intent of the American Public Health Association (APHA) Public Health Education and Health Promotion Section's Mayhew Derryberry Award was to recognize the contributions of outstanding behavioral scientists to the field of health education. The award was named in honor of Mayhew Derryberry, who, as a member of the U.S. Public Health Service, established the Division of Health Education in the Public Health Service. He assembled an outstanding group of scholars, including Godfrey Hochbaum, Andie Knutson, Howard Leventhal, and Irwin Rosenstock, who together made unique and lasting contributions to the field of health education. Later, Derryberry created the Experimental and Evaluation Service, where health education research was first initiated. In 1991, the APHA Public Health Education and Health Promotion Section changed the criteria for the Mayhew Derryberry Award. It is now given to a person who has made an outstanding contribution to the profession.

1981	GODFREY HOCHBAUM (deceased)
1982	MARSHALL H. BECKER (deceased)
1985	NOREEN M. CLARK
1991	JEANETTE SIMMONS

1992	KAREN GLANZ, FRANCES M. LEWIS, BARBARA K. RIMER
1993	KATE LORIG
1994	IRWIN M. ROSENSTOCK (deceased), NICHOLAS FREUDENBERG
1998	EUGENIA ENG
1999	DAVID A. SLEET
2003	MARTIN FISHBEIN

Index

Derryberry, M. (April 1938). Taking the public with you. *The Health Officer, 2,* 615–621. Reprinted with permission from W. B. Saunders Company.

Derryberry, M. (June 1938). The nurse as a family teacher. *Public Health Nursing, 30,* 357–365. Reprinted with permission from Blackwell Publishing (UK).

Derryberry, M. (July–August 1939). How to influence health behavior of adults. Reprinted with permission from W. B. Saunders Company.

Derryberry, M. (October 1939). The physician's and the nurse's part in health education. *American Journal of Public Health, 29,* 1109–1113. Reprinted with permission from the American Public Health Association.

Derryberry, M. (March 1941). Exhibits. *American Journal of Public Health, 31,* 257–363. Reprinted with permission from the American Public Health Association.

Derryberry, M. (January 1945). Methods of evaluating school health programs. *Connecticut Medicine, 9,* 19–22. Reprinted with permission from *Connecticut Medicine*.

Derryberry, M. (March 1950). Health education and public relations. *American Journal of Public Health, 40*(3), 251–252. Reprinted with permission from the American Public Health Association.

Derryberry, M. (1954). Health education aspects of sanitation programs in rural areas and small communities. *Bulletin of the World Health Organization, 10,* 145–154. Reprinted with permission from the World Health Organization.

Derryberry, M. (November 1957). Health education in transition. *American Journal of Public Health, 47*(11), 1357–1366. Reprinted with permission from the American Public Health Association.

Derryberry, M. (1958). Some problems faced in educating for health. *Professional Contributions, 6,* 78–87. Reprinted with permission from *Professional Contributions*.

Derryberry, M. (1960) Health education—Its objectives and methods. *Health Education Monographs, 8,* 3–9. Reprinted with permission from Northern California Society for Public Health Education.

Derryberry, M. (October 1960). Research: Retrospective and prospective. *International Journal of Health Education, 3*(4), 164–169. Reprinted with permission from International Union for Health Promotion and Education.

Derryberry, M. (May–June 1961). Better communications: An essential in today's public health. *Michigan's Health,* pp. 43–46. Reprinted with permission from Michigan Department of Community Health.

Derryberry, M. (May 1963). Research procedures applicable to health education. *The Journal of School Health, 33*(5), 215–220. Reprinted with permission from American School Health Association.

Derryberry, M. (1971). Education in the health aspects of family planning. *Pacific Health Reports, 2,* 16–50. Reprinted with permission from University of California, Berkeley.

Levy, J., Derryberry, M., & Mensch, I. (July 1942). A new technic of health education for use in baby stations. *American Journal of Public Health, 32*(7), 727–731. Reprinted with permission from the American Public Health Association.

McKeever, N., & Derryberry, M. (January 1956). What does the changing picture in public health mean to health education in programs and practice? *American Journal of Public Health, 46*(1), 54-60. Reprinted with permission from the American Public Health Association.

Palmer, G. T., & Derryberry, M. (May 1937). Appraising the educational content of a health service program. *American Journal of Public Health, 27*(5), 476–480. Reprinted with permission from the American Public Health Association.